D1370209

HEAD
INJURY

TEXAS TECH UNIVERSITY HEALTH SCIENCE CENTER LIBRARY

CONTRIBUTING EDITORS

MARLENE MORGAN, MOT, OTR/L
Director of Occupational Therapy
  Education and Training
Rehabilitation Institute of Chicago

RUSS HOLLANDER, MS, OTR/L
Assistant Director of Occupational Therapy
  Current Affiliation:
  Chicago Neurosurgical Center, Chicago, IL

CONTRIBUTING AUTHORS

JANET BISCHOF, BS, OTR/L
Senior Therapist
Rehabilitation Institute of Chicago

THERESA BUSH, BS, OTR/L
Senior Therapist
  Current Affiliation:
  Fairfax Hospital, Kirkland, WA

LORIE CRIPE, BS, OTR/L
Staff Therapist
Rehabilitation Institute of Chicago

JUDY HILL, BS, OTR/L
Clinical Specialist
Rehabilitation Institute of Chicago

RUSS HOLLANDER, MS, OTR/L
Assistant Director of Occupational Therapy
  Current Affiliation:
  Chicago Neurosurgical Center, Chicago, IL

MARLENE MORGAN, MOT, OTR/L
Director of Occupational Therapy
  Education and Training
Rehabilitation Institute of Chicago

CHRISTINE MORRISON, BS, OTR/L
Clinical Supervisor
  Current Affiliation:
  LaRabida Children's Hospital, Chicago, IL

JESSICA PRESPERIN, MBA, OTR/L
Senior Therapist
  Current Affiliation:
  Chicago area consultant

VINOD SAHGAL, MD
Director, Brain Trauma Program
Rehabilitation Institute of Chicago

ANITA VAN DAM-BURKE, BS, OTR/L
Staff Therapist
Rehabilitation Institute of Chicago

DOROTHY VEZZETTI, MS, OTR/L
Staff Therapist
Rehabilitation Institute of Chicago

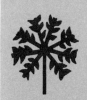

Rehabilitation
Institute of
Chicago
PROCEDURE
MANUAL

HEAD

INJURY

**A GUIDE TO
FUNCTIONAL
OUTCOMES
IN
OCCUPATIONAL
THERAPY**

KAREN M. KOVICH, OTR/L
Senior Author & Editor
Clinical Supervisor
Buchanan Family Foundation Fellow

DIANE E. BERMANN, MOT, OTR/L
Senior Author & Editor
Senior Therapist
Buchanan Family Foundation Fellow

SHARON INTAGLIATA, MS, MPA, OTR/L
Occupational Therapy Series Editor

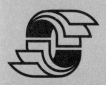

AN ASPEN PUBLICATION®
Aspen Publishers, Inc.
Rockville, Maryland
Royal Tunbridge Wells
1988

Library of Congress Cataloging-in-Publication Data.

Kovich, Karen M.
Head injury: a guide to functional outcomes in
occupational therapy/Karen M. Kovich, Diane E. Bermann.
p.   m.--(The Rehabilitation Institute of Chicago publication)

"An Aspen publication."
Includes bibliographies and index.
ISBN 0-87189-762-8
1. Brain damage--Patients--Rehabilitation. 2. Occupational therapy. I. Bermann,
Diane E. II. Title. III. Series. [DNLM: 1. Brain Injuries--rehabilitation.
2.. Head Injuries--rehabilitation. 3. Occupational Therapy. 4. Physical Therapy.
WL 354 K877h]
RC387.5.K68   1988   617'.481044--dc19
DNLM/DLC
for Library of Congress
88-2181
CIP

Copyright © 1988 by Aspen Publishers, Inc.
All rights reserved.

Aspen Publishers, Inc. grants permission for photocopying for personal or internal use,
or for the personal or internal use of specific clients registered with the Copyright
Clearance Center (CCC). This consent is given on the condition that the copier pay a
$1.00 fee plus $.12 per page for each photocopy through the CCC for photocopying
beyond that permitted by the U.S. Copyright Law. The fee should be paid directly to the
CCC, 21 Congress St., Salem, Massachusetts 01970.
0-87189-762-8/88 $1.00 + .12.

This consent does not extend to other kinds of copying, such as copying for general
distribution, for advertising or promotional purposes, for creating new collective works,
or for resale. For information, address Aspen Publishers, Inc.,
1600 Research Boulevard, Rockville, Maryland 20850.

Editorial Services: Mary Beth Roesser

Library of Congress Catalog Card Number 88-2181
ISBN: 0-87189-762-8

Printed in the United States of America

1 2 3 4 5

MED
WL
354
K849h
1988

Table of Contents

Series Preface

In recent years, occupational therapy has entered a dynamic new phase in its development as a health care profession. As advances in medical technology have enabled people to survive increasingly more catastrophic illnesses or trauma, we have been faced with many new demands. These demands have challenged us to learn new techniques and specialized skills to keep pace with the rapid changes taking place throughout the field of rehabilitation. Although these scientific advancements have had a significant impact on the rehabilitation treatment process, the basic tenets of our profession have not changed. As occupational therapists, we continue to assist individuals to engage in meaningful and productive activity. The role has been and will continue to be a critical component in the effort to enhance the health and well-being of our patients and to aid them in returning to the mainstream of society.

Since the Rehabilitation Institute of Chicago was founded in 1954, our Occupational Therapy Department has grown considerably in size. Along with the growth in numbers has come an evolution in the theoretical approaches, technology, and specialization of skills being used in our clinic. Accordingly, it was felt that developing uniform standards of clinical care would help to ensure a consistent and comprehensive approach to our occupational therapy treatment of patients with similar diagnoses.

Our department's Quality Assurance Committee encouraged the development of these standards. The committee recommended that the standards be written in a format that would facilitate our monitoring of the appropriateness and effectiveness of our treatment programs in an ongoing manner. The format developed focuses on (1) systematically identifying significant behavioral indicators in the recovery process, and (2) defining and describing the concepts, evaluation protocol, and treatment planning methods relevant to each patient's condition.

This volume describes our treatment approach to the head-injured patient and is the second in a series of three volumes to be completed by the Occupational Therapy Department at the Rehabilitation Institute of Chicago; the remaining volume will be devoted to standards for the treatment of stroke. The standards that serve as the foundation of each volume were compiled by clinical supervisors and senior staff members with input from our entire department; therefore, each volume represents a culmination of the ideas and efforts of many talented occupational therapists who have devoted their clinical expertise and creative wisdom to our department. The process of developing and refining these standards has solidified our collective rationale for treatment. The standards have been useful to us in orienting new staff and students to general treatment techniques as well as to therapeutic procedures that may be unique to our facility. They have also enabled us to begin to measure the results of our efforts in relation to the functional achievements of those we serve.

Our objective in producing these manuals for dissemination outside the Institute is to share the results of our efforts in a format that will be useful to other practicing clinicians. In recognition of the fact that every patient presents a unique neurological, psychosocial, and motivational picture, our standards are not meant to be prescriptive. Rather, they have been written in a way that will enhance the clinical problem solving and judgment that is the foundation of professional practice. It is our hope that occupational therapy students and clinicians will use these manuals as resources to supplement their own treatment planning processes.

Sharon Intagliata, MS, MPA, OTR/L
Director of Occupational Therapy
Rehabilitation Institute of Chicago

THE REHABILITATION INSTITUTE OF CHICAGO PUBLICATION SERIES

Don A. Olson, Ph.D., Series Coordinator

Spinal Cord Injury: A Guide to Functional
    Outcomes in Physical Therapy Management

Lower Extremity Amputation: A Guide to Functional
    Outcomes in Physical Therapy Management

Stroke/Head Injury: A Guide to Functional
    Outcomes in Physical Therapy Management

Clinical Management of Right Hemisphere Dysfunction

Clinical Evaluation of Dysphagia

Spinal Cord Injury: A Guide to Functional
    Outcomes in Occupational Therapy

Spinal Cord Injury: A Guide to Rehabilitation Nursing

Speech/Language Treatment of the Aphasias: An
    Integrated Clinical Approach

Preface

This book was written to serve as a guide in the occupational therapy management of head-injured individuals. The content reflects those areas addressed by the Occupational Therapy Department at the Rehabilitation Institute of Chicago (RIC). Generally, the severity of head injury ranges from mild to severe. At RIC, the head injury program treats primarily moderately to severely involved patients. As an acute rehabilitation facility, we must be prepared to treat a variety of physical and cognitive deficits resulting from head injury regardless of the severity of the injury. Rather than presenting detailed material focused on a specific area or level of recovery, this guide presents a comprehensive approach to the treatment of a variety of deficits. Included are those frames of reference and techniques that we as a department have found useful and effective in the treatment of head-injured patients. It does not attempt to cover all possible options available to occupational therapists today.

Throughout the text the importance of a multidisciplinary team approach and family involvement is emphasized. It is clear that head injury affects not only the individual but the family and friends as well. To meet the varied needs of the patient as well as significant others, a team approach is crucial to successful rehabilitation and reintegration into the community. The treatment techniques presented in this guide must be integrated with those of other professionals on the treatment team.

In general, this text reflects a developmental approach to many aspects of treatment. Many of the handling techniques used at RIC and described in the text are strongly influenced by a neurodevelopmental treatment approach. These techniques used by our therapists have proved successful in the remediation of motor deficits. This information is also representative of the authors' training.

It is our intent that this guide will prove useful to students and therapists less familiar with the diagnosis of head injury. For the more experienced clinician, it may assist in clinical problem solving and serve as a framework for developing quality assurance systems. The information and format in which it is presented may also assist in the development of new programs to effectively treat this population.

Diane Bermann
Karen Kovich

Acknowledgments

This book reflects the combined efforts of many individuals. We wish to thank The Buchanan Family Foundation for its financial support of this project. We acknowledge the efforts of the contributing authors, editors, and the occupational therapy staff at the Rehabilitation Institute of Chicago who assisted in reviewing the manuscripts in the early stages. The standards of care listed at the end of many units evolved through the energy of several therapists. The assistance and perseverance of Kathy Okkema in the final stages as we worked to complete the standards was invaluable. Other therapists who contributed to the standards are Mary Grimm VanNest, Mary Andree, Audrey Yasukawa, and Sheryl Kantor. We wish to thank the people who consented to be photographed, as well as Oscar Izquierdo and Jerry Gibson of the RIC Biomedical Media Department for their technical assistance in taking those pictures. We note Sandra Haynes for her patience in typing the many revisions of the manuscript. We wish to acknowledge the encouragement provided by Ruth Ann Watkins, Vice President of marketing at RIC, and Shari Intagliata, Director of Occupational Therapy at RIC. We extend our gratitude to the RIC occupational therapy staff who have used and refined the techniques described in this book and contributed to our body of knowledge.

It is with special regard that we thank our families and friends, especially John, Elise, Kathryn, John, Emilie, Debbie, and Mary. Their personal support and concern helped us through the many stages of development required to complete this book.

Finally, it is the patients and their families who have taught us about the many aspects of head injury that we thank. Their road to recovery may have been long, yet their hope and perseverance has been inspiring to us all. It is to them that this book is dedicated.

Diane Bermann
Karen Kovich

How to Use This Manual

Diane Bermann, OTR/L
Karen Kovich, OTR/L

This manual reflects the philosophy of the Department of Occupational Therapy (OT) at the Rehabilitation Institute of Chicago (RIC) on the treatment of head-injured patients. It incorporates our first-hand experiences treating these patients and touches on the theoretical basis for selected treatment. A developmental perspective can be noted throughout the text. In some cases, we recommend that lower-level skills be accomplished first. Some goal areas are not addressed until the patient reaches a certain level of functioning.

The manual is divided into five parts, with related units in each. Part I gives general information about head injury (HI). The units on evaluation, goals, and treatment planning discuss specific problems encountered when working with head-injured patients.

Part II, "Behavioral Components," links psychosocial, sensory-perceptual, and cognitive issues. Behavior is often reflected in the patient's social interactions. These interactions, in turn, are influenced by how the individual perceives the world and his ability to function in it.

Part III encompasses the physical aspects of managing the head-injured patient. It includes techniques to manage abnormal muscle tone and to facilitate functional movement through handling, positioning, splinting, and casting interventions.

Part IV, "Daily Living Skills," deals with the performance of functional tasks given the potential behavioral, sensory-perceptual, cognitive, and motor deficits associated with HI. The units encompass functioning from basic self-care through community re-entry skills. The unit on technical aids may help open new avenues of functioning to the severely physically involved patient and briefly touches on the use of computers as a therapeutic tool.

Part V, "Special Issues," combines three important areas of treatment. The first is the therapeutic use of groups by the occupational therapist. It describes the types of groups that are appropriate for patients functioning at different levels. Discharge placement sometimes presents special problems for the family and team. Some problems involving discharge planning are discussed in the unit. The pediatric unit briefly addresses those issues unique to the younger population that are not addressed in other units.

Five levels of responsiveness after HI are described in the chart below. The behavioral descriptors relate primarily to sensory-perceptual, cognitive, and communicative issues because motor performance does not always correlate with the patient's level of arousal. These five levels enable the occupational therapist to classify a patient's level of responsiveness based on a relatively brief observation period and help her decide which evaluations are appropriate, what aspects may need to be modified, and which can be postponed. Table 2-1 in the evaluation unit summarizes priority evaluations based on these descriptive levels. The therapist can then begin identifying the patient's assets and limitations.

Levels of Responsiveness

1. Minimally responsive

   - may show nonpurposeful movement patterns or automatic response to primary sensory stimuli
   - may show inconsistent periods of eye opening
   - unable to communicate needs
   - no awareness of or participation in basic living tasks
   - may exhibit severe alterations in muscle tone causing abnormal posturing

2. Awakening

   - begins to show purposeful response to primary sensory stimuli
   - begins to attend to environmental input and presence of familiar others

- begins to use simple communications for basic needs (i.e., yes/no response)
- participates in activities of daily living (ADL) program that focuses on performance of portions of basic living tasks
- begins to use available movement voluntarily and/or on command

3. Agitated

- exhibits extreme reactions to internal or external sensory stimuli
- ability to attend to tasks selectively varies with level of agitation
- ability to communicate needs varies with level of agitation
- ability to participate in basic living tasks or allow care to be performed varies with level of agitation
- quality of movement varies with level of agitation

4. Alert confused

- shows purposeful response to controlled multisensory stimuli
- shows ability to attend to simple and/or familiar tasks
- begins to control environment using available language and motor skill
- participates in ADL program that focuses on performance of basic living tasks (e.g., feeding, self-care)
- demonstrates difficulty learning techniques to compensate for motor deficits

5. Alert oriented

- shows purposeful response to multisensory stimuli
- may demonstrate concrete cognitive processes when performing complex and/or unfamiliar tasks
- consistently interacts with and controls environment using available language and motor skills

- participates in ADL program that focuses on basic living tasks, homemaking, and community reintegration
- may be able to compensate for motor deficits using adaptive techniques

A chart summarizing our standards of care is included at the end of each treatment unit. These charts list major long-term goals (LTGs) that are applicable to all levels of patients. These suggestions can be modified to meet individual needs. Under each LTG are functional indicators designed to assist the therapist in selecting the most appropriate LTG. The second column lists sample short-term goals (STGs). They are listed sequentially to help break the LTGs into steps attainable within a 2-week period, and examples of how they can be individualized is provided by the italicized variables. For further information on the use of these charts, refer to Unit 3.

The units on orthotics, positioning, and technical aids, along with Part V, do not have standards of care charts. There may be times when specific goals will be set in these areas, but in most cases they are the means used to achieve functional goals. The units in Part V do not address specific patient goals and, therefore, no standards of care are included.

Throughout the book, "he" is used to refer to the head-injured patient rather than "he/she" for ease in reading. "She" is used to refer to the therapist.

The text is problem-oriented and describes treatment in a developmental progression. Depending on the unit, goal areas or problem areas are in bold type to assist the reader in finding specific information. Examples of specific treatment and additional ideas are included in the text but are certainly not limited to what is stated here. Our hope is that these guidelines will enable therapists to create treatment plans specific to the needs of each patient.

Part I

Introduction

Medical Aspects of Head Injury

Vinod Sahgal, M.D.

Head injury (HI) is one of the major diagnoses in rehabilitation centers throughout the country. A wide range of estimates is available for measuring its epidemiology in the United States. In predominantly white populations, there are 200 to 250 HIs per 100,000 population; among non-whites in large cities, the incidence increases to 400 per 100,000 (Anderson & McLaurin, 1980; Miner & Wagner, 1986; Whitman, Coonley-Hoganson & Desai, 1984).

The majority of studies report that men are two to three times more likely to experience a HI than women, depending on the age of the individual (Jennett & Teasdale, 1981; Kraus, Black & Hessol, 1984; Miner & Wagner, 1986). The peak ages of vulnerability are 15 to 24 years, followed by 0 to 4. By the age of 50, the incidence falls rapidly but increases again over 65 years of age (Whitman et al., 1984).

Motor vehicle accidents are the leading cause of HI and account for 25 percent to 30 percent of those hospitalized (Jennett & Teasdale, 1981; Miner & Wagner, 1986; Rosenthal, Griffith, Bond & Miller, 1983). Falls are the second cause, accounting for 25 percent to 30 percent. Gunshot wounds and other interpersonal violence account for 7 percent to 40 percent, varying with population and location (Jennett & Teasdale, 1981). A study from the University of Virginia indicated that alcohol was involved in 72 percent of all HIs during a 2-year period (Rosenthal et al., 1983).

These observations suggest that 0.2 percent to 0.3 percent of the population of the United States are at risk for a HI each year, or 500,000 new cases annually; of these, 30 percent are either fatal or severe (Frankowski, Arnegars, John & Whitman, 1985). Since the life expectancy of patients who survive either severe or moderate brain damage is 20 to 30 years, and patients who suffer mild injuries live a normal life span, the economic, sociologic, and community-related impacts of HI are significant. Regardless of which statistics are used, it is clear that HI is a major problem facing today's health care system.

MECHANISMS OF HEAD INJURY

The severity of HI depends not only on the nature of the injury but also on the location, direction of impact, and magnitude of the force that affects the brain and the skull. Brain damage can be classified into two types: (1) primary brain damage, which occurs at the moment of impact; and (2) secondary brain damage, which occurs as a result of subsequent pathologic processes.

Primary Brain Damage

Cerebral concussion injuries are associated with neurologic dysfunction without objectively demonstrable cranial or cerebral pathologic conditions. Concussion usually involves a loss of consciousness of 15 minutes to 1 hour, followed by a brief period of post-traumatic amnesia (PTA). The duration of both the loss of consciousness and the PTA are used to determine the severity of the damage. Clinical symptoms or complaints after concussion often include persistent headaches, dizziness, lack of coordination in the hands and fingers, and diminished mental processes such as impairments in concentration, calculation, or memory.

Cerebral contusions are associated with neurologic dysfunction with one or more objectively demonstrable findings. The damage may be focal or diffuse. Focal damage is often confined to the tissue surrounding the site of impact on the skull and can be superficial or deep. It also occurs when the brain is subjected to sudden and extreme acceleration or deceleration or in the presence of a closed blunt injury, causing the brain to impact the skull. Cerebral contusions are most frequently seen in the frontal lobes and under the surfaces of temporal lobes due to the irregular surface structure of the anterior and middle cranial fossa. Damage to the occipital pole can occur but is less common. The damage at the site of impact is known as the ''coup injury.'' The damage at the opposite side is termed the ''contra-coup injury.'' When the frontal area of the head is struck, the result is most often a coup injury; a blow to the back of the head produces a coup and a contra-coup injury due to the shearing effect against the structural irregularities of the skull.

Diffuse brain damage usually occurs from a high-velocity acceleration or deceleration injury that produces movement of the brain inside the skull. The result is widespread shearing of axons in the white matter that is not confined to one location. The patient is often deeply comatose, demonstrating decerebrate posturing.

Cerebral lacerations are always associated with an open head injury and involve discontinuity of the cerebral substance. They may also cause damage to the scalp, skull, or meninges.

Secondary Brain Damage

Secondary damage refers to the events that occur in the brain as a result of the primary lesion. The most common are intracranial hematoma, cerebral ischemia and anoxia, hydrocephalus, intracranial infection, and post-traumatic epilepsy.

Intracranial Hematoma

A subdural hematoma usually results from a blunt injury that causes tearing of the veins in the subdural space. These veins drain the cerebral venous blood into the sinuses from a low-pressure channel. The result is a slow accumulation of blood in the subdural space. The blood forms a clot, which grows over time. The most common sites of subdural hematoma are the frontal, parietal, occipital, and interhemispheric regions. Common symptoms include headache, dizziness, drowsiness, lethargy, and confusion, along with focal neurologic deficits such as dilated pupils, hemiparesis, and incontinence. If not diagnosed and treated early, it is generally fatal.

Epidural hematoma is a more malignant condition because it is caused by an arterial bleed in the epidural space. It commonly involves a rupture of the middle meningeal artery associated with skull fracture. This is associated with loss of consciousness, followed by a lucid interval of minutes to hours, after which the patient demonstrates headache, nausea, vomiting, and increasing stupor to a comatose state. Prompt recognition and management almost always result in a good outcome.

An intracerebral hematoma results from arterial, venous, or capillary bleeding within the substance of the brain. The bleeding is mostly restricted to the white matter with the most common sites being the frontal, temporal, and occipital lobes. On many occasions the isolated hematomas are associated with diffuse pinpoint bleeds throughout the white matter and pons. Brainstem hematomas are also rather common.

Cerebral Ischemia and Anoxia

Glucose is the most significant energy source for neuronal function. Its use is dependent upon the presence of oxygen, which is supplied to the brain by arterial blood. In severe to moderate HI, cerebral swelling often results in increased intracerebral pressure, which may cause a relative lack of oxygen, resulting in deficient energy production from substrate use. If uninterrupted, this sequence of events can result in irreversible damage. The most recent acute therapeutic interventions are thus designed to control cerebral edema, maintain the oxygen and blood supply, and restrict the secondary damage.

Intracranial Infection

The intact dura normally provides an effective barrier to intracranial infection from the various nasal sinuses. When the continuity of the dura is compromised or there is communication between the subdural space and the cranial air sinuses, bacterial infection can occur. The most common infection is meningitis;

frontal and temporal lobe abscesses also occur frequently. Ventriculitis and cerebritis may be seen in patients requiring shunts for the treatment of hydrocephalus.

Hydrocephalus

Obstructive hydrocephalus occurs when the normal pathway for the flow of cerebral spinal fluid is interrupted or blocked. When this occurs, the ventricles expand into the area occupied by the white matter. The patient may complain of headache, nausea, vomiting, loss of normal gait, and urinary incontinence. A shunt can be surgically placed to prevent the ventricles from expanding. A favorable therapeutic response can be expected in only 25 percent of these patients.

Communicating hydrocephalus occurs in the presence of severe brain damage where the ventricles expand to occupy the space left by the deterioration of the white matter. The cerebral spinal fluid flow is not obstructed and demonstrates normal pressure; therefore, shunting may not be effective on this type of hydrocephalus.

Post-traumatic Epilepsy

Early onset epilepsy occurs in the first week after injury; late onset epilepsy occurs after the first week. In late onset epilepsy, approximately 75 percent of patients will have their first seizure within the first year and the remaining 25 percent within 4 years (Frankowski et al., 1985). The incidence of early onset epilepsy in adults is 5 percent in nonmissile injuries and increases to 11 percent in children under 1 year of age (Frankowski et al., 1985). The incidence of late onset epilepsy in patients with blunt injury is 5 percent (Frankowski et al., 1985). The risk of post-traumatic epilepsy increases with the duration of PTA, intracranial hematoma, fracture of the skull, or discontinuation of the meninges.

The following anticonvulsants, in order, are the mainstay of antiepileptic therapy: diphenyl-hydantoin (Dilantin), carbamazepine (Tegretol), phenobarbital, primidone (Mysoline), valproic acid (Depakene), and clonazepam (Klonopin). The merits of monotherapy and the disadvantages of polytherapy cannot be overemphasized in the treatment of seizure disorders since the side effects impact performance. The effects of diphenyl-hydantoin and phenobarbital on cognitive function have been the focus of many investigations. They have shown that both impair cognitive function; carbamazepine has the least effect on cognitive function (Committee on Drugs, 1985). The most common side effects of anticonvulsants that compromise cognition are confusion, drowsiness, decreased attention span, ataxia, and altered motor performance. Thus, the patient's poor participation and performance may be a result of medication and should be reported to the physician immediately.

CLINICAL PICTURE

Altered Levels of Consciousness

Altered consciousness is the most consistent result of acceleration/deceleration injuries to the skull, the duration of which can indicate the degree of damage. Jennett and Teasdale's (1981) definition of *coma* used by the National Data Bank Survey states that "eye opening does not occur, no comprehensible speech is detected and the extremities move neither to command nor appropriately to localize or ward off noxious stimuli."

Continuous monitoring of levels of consciousness during the acute recovery period can reveal improvement in brain function or the presence of a secondary complication. Because such monitoring is necessary, there arose a need to develop a consistent means by which a variety of medical personnel could rate and record the patient's level of consciousness and compare it with previous levels. The Glasgow Coma Scale (GCS), developed by Jennett and Teasdale (1981), has become a widely used measure of level of consciousness after traumatic brain injury. With this scale, an individual is rated in the areas of eye opening, motor, and verbal response (Table 1-1). The scale also attempts to use levels of consciousness to assist in determining the severity of injury and in predicting the outcome.

The reticular activating system is a structure lying within the brainstem that is responsible for the state of arousal in humans. It controls the cycles of wakefulness and sleep, and our threshold to environmental stimuli. Consciousness has two aspects: arousal and alertness. Arousal refers only to having the eyes opened and being in a state of wakefulness. Alertness requires higher cortical functioning and implies a knowledge of one's self and surrounding environment, and the ability to make meaningful and adaptive responses. Full consciousness implies both arousal and alertness.

After severe injury, loss of consciousness occurs when the reticular activating system can no longer

TABLE 1-1   Glasgow coma scale

Eye opening		
Spontaneous	(E) Eye	4
To speech		3
To pain		2
Nil		1
Best motor response		
Obeys	(M) Motor	6
Localizes		5
Withdraws		4
Abnormal flexion		3
Extensor response		2
Nil		1
Verbal response		
Oriented	(V) Verbal	5
Confused conversation		4
Inappropriate words		3
Incomprehensible sounds		2
Nil		1
GCS (E + M + V) = 3 to 15		

Source: From *Management of Head Injuries* by B. Jennett and G. Teasdale, 1981, Philadelphia: F.A. Davis Company. Copyright 1981 by F.A. Davis Company. Reprinted by permission.

transmit impulses to the cerebral hemispheres, possibly due to increased intracranial pressure, cerebral ischemia, diffuse cerebral edema, and physical damage to nerve fibers. The patient in an altered state of consciousness can be classified into one of three categories:

1. *The vegetative state* is one of wakefulness but minimal responsiveness. The patient offers no comprehensible motor or verbal response, maintains blood pressure and respiration without assistance, and has clear wake and sleep cycles. The motor system demonstrates quadriplegia with pseudobulbar palsy. Spontaneous and purposeful movements are generally absent.
2. *Akinetic mutism* is a state of wakefulness in which patients appear to follow with their eyes and may speak in monosyllables but are incapable of sophisticated cognitive, verbal, or motor responses.
3. *The locked-in syndrome* usually occurs as a result of damage to the region of the ventral pons, interrupting the majority of motor pathways. The patient usually demonstrates full cognitive awareness but is extremely limited in motoric and verbal response. These patients most often use head or eye movement to communicate.

Post-traumatic Amnesia

PTA is defined as the interval between the occurrence of the head injury and the return of full consciousness and continuous memory of ongoing events. It can be used to determine the severity of damage and is discussed further in "Predictors of Outcome."

Respiratory Function

Impaired respiratory function is common after severe HI, especially in the unconscious patient. Lack of adequate oxygen in the blood can lead to cerebral anoxia, which may further damage the brain. Abnormal breathing patterns may be a result of damage to the areas of the brain controlling autonomic function, specifically the brainstem. Respiratory function can also be impaired secondary to damage to the airway or lungs, or obstruction of the airway by the tongue or body fluids.

If prolonged ventilation is required, a tracheostomy tube is used. This involves placing a tube just above the sternal notch that inserts into the trachea, allowing respiration at that point and bypassing oral or nasal air intake. In cases of severe HI, patients often require the tracheostomy on a long-term basis. Hypostatic and aspiration pneumonias are common. In an informal study of 400 HI patients over a 4-year period at the Rehabilitation Institute of Chicago (RIC), pneumonias accounted for approximately 40 percent of medical complications.

Nutrition

The unconscious patient requires a nasogastric tube to insure adequate nutrition. Often, patients who are conscious may continue to require tube feedings secondary to a lack of oral motor control. A nasogastric tube is placed through the nose and esophagus into the stomach and is used to provide a liquid diet and to insure proper caloric intake. When it becomes clear that a patient will require tube feedings on a long-term basis, a gastrostomy or jejunostomy tube is placed into the stomach or small intestine through a small incision in the abdomen. Feeding programs can be constant or at intervals throughout the day depending on the individual's nutritional needs. Any type of tube is often irritating to the patient and must be monitored so that it is not pulled out. An abdominal binder can be loosely fitted over the stomach to prevent this occurrence.

Altered Sensation

HI may result in loss or impairment of one or all tactile modalities of pain, temperature, pressure, touch, or position sense. Depending on the location and type of lesion, the impairments are often found in a hemisensory distribution but may be found throughout the body. Often, HI results in loss or distortion of other primary senses of vision, olfaction, taste, and hearing.

Visual deficits occur from damage along the visual system including the retina, cranial nerves, or occipital lobe. Among the visual impairments seen after HI are field cuts, nystagmus, diplopia, ptosis, cortical blindness, and tracking disorders.

Hearing disorders most frequently occur from damage to peripheral structures, such as the tympanic membranes, or from more centrally located structures, such as the auditory nerve or temporal lobe. Resulting problems include partial or complete deafness, tinnitus, or an inability to process auditory stimuli.

Loss or distortion of the sense of smell is common due to the proximity of the olfactory nerve to the boney irregularities on the frontal portion of the skull. Deficits in the senses of smell and taste may be much less apparent than those in the other primary senses.

Altered Cognitive and Behavioral Function

Intellectual deficits in memory, judgment, comprehension, attention, and concept formation; language disabilities; and lack of drive are common mental sequelae. Functional deficits secondary to focal lesions of the nondominant hemisphere (frontal, temporal, parietal, and occipital lobe syndromes) are also sequelae. These syndromes have been well described in standard neurology and neurobehavior texts. It is important that they be recognized due to their great impact on functional capabilities.

The most difficult problem is to differentiate organic functional deficits and behavioral or psychological responses. The most useful observation in this regard is gross discrepancies in the performance of various therapeutic activities. When a patient demonstrates difficulty in one or two activities but in no others, organic deficits should be suspected, with the discrepancies related to the demands of the various activities. When problems arise in participation in all activities, they are most likely behavioral. This distinction is extremely important because repetitive efforts may improve par-

ticipation in the former; in the latter, participation and performance often deteriorate.

The therapeutic participation problems are divided into the two categories of aggressive and apathetic behavior. Both are generally managed with environmental manipulation and psychotropic drugs such as haloperidol (Haldol), phenothiazines, lithium, and tricyclic antidepressants. In treating apathetic behavior, various analeptic drugs such as methylphenidate hydrochloride (Ritalin) have been tried, but the responses have been variable.

Altered Motor Performance

Motor impairments resulting from HI can take many forms such as paralysis; paresis; abnormal muscle tone, such as spasticity or rigidity; and movement disorders, such as ataxia or loss of range of motion (ROM). These impairments may be diffuse, involving the trunk and all extremities, or localized to one side or extremity depending on the extent and location of the brain damage.

Spasticity presents as a hypertonic state manifested by an increased resistance of the muscle to passive stretch. It is commonly found in patterns throughout the trunk and extremities and, depending on the severity, may greatly limit volitional movement.

Rigidity produces bidirectional resistance to movement and is a hypertonic state resulting from damage to basal ganglia or is associated with decerebrate or decorticate postures. Decerebrate rigidity is demonstrated by abnormal extensor tone in the upper and lower extremities; decorticate rigidity is characterized by patterned flexion of the upper extremities and extension of the lowers.

Abnormal postural reflexes often emerge after HI. They were previously integrated into the central nervous system (CNS) during development but reappear due to loss of inhibition of higher cortical control. These reflexes affect muscle tone and volitional movement.

Ataxia is a movement disorder arising from damage to the cerebellum or to the pathways transmitting proprioceptive information. It can occur in the head, neck, trunk, and extremities and results in an inability to coordinate the speed and direction of movement.

Severe spasticity or rigidity along with prolonged periods of immobility often results in joint contracture and loss of ROM in the extremities. An informal study of 400 HI patients seen at RIC over a 4-year period indicated a 75 to 80 percent incidence of joint contracture, with 87 percent showing multiple joint involvement. The hips were involved in 81 percent, and the shoulder and ankles in 76 percent. Elbow contracture was present in 44 percent.

Heterotopic ossification, also called ectopic bone, is common in HI. Although the etiology is uncertain, abnormal calcification occurs in and around the joint space. As this calcification grows, joint range becomes increasingly compromised, with pain occurring due to swelling of the surrounding area. While passive ROM movements may help maintain joint range, they will not improve range that has already been lost secondary to the ectopic bone. The calcification must be surgically removed when mature in order to increase joint range.

PREDICTORS OF OUTCOME

The ability to predict functional outcome after HI is important not only to the patient and family but to the treatment team so they may determine realistic goals. Outcome depends on many factors, including the severity of the injury, the quality of medical care, and the extent of physical and mental deficits.

Severity of Injury

The severity of injury serves as a general indicator of outcome and can be determined by assessment of PTA and/or coma and the extent of actual brain damage. One such scale used at RIC is presented below.

- *Severe injury* occurs when loss of consciousness and/or PTA exceeds 24 hours or there is demonstrable cerebral contusion, laceration, or intracranial hematoma.
- *Moderate injury* occurs when loss of consciousness and/or PTA lasts for more than 30 minutes but less than 24 hours without cerebral laceration or intracranial hematoma. Cerebral contusion is usually present; skull fracture may or may not occur.
- *Mild injury* occurs when the loss of consciousness and/or PTA is less than 30 minutes without cerebral contusion, laceration, hematoma, or skull fracture. Cerebral concussion is generally observed.

These categories correlate well with the GCS. Severe injury was associated with a GCS of 3 to 8;

moderate injury with a score of 9 to 12; mild injuries with a score of 13 to 15 (Frankowski et al., 1985). In addition, the Glasgow Outcome Scale (GOS), developed by Jennett and Teasdale (1981), looks at resulting disability as measured by functional capabilities. By using a functional measurement, the interfacing physical and mental deficits are taken into account without having to look at each separately (Table 1-2).

Jennett and Teasdale (1981) showed that approximately 75 percent of the patients who suffered severe HI reached a good to moderate level of recovery, with 90 percent doing so within the first 6 months after injury. After this time, recovery often continues, but it may be insufficient to justify a change in rating on the GOS.

Quality of Medical Care

Medical attention at the time of injury and ongoing quality care throughout hospitalization are vital to optimize the patient's potential for recovery. This involves prompt recognition and treatment of complications and other medical problems, and meeting the specific needs of the individual through providing therapeutic intervention.

Extent of Physical and Mental Deficits

Deficits in mentation are the most consistent consequence of HI and contribute most significantly to overall functional disability. While physical deficits affect outcome the least, they are often the most amenable to therapeutic intervention. Among significant deficits

TABLE 1-2   Glasgow outcome scale

0–1	*Good recovery:* normal participation in social, vocational, and physical life
2–3	*Moderate disability:* independent but disabled (physical or cognitive) requiring an altered physical, social, psychological, or vocational environment for participation
4–5	*Severe disability:* totally dependent in managing normal or modified environment
6	*Vegetative state:* totally dependent with no awareness of the environment

Source: From *Management of Head Injuries* by B. Jennett and G. Teasdale, 1981, Philadelphia: F.A. Davis Company. Copyright 1981 by F.A. Davis Company. Reprinted by permission.

that limit functional outcome are contracture, ataxia, spasticity, and ectopic bone. Socially, the single most significant predictor of reintegration of head-injured individuals is their premorbid life style and adjustment.

Importance of the Team Approach

Deficits resulting from HI are medical, physical, functional, communicative, behavioral, cognitive, and social. Because of this, therapeutic intervention aimed at all of these areas necessitates working with a team of professionals including a physician; nurse; occupational, physical, and recreational therapists; vocational counselor; speech and language pathologist; rehabilitation engineer; psychologist; and social worker. This team approach is defined at RIC as a well-orchestrated, goal-directed use of professionals towards the betterment of the patient's medical, physical, functional, and social condition. The value of a team approach cannot be overemphasized. It facilitates communication among all team members to assist in setting the priorities of the rehabilitation process and in conveying a patient's level of function and expected outcome in all disciplines. It also enables the team to provide the patient and family with consistent information regarding recovery and how to carry over therapeutic inter-

vention into various aspects of the patient's day. Specific approaches to the management of the patient's disability are described in the following units.

REFERENCES

Anderson, D.W., & McLaurin, R.L., Eds. (1980). Report on the National Head and Spinal Cord Injury Survey. *Journal of Neurosurgery, 53* (Suppl.), S1–S43.

Committee on Drugs. (1985). Behavioral and cognitive effects of anti-convulsant therapy. *Pediatrics, 76,* 644–647.

Frankowski, R., Arnegars, F., John, F., & Whitman, S. (1985). Epidemiological and descriptive studies, part I. The descriptive epidemiology of head trauma. In Donald P. Becker & John T. Povlishak (Eds.), *U.S.-CNS Trauma Status Report, 1985.*

Jennett, B., & Teasdale, G. (1981). *Management of head injuries.* Philadelphia, F.A. Davis.

Kraus, J., Black, M., & Hessol, N. (1984). The incidence of acute brain injury and serious impairment in a defined population. *American Journal of Epidemiology, 119,* 186–201.

Miner, M.E., & Wagner, K.A. (1986). *Neurotrauma: Treatment, rehabilitation and related issues.* Boston: Butterworths.

Rosenthal, M., Griffith, E., Bond, M., & Miller, J. (1983). *The rehabilitation of the head injured adult.* Philadelphia: F.A. Davis.

Whitman, S., Coonley-Hoganson, R., & Desai, B.T. (1984). Comparative head trauma experiences in two socioeconomically different Chicago-area communities: A population study. *American Journal of Epidemiology, 4,* 570–580.

Evaluation

Diane Bermann, OTR/L

A complete evaluation is the basis of an effective treatment program for any patient. Evaluation provides information concerning the patient's status, areas of strength, and areas of limitation as well as a point from which one can measure progress. Accurate and precise information gathered from evaluations is used to formulate goals and to assist in selecting the types of treatment required to meet them. A major challenge in evaluating head-injured patients is facilitating their optimal performance when deficits of attention, level of consciousness, and communication exist and may affect the validity of test results.

A thorough occupational therapy (OT) evaluation provides the team with information necessary for the complete management of the head-injured patient. Evaluation includes:

- chart review
- psychosocial skills
- muscle tone
- reflexes
- movement disorders
- strength
- head control
- postural adaptation and balance
- sensation
- range of motion (ROM)
- upper extremity control
- hand functioning and coordination
- sensory-perceptual and cognitive skills
- activities of daily living (ADL)
- community living skills

Evaluations that use simulations of functional tasks and actual task performance provide essential information concerning the patient's potential for return to independent living. The performance evaluation may be especially important for a patient functioning at a high skill level. Although the patient may suffer minimal physical and verbal deficits, performance may deteriorate during tasks performed in a multistimulus environment. The OT evaluation also assists the team by assessing the impact of sensory and perceptual deficits on the performance of daily living tasks and by identifying channels through which the patient learns best.

Evaluation of the head-injured patient may present unique challenges. Problems that may interfere with traditional evaluation techniques requiring patient participation include:

- altered levels of consciousness
- limited reliability of communication
- distractability or attentional deficits
- agitation
- memory deficits
- pain behaviors
- inability or refusal to participate
- denial of deficits

Suggestions for handling these problems will be addressed as they apply to specific evaluations.

Observation skills and the ability to analyze task components are major assets of the occupational therapist in evaluating patients. It is the close observation of a patient's response to stimuli that will assist her in evaluating the patient with a low level of arousal. Keen observation is needed to grade responses to stimuli and to monitor changes. Similarly, it is the therapist's observational skills that contribute to the evaluation of skill performance in the higher functioning patient. Observation and task analysis are key to evaluating the causes of poor patient performance. Poor performance may be caused by impaired sequencing, motor planning, problem solving, or combinations of other cognitive, perceptual, or physical limitations.

The therapist may be required to evaluate patients at any point in their recovery. Certain behaviors associated with head injury (HI) make evaluation difficult. Other behaviors make components of the evaluation inappropriate for a particular patient. For example, evaluation of patients who are minimally responsive to the environment focuses on their level of arousal, sensory awareness, and sensorimotor components of ROM, muscle tone, and postural adaptation. Psychosocial aspects of evaluation relate more to the family or significant other, and ADL evaluations are not indicated.

At the other end of the continuum, the evaluation of patients who are oriented to their surroundings is very different. It is essential to evaluate their psychosocial adjustment; cognitive skills; complex sensory-perceptual, and sensorimotor skills; and their effects on ADL performance. Table 2–1 may be helpful in prioritizing the components of the OT evaluation for patients displaying these behaviors.

COMPONENTS OF THE OCCUPATIONAL THERAPY EVALUATION

Chart Review

A chart review is the first step in evaluating the patient. Information gathered from the chart includes the patient's medical history, history of the current illness, medical course of treatment, and current medical status. The medical history will indicate pre-existing conditions that may affect evaluation and treatment. For example, a previous fracture may have resulted in a ROM limitation unrelated to the current injury. The history of the current illness or injury and the medical course of treatment provide information concerning the incident and the acute phase of treatment. Information may include the patient's coma duration and complications. The chart also provides information concerning the patient's present status including medications received and precautions that may affect care. Information from the chart most important for evaluation and treatment includes:

- personal information such as age, marital status, family configuration, residence, and work history
- date of onset and cause of injury
- coma duration
- lifesaving medical procedures performed such as a tracheostomy, ventricular-peritoneal or other shunt, insertion of gastric or other feeding tube
- complications during acute phase that may affect recovery such as infections, hydrocephalus, or seizures
- concurrent injuries, such as fractures, and associated precautions

Psychosocial Evaluation

Evaluation of psychosocial issues is accomplished through interview and observation. If the patient is alert and can communicate verbally, one first determines his level of orientation. Although orientation is more cognitive in nature, it needs to be evaluated first in order to determine the patient's reliability in providing psychosocial information. Once orientation is established, the therapist continues the interview to determine the patient's premorbid life style, interests, leisure activities, and work and family roles. Information should be verified by the medical chart or family members. Leisure and role checklists (Oakley, 1981) are available to assist in the interview process. If this information cannot be ascertained from the patient, then family members, significant others, and the social worker can be interviewed. Meeting with family members on a regular basis establishes a means of evaluating the level of family involvement, their understanding and expectations, and their coping skills, learning styles, and abilities. Meetings involving the entire team are useful for setting appropriate goals and ensuring a consistent approach.

Evaluation of the patient's behavior, such as sustained attention, level of arousal, agitation, and social

TABLE 2-1 Recommendations for component skill and ADL evaluation

	Minimally responsive	Awakening	Agitated	Alert confused	Alert oriented
Psychosocial					
Participation in treatment	—	1	1	1	1
Social interaction	—	2	1	1	1
Interest identification and role changes	—	—	2	1	1
Cognitive					
Arousal/attention	1	1	1	1	1
Memory—recent	—	1	1	1	1
Memory—remote	—	1	1	1	1
Initiation	—	2	2	1	1
Sequencing	—	—	2	1	1
Safety/judgment	—	—	1	1	1
Problem solving	—	—	2	1	1
Awareness of errors	—	—	2	1	1
Ability to follow commands	1	1	1	1	1
Sensory/perceptual					
Tactile sensation	1	1	2	1	1
Visual response	1	1	2	1	1
Auditory response	1	1	2	—	—
Body awareness	—	1	2	1	1
Visual perceptual	1	1	2	1	1
Motor planning	—	2	2	1	1
Sensorimotor					
Range of motion	1	1	2	1	1
Muscle tone	1	1	2	1	1
Head control	1	1	2	1	1
Postural adaptation	—	1	1	1	1
Upper extremities use	—	1	1	1	1
Hand function	—	1	2	1	1
Endurance	—	2	2	1	1
ADL					
Self-care	—	1	1	1	1
Home management	—	—	—	2	1
Community integration	—	—	—	2	1
Leisure	—	—	1	1	1
Prevocation/vocation	—	—	—	2	1

Rating: 1 = Evaluation a priority
   2 = Evaluation may require modification or may be difficult to perform
   — = Evaluation not indicated

appropriateness, in various situations can be performed by structuring the environment. Observations can include the amount of redirection cueing or correction needed for the patient to complete a task or the emergence of inappropriate social behaviors in various situations such as:

- low-stimulation environments with limited auditory and visual distractions
- multistimulus environments similar to normal living or treatment situations
- therapeutic sessions including gross motor, table-top, cognitive activities, and overlearned, automatic ADLs
- one-on-one interactions between patient and therapist
- group situations
- social interactions with the family

The patient's behaviors in these situations will assist the therapist in deciding the appropriate types of treatment, the level of challenge the patient can tolerate, and the amount of input required from the therapist to produce the desired behavioral response. Socially acceptable behaviors can be reinforced early in the evaluation and treatment progression and unacceptable behaviors discouraged.

It is important to assess the patient's awareness of his abilities and limitations. It may not be possible to address this issue adequately in an initial evaluation, but it is appropriate in the ongoing evaluation and treatment. The higher functioning patient with few physical impairments will often deny the existence of deficits. It is much easier for both the patient and the family to recognize physical deficits than cognitive and perceptual deficits. There are times when the team will find it necessary to allow the patient to fail in a structured evaluation situation to point out specific deficits to the patient and family. This should be done early enough in the treatment program to allow the patient and therapist to build on the strengths of the individual in order to develop the skills necessary for task success before discharge.

Sensorimotor Evaluations

The sensorimotor evaluations usually require the least adaptation. With the exception of sensation, the evaluations are relatively passive, requiring the patient's cooperation more than his participation. In addition, many of the responses the therapist will be looking for are spontaneous, such as postural adaptations.

Muscle Tone, Reflex Activity, Movement Disorders, and Strength

Normal muscle tone, integrated reflexes, and sufficient muscle strength are necessary for movement and function. Evaluations are described here in isolation, but in function they are integrated components, and the influence of one may affect the evaluation of another. These sensorimotor components are evaluated to help determine the underlying causes of dysfunction in head control, postural adaptation, upper extremity control, and hand functioning necessary for completion of ADL and to help plan remediation. Key factors that help predict the patient's potential for motor learning and skill development are the ability to control abnormal muscle tone and the patient's sensory status. Even

when movement is possible, function can be impaired due to poor sensory processing.

Abnormal muscle tone can be severe; spasticity, rigidity, and flaccidity can all be encountered. Abnormal movement patterns such as ataxia may also be present. Muscle tone is the resistance a muscle offers to passive stretch. Many factors contribute to changes in muscle tone, including physical and emotional stress, body position in relation to gravity, and the environment (Bobath, 1978). Because of this, muscle tone should be assessed with the patient in various positions including supine, sidelying, sitting, and standing.

Evaluation of the scapula and trunk musculature should not be overlooked because they have a profound influence on upper extremity function. Palpation, visual examination, and passive movement are effective in assessing abnormal tone in the trunk (Figures 2–1 and 2–2). Shortening of one side of the trunk combined with resistance and downward rotation of the scapula with resistance to passive movement usually indicates spasticity. Rigidity in trunk musculature is indicated by lack of rotation in either the upper or lower trunk. Flaccidity in the trunk is indicated by shortening of one side or floppiness in the trunk with no resistance to passive movement. Decreased tone in the scapular musculature often results in excess scapular movement and/or winging of the scapula.

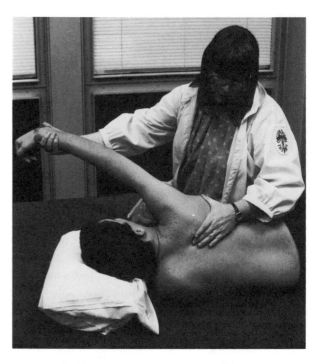

Figure 2–1 The scapula should rotate upward when the humerus is flexed above 90°.

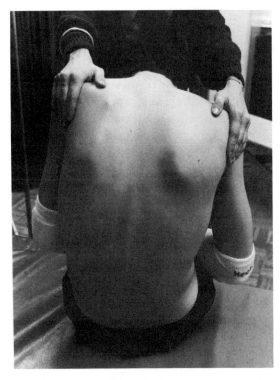

Figure 2–2 Note the shortening of the right side of this patient's trunk. Palpation is necessary to determine the type and intensity of the abnormal tone.

As some patients attempt to move from position to position, abnormal patterning may be observed. This may be attributed to abnormal tone, but the tonal influences of reflex activity should not be overlooked. Reflexes are evaluated for their presence and effects on muscle tone and movement patterns. Primitive reflex activity in the adult is considered an abnormal response. Common reflex influences that emerge after HI include:

- tonic labyrinthine reflex (TLR) prone and supine
- asymmetric tonic neck reflex (ATNR)
- symmetric tonic neck reflex (STNR)
- positive supporting reaction
- grasp reflex

Often, the therapist can detect the reflex influence without formal testing, but there are occasions when specific testing may be required to clarify the clinical picture.

The TLR is tested by placing the patient with his head in midline. The presence of the TLR is indicated in supine by increased extensor tone or extension of the extremities. Presence of the TLR in prone is indicated

by increased flexor tone or flexion of the extremities (Fiorentino, 1973). It reduces the patient's ability to cope with gravitational pull in all directions and strongly influences head and trunk control.

The ATNR (Figure 2–3) is tested by actively or passively rotating the head 90 degrees. If this reflex is present, limbs on the patient's face side will extend, while those on the skull side will flex. This reflex can be tested with the patient in supine, sitting, or quadruped positions. In some cases, movement into flexion and extension does not occur, but changes in muscle tone can be noted. This can interfere with hand to mouth function and eye-hand coordination.

The STNR is tested by flexing and extending the patient's neck. When the neck is flexed forward, the upper extremities will flex and the lower extremities will extend if this reflex is present. When the head is extended, the upper extremities will extend and the lower extremities will flex. This reflex can be tested with the patient prone over a bolster or in the quadruped or sitting position. Mild reflex influence may produce tonal changes rather than movement of the extremities. This often affects the patient's ability to move from position to position.

The positive supporting reaction is tested by stimulating the ball of the foot. It is best to test by placing the patient in an upright position, but the patient can sit if unable to stand. When the ball of the foot makes contact with the floor, it causes an increase in extensor tone in the leg and plantar flexion resulting in rigid extension of the leg with weight on the toes preventing normal weight bearing.

The grasp reflex (Figure 2–4) is tested by applying pressure in the palm of the patient's hand from the ulnar side. The reflexive response is mass finger flexion and

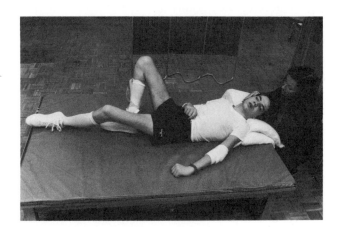

Figure 2–3 This patient's upper extremities are influenced by the ATNR in the supine position.

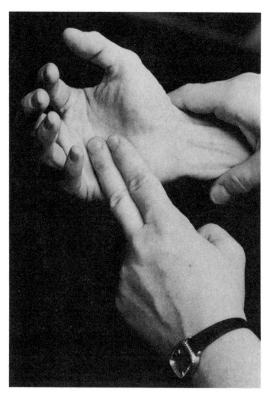

Figure 2–4 The grasp reflex can be tested by placing a firm object or the tester's fingers in the patient's palm. The pressure on the palm produces sustained mass finger flexion.

grasp of the stimulus that prevents release of the object, affecting hand function.

Other reflexes may be present and, if suspected, can be tested. Trombly (1983) and Fiorentino (1973) provide lists of reflexes, test positions, and responses. Test positions and the intensity of response are noted for all reflexes tested. In extreme cases, damage to the brainstem can produce decerebrate rigidity. Typical posturing of decerebrate rigidity is hyperextension of the neck, extension of the lower extremities, extension and internal rotation of the upper extremities, and flexion of the wrists. The presence of decerebrate rigidity for an extended period would indicate limited functional goals. Decorticate rigidity may occur with severe cortical damage. It produces extension of the lower extremities and flexion of the upper extremities (Chusid, 1976). The influences of abnormal tone and reflexes will affect the head-injured patient's potential for functional use and control of his extremities.

Upper extremity muscle tone is tested by quickly stretching or lengthening a muscle and determining the amount of resistance encountered. For example, when testing elbow flexors, the patient's arm is quickly moved into extension to elongate the flexors passively.

The reverse is done to test elbow extensors. When spasticity is present in the upper extremities, there is a range of free movement, then a strong contraction of the muscle in response to stretch followed by free movement as the muscle relaxes. This is referred to as a "clasp-knife phenomenon." Spasticity is graded minimum, moderate, or severe depending on the point at which the stretch reflex is elicited. Minimum spasticity is defined as resistance to passive stretch occurring in the last third to quarter (Trombly, 1983) of the available ROM. Spasticity is moderate when resistance occurs in the mid-ranges of the available arc of movement and is severe when resistance occurs in the first quarter (Trombly, 1983) to third of the available range. Each joint should be evaluated separately as some muscles may have severe spasticity and others minimal abnormalities. When muscles cross multiple joints, one joint is stabilized, and the stretch reflex is elicited by moving the other joint.

When rigidity is present in a muscle group, resistance is encountered throughout the entire arc of movement. In cog wheel rigidity, there is alternating resistance and relaxation throughout the entire ROM.

Flaccidity exists when there is no resistance to passive stretch. Limbs that are flaccid feel limp and floppy. The type, grade, and location of abnormal tone are recorded. If spasticity is elicited during the evaluation, attempts should be made by the therapist to normalize the muscle tone after testing, as described in Unit 6.

Ataxia and tremors are disorders of motion that may affect functional performance when cerebellar damage has occurred. Intention tremors occur during activity, intensify at the endpoint of the movement pattern, and are usually absent at rest. The therapist should evaluate the joints involved. Often a proximal tremor affects distal control, and stabilization of the joint will improve the patient's performance. Ataxia is defined as muscular incoordination that is manifested when voluntary muscular movements are attempted (Clayton, 1985). Ataxic movements can be noted in the upper extremities, and when present in the trunk, may cause a wide-based staggering gait in which patients fix their upper extremities in an attempt to maintain stability.

Muscle weakness can be a factor in evaluation and is often evident in neck extensors. Some patients display minimal physical involvement and may exhibit the debilitating effects of bedrest or inactivity. For these patients, a functional muscle test that grades muscle groups will provide the necessary baseline information. Apparent weakness may be due to hypotonia. A specific manual muscle test may be indicated to assess for peripheral nerve injuries when suspected. Muscle testing is not performed on the patient who exhibits spasticity because the abnormal tone masks the actual strength of the muscle, and the application of resistance can increase the level of spasticity. At times it may be necessary to determine the presence of a peripheral nerve injury in an extremity with abnormal muscle tone. In these instances, observation of movement at each joint will provide information concerning gross muscular innervation.

Head Control, Postural Adaptation, Balance, and Equilibrium

Effective head control allows for proper visual orientation and assists in communication, feeding, and interaction with people and things in the environment. It can be affected by abnormal muscle tone, reflexes, movement disorders, and muscle weakness. The causes of deficient head control may be varied and are determined by evaluation. Head control is usually assessed with gravity eliminated in supine and against gravity in prone or sitting positions. Movement patterns assessed include:

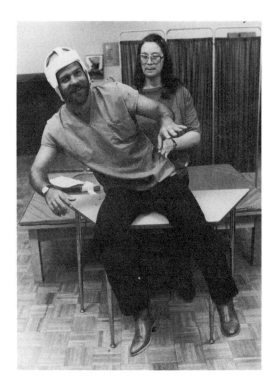

Figure 2–5 Testing equilibrium responses in seated position. Note the lack of rotation in the patient's trunk.

- lateral head movement
- flexion and extension
- rotary movements
- vertical head control against gravity

Limitations noted during the assessment include:

- asymmetry
- ROM limitations
- lack of movement, partial movement, or abnormal movement patterns
- endurance
- abnormal muscle tone

Remediation of poor head control reflects the underlying causes.

Spontaneous postural adaptation and equilibrium responses are essential for function in any nonsupported posture. Postural adaptation is a combination of automatic reactions of the trunk and limbs in response to gravity. These include righting, equilibrium, and spontaneous adaptation of muscles to changes in posture (Bobath, 1978). Balance and equilibrium reactions are tested in all developmental postures such as sitting, kneeling, half kneeling, and standing, if able (Figures 2–5 through 2–7). The patient is assessed for the following:

- the ability to maintain the test position without upper extremity support
- the ability to shift weight actively and reach out to sides, front, and back while in the test position
- the ability to regain midline position when the center of gravity is displaced by the therapist
- the ability to posturally adapt in relation to objects and during tasks

To assess this, the therapist places her hands on the patient's trunk, shoulders, or pelvis and gently applies pressure with one hand to 'tap' the patient off center. The therapist then catches the patient with her other hand. The therapist continues to alternate tapping and catching as the patient is moved further away from midline. The therapist observes the patient's responses, and when the patient's maximum level of displacement occurs, he is allowed to return to midline. Patients are not permitted to use upper extremities to stabilize or support themselves. For example, the normal response

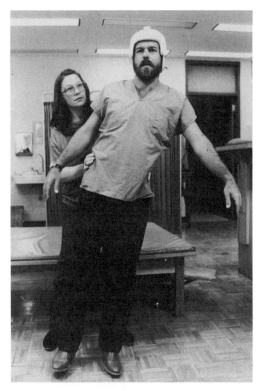

Figure 2–6 Testing equilibrium responses in standing. Note the extension in the trunk and extremities in an attempt to stabilize.

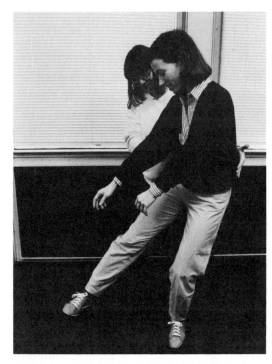

Figure 2–7 A normal balance and equilibrium response in standing. Note the trunk rotation and flexion used to accommodate the weight shift.

to the challenge of displacement to the right side in sitting or standing would be:

- head returning to left for maintaining midline position
- shortening of the left side of the trunk
- elongation of the right side of the trunk
- extension and abduction of the left arm
- extension and abduction of the left leg
- return to midline position

The process would be repeated to the left side and forward and backward. In a normal response, the head should approach or maintain midline. The patient's ability to reach a high shelf, low shelf, and across midline adds a functional component to the evaluation and assesses the patient's spontaneous adaptation during activity. Quality of response, timing, and the triggering of abnormal movement patterns during testing are noted. Responses that can be recorded are:

- *normal:* adequate level of response and timing
- *delayed:* timing of response is delayed or patient demonstrates over-reaction to amount of displacement encountered
- *emerging:* responses elicited only in extreme ranges of displacement or primitive responses such as protective extension are shown at less than extreme ranges
- *absent:* no spontaneous response to displacement

Transitional movements are those movements required to change from one position to another. Transitional movement patterns should be observed, especially in the patient with minimal physical impairments where subtle deficits in the quality of movement may be noted. The ability to move independently from supine to standing with and without upper extremity support can be used to evaluate transitional movement. Smooth coordinated movement patterns require an integrated postural adaptation system. Postural adaptation is an evaluation of patient response to gravity, movement, and activity.

Sensation

Upper extremity sensation is evaluated for two reasons. The first is to determine the patient's potential for safety awareness, and the second is to assess his potential for spontaneous use of the extremity. Sensation is usually not assessed in the minimally responsive or awakening patient except in gross responses referred to in the sensory awareness evaluation. The therapist must use clinical judgment in deciding if the confused or agitated patient can adequately focus his attention on the evaluation to provide a reliable response. Testing is done with the patient's vision occluded using a shield or blindfold, or by allowing him to close his eyes. For nonverbal patients, word or picture cards can be used in conjunction with eye gaze or pointing.

Superficial sensations evaluated are sharp and dull or temperature discrimination and light touch. These are associated with safety awareness. If superficial sensations are intact, localization to touch and two point discrimination are assessed. Position sense and kinesthesia are evaluated to help predict the patient's potential for spontaneous upper extremity use. Superficial sensations are rated intact, impaired, or absent and can vary proximally to distally or along peripheral nerve distributions. Any hypersensitivity to stimulation is graded as impaired.

Range of Motion

Goniometric ROM measurements are taken initially as a baseline from which to monitor changes. In patients with abnormally high tone, general relaxation should be attempted before measuring to reduce the potential for pain and to insure recording of the patient's maximum available range. Measurements of shoulder, elbow, wrist, and hand are recorded when limitations are suspected. The therapist notes the patient's position when measurements are taken, sitting or supine, and notes muscle length and joint mobility. This is important when muscles span two joints such as the wrist and fingers. X-ray tests should be requested if heterotopic bone formation is suspected at any joint. If limitations exist at the elbow, wrist, or hand, further evaluation for casting intervention may be indicated (see Unit 7 for specific criteria). Pain is sometimes associated with the end ranges. The patient may have become protective of the extremity or may focus on the pain. In some cases, the patient can be distracted from the pain by an activity requiring spontaneous movement or by involvement in a cognitive task. While the patient is distracted, the therapist may be able to take a measurement. If limitations are suspected in the neck, measurements can be taken. Specific ROM measurement techniques are not reviewed since numerous references to them exist (Trombly, 1983).

Upper Extremity Control

The shoulder girdle is a complex structure that serves as a basis for upper extremity control. The movements of the scapula, clavicle, and humerus must be evaluated as a working unit. For example, as the humerus is flexed, the scapula slides along the rib cage, protracts slightly, and upwardly rotates as the clavicle rotates on its axis. The muscles attached to these bones work in a coordinated manner to provide the proximal stability necessary for arm placement against gravity and to allow for distal function. The previous evaluation of muscle tone should provide information related to decreased functional use caused by problems of the shoulder girdle.

We consider arm placement to be the ability to move and use a limb functionally. Factors previously evaluated that affect arm placement include muscle tone, ROM, muscle strength, trunk control, presence of abnormal reflexes, and movement disorders. Synergy patterns also influence functional arm placement. If the patient's arm moves in mass patterns of flexion and extension, it is considered to be moving in synergy patterns. Synergistic movement is usually not functional. Brunnstrom (1970) described stages of synergies, and although they are more closely related to stroke patients, some head-injured patients exhibit them. For evaluation purposes, these stages can be used or described:

- *stage 1:* flaccid
- *stage 2:* synergies developing with flexor spasticity
- *stage 3:* mass flexion or extension when patient is asked to move arm, with increasing spasticity
- *stage 4:* some movement deviating from synergy
- *stage 5:* patient independent of basic patterns
- *stage 6:* isolated joint movement, near normal coordination, and no spasticity

If arm placement against gravity is not possible, evaluation begins with the patient in a gravity-eliminated position such as supine or sidelying. In supine, the evaluation of function includes the patient's ability to:

- hold the arm at 90° shoulder flexion (Figure 2–8)
- hold the arm above 90° shoulder flexion with and without external rotation (Figure 2–9)

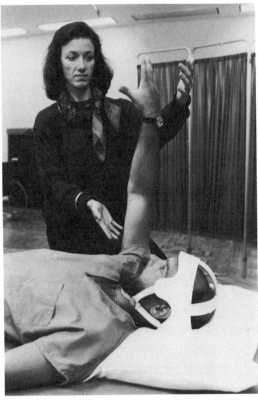

Figure 2–8 Evaluation of arm placement in a gravity-eliminated position.

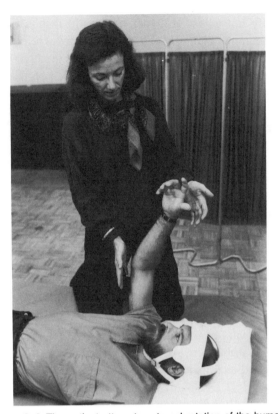

Figure 2–9 The patient attempts external rotation of the humerus.

- hold the arm below 90° shoulder flexion with and without external rotation
- move the arm between two points in space
- control the arm from 90° shoulder flexion down to the side of the body
- move the arm from adduction into abduction
- move the arm from 90° abduction to adduction
- with the humerus at 90°, flexion of the elbow to touch the top of the head or opposite shoulder, extension of the elbow, extension of the wrist, flexion and extension of the fingers (Figure 2–10)

If arm placement against gravity is possible, the patient's performance is evaluated as to control, timing, tonal, or synergistic influences when asked to touch the:

- top of the head
- back of the neck
- mouth
- small of the back
- lap
- feet

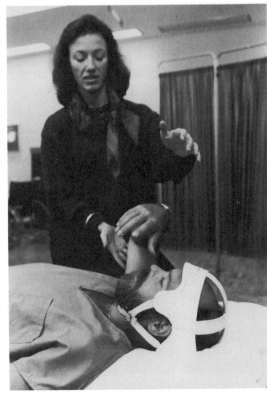

Figure 2–10 The patient attempts isolated elbow flexion and extension in the supine position.

Statements concerning spontaneous use of the upper extremities in unilateral and bilateral tasks are included in the evaluation.

Hand Function and Coordination

Hand function is a combination of strength, control, and manipulation skills. Its evaluation requires observation, measurement, and analysis of movement patterns. Grasp patterns can be evaluated informally by presenting objects of various sizes and shapes and observing how the patient picks them up and manipulates them. Abnormal patterns of movement should be noted such as inefficient wrist position, synergy patterns, influences of abnormal tone, or tremors. Common wrist-hand deficits noted post head injury that limit skilled object manipulation include:

- difficulty extending wrist and fingers simultaneously, which may be caused by tendon tightness
- hyperpronation during grasp, which may be caused by reflexive patterning
- difficulty releasing objects without flexing the wrist, due to poor finger extension

Diadochokinesia or rapid alternating movements such as turning the palm up and down can be evaluated by counting the number of repetitions possible in 10 seconds and evaluating the quality and rhythm of the movement patterns. In the absence of spasticity, grip and pinch strengths using a dynomometer and a pinch meter can be recorded and compared with established norms. The 9-hole peg test (1971) may be used as a quick evaluation tool to assess coordination and may also be compared with norms. For the patient with minimal physical impairment, more involved hand function tests may be indicated, especially if vocationally important. Tests available include The Minnesota Rate of Manipulation Test (1946), Purdue Pegboard (1948), and Crawford Small Parts Dexterity Test (1956).

Evaluation of the sensorimotor status of the agitated patient may present special problems. The patient may not be able to attend to or tolerate the structured evaluation. Frequent rest periods or breaks may help. If not, observation of the patient's performance of functional tasks can be used to assess the patient in general terms. When the agitated patient becomes able to tolerate short periods of evaluation, the therapist should prioritize the evaluations that provide the most essential information needed for establishing goals and planning treatment.

Sensory-Perceptual and Cognitive Functions

Sensory-perceptual and cognitive functioning span a wide range of levels in the head-injured population. At the lowest level of evaluation, the therapist is recording the response or lack of response to a single stimulus. At the highest level, the therapist is observing the patient solving complex problems in sophisticated daily living tasks. The types of evaluations performed will depend on the level of functioning observed.

Patients at the lowest range of function are sometimes categorized as comatose, semicomatose, or vegetative. Evaluation of this patient may occur very early post injury or later if the injury was severe and the patient's progress slow.

The patient may open his eyes periodically, but there is usually no apparent focusing or tracking, and response to voice commands is infrequent. Gradually, the patient may begin to demonstrate more adaptive responses to stimulation. As function improves, the individual will track visually and may be able to respond to simple verbal commands.

Sensory awareness evaluation of the patient is important and involves rating the responses to various stimuli. Responses are usually graded as (1) no response, (2) generalized response, or (3) localized response. A generalized response is not specific to the type of stimulation presented. When presented with a single stimulus, the patient may show a whole body response, such as flexed posturing, or an autonomic nervous system response, such as increased respiration. A localized response is more stimulus specific, such as withdrawing an arm when pricked with a pin or turning the head in response to auditory input. Latency of response is common in the early stages, with some patients taking up to 2 minutes to process information and produce a response. Latency of response should be recorded as well as consistency of response, which can be reported in percentages.

The therapist evaluates responses to input in all sensory systems: tactile, auditory, vestibular, visual, olfactory, and gustatory. Care should be taken to allow enough time for the patient to respond before restimulating or changing the stimulus (Farber, 1982). Responses to stimulation can be recorded narratively or in chart form. When referring to a chart, it may be easier to compare responses, but a narrative may better expand on the quality of responses. It is important to rate variations in response that may be related to time of day or to the presence of family members. At this stage of recovery, treatment is often combined with continued evaluation, as the therapist notes the patient's response to all treatment attempts. Types of stimulation and possible responses are expanded in Unit 5.

Patients who are confused or agitated may be looking around, but they may not be able to process environmental information adequately. This is a major factor contributing to confused and agitated states. The agitated patient may not be able to process all of the incoming sensory stimulation and filter out the nonessential information in order to produce an adaptive response. Often, by reducing the amount of environmental stimuli, the patient's agitation will subside long enough to participate in a few simple evaluation tasks.

If changing the environment does not decrease the agitation, one may choose to evaluate the effects of relaxation techniques such as rolling, slow rocking, or wrapping the patient in a blanket for the effects of neutral warmth (Farber, 1982) (see Unit 6 for details of treatment). Pacing, being allowed to move freely, or propelling a wheelchair for a short time can be evaluated for their effectiveness in reducing agitation and in producing the calmer state needed for accurate evaluation. Restraining the patient usually produces an adverse reaction, making evaluation impossible, and is only used to prevent self-inflicted injury.

Orientation

Once the patient is calmer, short periods can be used for further evaluation. Basic orientation can be assessed using an interview and includes orientation to:

- person (self and information about self)
- place (hospital, city, state)
- time (month, day, year, and time of day)
- recognition of others (family, physician, therapists)
- reason for hospitalization
- events immediately preceding injury
- ongoing day-to-day events

If the patient cannot provide this information, it should be supplied by the therapist in a nonthreatening manner to reduce frustration.

Sensory-Perceptual

The therapist can use functional tasks such as hygiene and dressing as part of the evaluation. Analysis of task performance will provide information concerning attention to task, ability to cross midline, motor planning, sequencing, sense of position in space, visual processing, and directionality. For example, the patient's inattention to task may reflect a decreased level of arousal or problems with sustained attention. Shaving one side of the face may indicate visual field problems, neglect, or inability to cross midline. Difficulty dressing may reflect any of several problems including figure-ground discrimination problems, position-in-space deficits, or motor planning disturbances. To further pinpoint the deficit area, the therapist may have the patient select an object from a cluttered drawer. Inability to do this may indicate that there is a figure-ground problem, affecting visual perception. Simple puzzles of differing size and shape may provide visual spatial information. The patient's topographic orientation in the hospital can also be used to assess high-level perceptual skills, such as his ability to locate his room and his area within the room, and to identify personal belongings. Confused and agitated patients may not be able to participate actively in a formalized, cognitive-perceptual testing situation. Observations by the therapist must be as objective as possible while addressing functional performance and the environmental effects on performance.

Patients who are alert and oriented to their surroundings with few physical impairments are more receptive to formal testing than are other patients. They may continue to have problems with attention but should be able to tolerate a more inclusive test battery. Formal and informal assessments can be performed to evaluate tactile processing, motor performance, and visual perception (Chapparo & Ranka, 1980). Tests that provide information on tactile processing include:

- finger identification, including bilateral simultaneous stimulation
- localization to touch
- stereognosis
- kinesthesia
- graphesthesia

Evaluations of motor performance include:

- imitation of nonhabitual postures
- imitation of nonhabitual rhythmic sequences

- imitation of familiar tasks, using only gestures
- motor accuracy or tracing tasks

Evaluations of visual perception include:

- visual screening—including color, shape recognition, depth perception, occular motor ROM, visual pursuit, fixation, and scanning—may be appropriate before testing all areas
- Hooper Visual Organization Test (1958)
- Symbol Digit Modalities Test (1973)
- Sherman Mental Impairment Test (1956)
- Motor-Free Visual Perception Test (1972)
- mazes

Strengths can be determined by evaluating all areas. The findings are then used in the patient's treatment program to maximize performance. The treatment plan also includes strategies to facilitate skills in deficit areas.

Cognition

The ability to process and organize sensory information is the foundation for higher-level cognitive skills. It is difficult to make a sound cognitive decision based on faulty processing of the environment. The psychologist provides information on cognitive functioning to the team based on neuropsychological testing of the patient. Cognitive skills are evaluated by the occupational therapist primarily by assessing performance of selected functional tasks. When observing the patient's performance of a meal preparation task or the completion of a woodworking project, the therapist notes:

- selective attention (distractability)
- organizational skills
- short-term memory
- sequencing
- problem solving
- speed and accuracy of performance
- safety and judgment

For example, in meal preparation, the patient may have difficulty attending to several aspects of the task simultaneously. This may be due to attentional problems, organizational deficits, or memory problems. If the patient must refer to a recipe numerous times, memory deficits may be the key factor. This, combined with the patient's forgetting to turn the stove off, would compromise the patient's safe performance of hot meal preparation. Further, if the patient fails to recognize the problem, his judgment would be questioned.

Basic survival skills in reading and money management can be assessed using games or simulations and community trials. The use of consequence cards and situation cards may aid in evaluating more abstract problem solving. The therapist should be cautious interpreting these data since there are often differences between verbal abilities and performance skills. If the patient is severely physically involved and cannot perform tasks, his verbal responses will provide some information concerning his level of cognitive functioning.

The patient who is alert with severe physical limitations and communication deficits poses different problems in sensory-perceptual, and cognitive evaluation. First, it must be established that the nonverbal patient can comprehend language. The team may work together to establish reliable ''yes'' and ''no'' responses. By setting up testing situations where the patient must pick one of several alternatives either by pointing, eye gaze, or a ''yes'' or ''no'' response, information on sensory-perceptual, and cognitive functioning can be gathered.

Orientation questions can be rephrased to require a ''yes'' or ''no'' response as can short-term and long-term memory assessments, such as ''Was your last meal lunch?'' or ''Were you born in Seattle?'' Picture cards can be used to assess the patient's ability to categorize and sort items. Sequencing skills may be assessed using picture sequence cards. Categorizing items implies an understanding of the relation between objects and their properties. Sequencing events requires the ability to understand the concepts of ''before'' and ''after.''

The Motor-Free Visual Perception Test (1972) can be modified to a ''yes'' or ''no'' response to assess basic visual perceptual skills by the therapist pointing to each possible answer. Standardized scores cannot be used if administration is modified in this way.

Given severe physical and verbal limitations, the sensory-perceptual, and cognitive evaluations will not be so thorough as those of the less-involved patients, but the information gathered is essential for establishing the potential of the individual to use various alternative communication devices, environmental control devices, and possibly computers in a functional manner.

Daily Living Skills

Daily living tasks include self-care, homemaking, leisure, prevocational, educational, and community-living skills. Their performance is usually the long-term goal of treatment. Effective psychosocial, cognitive, sensory-perceptual, and sensorimotor skills are necessary for the patient to participate optimally in ADL tasks.

Information gathered in the psychosocial evaluation relates to the specific tasks the individual will need to perform in order to resume aspects of his previous roles. Physical deficits may be obvious, and adaptations may be helpful in making the patient independent in certain tasks. However, in many cases it is the sensory-perceptual, cognitive, and behavioral components of the patient's performance that are more difficult to evaluate and ultimately affect his ability to function independently.

Basic self-care skills of feeding, dressing, grooming, and bathing are of primary concern and are evaluated as soon as possible. Oral feeding is often an important goal for patients who require tube feedings to meet their nutritional needs.

The ability to suck, swallow, chew, or control food may be impaired after HI. A thorough evaluation of oral motor control is completed in order to identify specific deficits that interfere with feeding. This evaluation serves as the basis for a graded feeding program that maximizes patient independence and minimizes the possibility of choking or aspiration. It may be completed by an occupational therapist or a speech and language pathologist; at RIC, the latter are primarily responsible. However, because OT is closely involved with feeding training and, in many facilities, is responsible for the treatment of oral motor disorders, a brief outline of assessment is provided. The reader is referred to the reference list in Unit 9 for more information on this topic.

Evaluation of internal and external oral functioning includes assessment of:

- tongue movement, including protraction, retraction, elevation, depression, and lateralization
- presence or absence of the bite reflex
- lip movement and the ability to suck
- the swallowing mechanism
- sensory sensitivity of the mouth and perioral areas
- muscle tone and control of oral musculature

In some facilities, the effectiveness of the food intake system is further evaluated using a "cookie swallow test" or videofluoroscopy. This process involves a video X-ray film of the patient's head and neck while swallowing a small amount of barium. Oral motor function is observed, and recommendations for feeding training are made.

It is best to evaluate performance of self-care at the times of the day these activities normally occur. This helps orient the patient and makes the activity more meaningful. Homemaking, leisure, and prevocational skills can be assessed during therapy when appropriate for the patient. Evaluation should specifically address how the patient performs each task. Factors to consider include:

- Which aspects of the task can be performed adequately?
- Which aspects require assistance?
- What kind of assistance is required?
- Can the assistance be graded?
- Can the patient sequence the task?
- Can the task be completed in a reasonable amount of time?
- Is cueing helpful to the patient (visual, manual, or verbal)?
- Is safety an issue?
- Is equipment required?

Components of all previous evaluations affect the functional performance of the head-injured individual. It is the therapist's responsibility to determine which factors are affecting the patient's performance: motor, sensory, cognitive, and/or perceptual. It is then possible to judge whether the patient's functional outcome can be improved by therapeutic intervention and to decide what type of intervention should be used.

Once the patient's performance is observed, it can be rated and goals established for the individual skills of feeding, upper and lower extremity dressing, grooming, and bathing. The following continuum is currently used at RIC (see Unit 9):

- independent
- independent with equipment or adaptive environment
- independent with set-up

- minimal assistance (patient performs 75% or more)

- moderate assistance (patient performs 50% to 75%)

- maximal assistance (patient performs 25% to 50%) (also includes dependent, but can direct care)

- dependent (patient performs less than 25%)

- not applicable, or patient not responsible for task

Community integration skills are evaluated in patients whose physical and cognitive status indicates potential for skill development. Skills include use of communication devices, topographic orientation, use of money, use of transportation, and time management. In the clinic, evaluation may be done by simulation of the activity. Once skills are acceptable in the structure of the clinic, evaluation of skills progresses to task performance in the community. Information gathered from the performance evaluations will help the team assess the patient's potential for successful independent living or determine necessary modifications. Often, the evaluation of community living skills provides important bottom-line information for family and employers.

Complete evaluation and re-evaluation of head-injured patients is an integral part of their management. It is difficult to separate evaluation and treatment since the therapist is always evaluating the effectiveness of the selected treatment techniques and the patient's responses. A good evaluation is the necessary foundation of sound goal formation and effective treatment planning. Ongoing evaluation is necessary in order to obtain information needed for documenting patient progress and the effectiveness of OT interventions.

REFERENCES

Ayres, J.A. (1972). *Sensory integration and learning disorders*. Los Angeles: Western Psychological Services.

Bobath, B. (1978). *Adult hemiplegia: Evaluation and treatment* (2nd ed.). London: William Heinemann.

Brunnstrom, S. (1970). *Movement therapy in hemiplegia*. Hagerstown, MD: Harper & Row.

Chapparo, C. & Ranka, J. (1980). *Patterns of sensory integrative dysfunction in adult hemiplegia*. Unpublished Research Project RT-20, Project R-112, Rehabilitation Institute of Chicago.

Chusid, J.G. (1976). *Correlative neuroanatomy and functional neurology* (16th ed.). Los Angeles: Lange Medical Publications.

Clayton, T. (Ed.). (1985). *Taber's cyclopedic medical dictionary* (15th ed.). Philadelphia: F.A. Davis.

Crawford Small Parts Dexterity Test. (1956). The Psychological Corporation, New York.

Farber, S. (1982). *Neurorehabilitation: A multi-sensory approach*. Philadelphia: W.B. Saunders.

Fiorentino, M.A. (1973). *Reflex testing methods for evaluating CNS development* (2nd ed.). Springfield, IL: Charles C Thomas.

The Hooper Visual Organization Test. (1958). Los Angeles: Western Psychological Services.

Kellor, M., Frost, J., Silverberg, N., Iversen, I. & Cummings, R. (1971). Hand strength dexterity. *American Journal of Occupational Therapy, 25*, 77–83.

Minnesota Rate of Manipulation Tests. (1946). Circle Pines, MN: American Guidance Service.

Motor-Free Visual Perception Test (MVPT). (1972). Novato, CA: Academic Therapy Publications.

Oakley, F. (1981). The Role Checklist. College Park, MD: Available from the author.

Purdue Pegboard. (1948). Lafayette, IN: Lafayette Instrument Co.

Sherman Mental Impairment Test. (1956). Los Angeles: Western Psychological Services.

Symbol Digit Modalities Test. (1973). Los Angeles: Western Psychological Services.

Trombly, C.A. (1983). *Occupational therapy for physical dysfunction* (2nd ed.). Baltimore: Williams & Wilkins.

Goal Setting and Treatment Planning

Karen Kovich, OTR/L

The purpose of rehabilitation is to restore an optimum level of function to an individual through therapeutic intervention. To do this, the therapist uses an ongoing process involving evaluation and interpretation of data to determine the needs of each patient. The therapist then synthesizes evaluation results, professional knowledge, experience, and resources with input from the patient and family to design a treatment program to meet those needs. This process is known as treatment planning.

The treatment planning process in occupational therapy (OT) is fundamental and is applied to a variety of diagnoses. It involves (1) gathering data, (2) interpreting the data to identify problem areas, (3) setting goals to address problem areas, (4) developing methods to achieve identified goals, (5) implementing the methods, and (6) re-evaluating to determine progress and the effectiveness of intervention.

GATHERING DATA

As stated in Unit 2, a formal OT evaluation of a patient's psychosocial, cognitive, sensory-perceptual, and motor skills, and activities of daily living (ADL) is only one source of data. Other sources include the medical chart, documentation from previous facilities, and the patient's family and friends. Family and friends may provide valuable information and insight into the patient's previous life style, roles, and interests. In addition, they can convey to the treatment team the patient and family's understanding and acceptance of the disability and their expectations regarding outcome. Other professionals provide information that may assist the occupational therapist in determining a course of action. These sources may include reports from nursing as to the times of day the patient is most alert or a report from the psychology department regarding the individual's potential for new learning.

Additional research in books and journals or by examining case studies should be done by the therapist to gain more in-depth knowledge of how a patient's clinical presentation compares with the classic picture. Completing this process allows the therapist to more effectively influence and predict the outcome.

INTERPRETATION OF DATA

Once the data from the OT evaluation are gathered, they are analyzed and integrated with those from other sources to gain a total picture of the patient's strengths and weaknesses. Due to the nature of head injury (HI), problem areas that become apparent are frequently a complex mixture of cognitive, sensory-perceptual, sensorimotor, and behavioral deficits. It is often difficult to determine which deficit or combination of deficits is responsible for a breakdown in functional skills. To do this, the therapist must complete a two-step process. First, each deficit must be identified and, second, its severity in relation to other deficits must be determined. The therapist then decides which areas can best be addressed through intervention in OT. As a result of this process, goal areas for each patient are defined.

SETTING GOALS AND ESTABLISHING PRIORITIES

Long-Term Goals

Once the evaluation information is integrated and specific problem areas are identified, the therapist may begin to predict an expected outcome level. Long-term goals (LTGs), which describe the level of function the patient will reach by the end of his hospitalization, are set first. While specific to patient function, they are more general than short-term goals (STGs) and define a functional endpoint. LTGs may need to be adjusted during the course of the patient's hospitalization.

In order to set LTGs, the therapist first looks at the components of a functional task and their interrelation. The minimum level of skill in those components necessary to meet an LTG are then identified. Additionally, adapted methods or equipment that may be used to compensate for deficits are considered. For example, a goal of independence in dressing implies that the patient has a minimum level of functioning in controlling his trunk, the upper extremities, problem solving, and sequencing. Developing skill in trunk control or upper extremity functioning, however, may depend on the patient's level of cooperation. By analyzing the required level of ability in these areas, the interrelation of skills, and the current level of functioning, the therapist can set LTGs.

In order to use the standards given at the end of the units to assist in setting LTGs, the therapist should review the indicators listed below each LTG to identify those that most closely describe the patient. The corresponding LTG can be used as is or modified to reflect the expected status at discharge. LTGs are listed for all component skills and specific functional tasks.

The achievement of goals and the success of the treatment program do not depend solely on the evaluation, treatment planning, and clinical skills of the occupational therapist. Involving the patient (if able), the family, and other team members is critical if they are to play an active role in the treatment process.

Short-Term Goals

Once LTGs are set and discussed with the patient and family, STGs can be developed to meet each LTG. STGs are more specific and reflect performance in and progress through the component skills necessary to meet the functional endpoint. The following example illustrates the relation between LTGs and STGs:

- LTG: independence in dressing in an unsupervised environment
- STGs:
  1. patient to demonstrate sustained attention for participation in treatment 10 minutes without cueing
  2. patient to demonstrate trunk balance sufficient for function in unsupported sitting for 10 minutes
  3. patient to develop overhead arm placement with one upper extremity sufficient for donning a pullover shirt
  4. patient to manipulate clothing fasteners independently 100 percent of the time

In this example, independence in dressing will be achieved only if the component skills identified by the STGs are mastered. While STGs may be worked on simultaneously, careful task analysis frequently shows a clear sequencing of skills that will aid the therapist in establishing priorities. In the example, trunk balance must be achieved before arm placement is possible, and overhead arm placement should be achieved first to enhance fine motor skills. The failure to achieve STGs in the projected length of time is frequently an indication that adaptive methods will need to be used by the patient. For example, if trunk balance sufficient for unsupported sitting is not achieved, dressing tasks may need to be modified to enable them to be done in supported sitting.

STGs should be written in objective and measurable terms. This allows the occupational therapist and others on the treatment team to measure progress accurately and to revise the treatment plan in a timely manner. Objective, measurable goals are most easily developed for physical limitations or for specific functional tasks such as drinking from a cup or writing. The challenge that faces the therapist in writing such goals for the head-injured patient lies in the fact that his performance is almost always affected by a combination of cognitive and behavioral deficits that may be difficult to measure independently and objectively. In these cases, goals must be qualified by identifying the specific behaviors or environmental considerations that are necessary for successful performance. These may include the amount of time or assistance required, the percentage of a task the patient is to perform, or specific descriptions of consistency and quality. These measurable and objective statements can then be upgraded to formulate new goals.

The standards given at the end of the units provide sample STGs for each LTG to be used for interim documentation. They contain italicized sections that can be modified to upgrade or downgrade the goals or to more clearly specify the desired behavior. For example, consider the following STG: "Patient will (*hold, pick-up*) _____ sized objects using (*lateral, palmer*) prehension." This may be customized by choosing the italicized descriptions most appropriate to the patient. The customized STG might then state: "Patient will pick up a 1-inch cube using lateral prehension." It is expected that other STGs will be needed to reflect each patient's needs and progress.

Mutual Goal Setting

Often, as a result of HI, deficits occur that impair an individual's ability to assist in formulating goals or to participate in treatment. Cognitive deficits, for example, may decrease the patient's insight into specific limitations. While the therapist can identify problem areas, some patients may strongly deny that they exist and, therefore, see no point in working on remediation. Others may admit to existing problems but, due to a lack of knowledge of the recovery process, set goals that are far beyond the therapist's expectations. In each case, it is important for the therapist to continue to discuss goals with the patient and to reinforce the factual information on which the professional goals are based. A goal area for such patients may be to enhance comprehension of their disability and the resulting deficits. When the patient cannot engage in realistic goal setting, the situation should be discussed with family members. This enables the family to provide the patient with consistent information on appropriate expectations of treatment.

In addition to determining mutual goals, discussing problem areas with the patient may bring to light differing priorities for the therapist and patient. A patient's priorities are determined by such things as life style,

level of education, culture, interests, roles, and responsibilities before the injury. In all cases, understanding the patient's priorities is important. They will affect his ability to see the significance of and participate in therapeutic activities. Therefore, in formulating goals, the therapist should address not only deficits caused by the HI but the patient's life style before the injury.

Family involvement in goal setting becomes especially important when the patient cannot actively participate. The feeling of loss for the family frequently becomes more profound when the patient cannot communicate with them. Despite the severity of the injury, the family often looks to the therapist to confirm their hope that the patient will return to a normal state of functioning. Although they may lack the objectivity to assist in realistic goal setting initially, it is important that they be given an explanation of the goal setting process, why specific goals have been set, and how treatment will proceed. All patient-related goals offered by the family should be acknowledged and addressed with professional discretion, or explanations given as to why they cannot be addressed at this time. This process is very important in educating family members in order to promote realistic expectations and to prepare them to become more effective participants in treatment.

FORMULATION AND IMPLEMENTATION OF THE TREATMENT PLAN

The treatment plan is composed of a series of principles and methods used to meet the desired goals. A principle for treatment is selected based on the underlying cause of the problem. Once the principles are selected, appropriate treatment methods are chosen. For example, after HI, a patient with spasticity in the upper extremity may develop an elbow flexion contracture. In this case, the principle for the basis of treatment is that maintained stretch on a muscle will elongate muscle fibers and allow for increased range of motion (ROM). Therefore, aggressive daily passive ROM or serial casting may be the therapeutic method applied to the problem.

Due to the nature of HI, it is often challenging to select appropriate methods of treatment. Frequently, the method of choice to remediate one problem may not be feasible because of deficits in other areas. For example, a patient may need to learn a one-handed dressing technique but, due to cognitive deficits affecting new learning or memory, may be unable to remember the technique from day to day. The therapist's ability to meet this challenge and to formulate effective methods is enhanced by her knowledge of activity analysis. By combining knowledge of activity with clinical experience, it is possible to select or adapt methods that address two or three deficit areas simultaneously. To follow up on the example, alternative solutions for this patient may include attempting to learn the new technique by daily repetition or compensating for the problem area by referring to written or pictorial instructions posted by the bed.

The treatment plan should include methods that address all problem areas related to OT as defined through the data analysis. Throughout treatment, priorities continue to emerge as the therapist proceeds developmentally with the plan, working on basic skills first and moving to the more complex. Each treatment plan should relate specifically to an STG. To ensure consistency, each method should include information on specific activities to be completed, positions and tools used, the structure of the environment, the role of other individuals, guidance required, time of day, and whether the treatment will be individual or in a group.

Due to the range of severity of clinical symptoms seen in head-injured patients, the role of the therapist as an active participant in the treatment session may vary. When treating a minimally responsive patient, the therapist assumes a very active role. Because the patient has little ability to participate actively, most techniques are performed solely by the therapist. At the other extreme, an alert oriented patient working on independent living skills may need the therapist to be less active, providing only minimal verbal cueing to optimize functioning and/or give feedback on performance.

As methods are implemented, it may be necessary to adapt a chosen activity to gain the desired therapeutic effect. This is frequently the case with head-injured patients due to the subtlety and fluctuation of cognitive and behavioral deficits. Factors that can be modified to meet the patient's needs in these cases are often external, such as the number of cues or the amount of supervision given, the amount of time the patient is required to work, or the number of steps in the task being performed (see Unit 9).

A common problem seen in HI is the patient's refusal or inability to participate due to agitation or other behavioral problems. This may occur in all therapies or, more specifically, in those that work on deficit areas that are the most frustrating for the patient. Agitation or frustration may also occur when the patient does not see the therapeutic value of an activity because it addresses a deficit area indirectly. For example, patients may be unable to see that participating in meal preparation helps to develop problem-solving skills. If a patient becomes agitated or refuses to participate, the therapist should determine what provoked or preceded the incident and try to modify the task to make it less demanding. It may also be beneficial for the therapist to choose a different task that the patient will be less resistant to but that offers the same therapeutic benefits. When a patient first begins to display agitation and refuses to participate, a plan to deal with the behavior should be developed by the treatment team (see Unit 5). In this way, the behavior will be dealt with consistently by all disciplines and family members. This approach enables the patient to gain the maximum benefit from treatment.

RE-EVALUATION AND DOCUMENTATION OF PROGRESS

Throughout treatment, an ongoing process of observation and evaluation should occur in order to determine the effectiveness of the total plan. The therapist must determine if the STGs are being achieved in the projected time. Progress is measured through observation of patient performance and re-evaluation on specific tests. This allows the therapist to compare a patient's current status with his baseline measure of functioning.

Progress may be very slow and difficult to measure. This may be due to a number of factors including the severity of the injury, the time elapsed since onset, or the subtle ways in which cognitive and perceptual deficits affect function. Despite these complicating factors, the need for documentation strongly supports the writing of STGs in measurable and objective terms. Many times it is in the quality or consistency of performance, the time or amount of cueing required, or changes in the level of alertness, attention, or concentration that the therapist will use in noting progress. If these factors have been described in measurable terms, the therapist will be able to document progress in a task even if the change is not significant enough to affect functional performance. Complete, objective, and measurable documentation has also become increasingly important to justify private and public reimbursement.

The information gained through observation, re-evaluation, and objective measurements of progress may necessitate revision of the treatment plan, including methods, STGs, or LTGs. The complexity or duration of an activity may need to be increased to keep it challenging and therapeutic or may need to be decreased if other problems develop such as increased agitation or medical complications.

STGs change continually as a patient attains the component skills. Grading STGs may involve changing the level of performance of a component skill or adding a new skill to the plan. LTGs are revised and upgraded less frequently once the patient has mastered the component skills necessary to increase his level of functioning. If a patient cannot achieve a goal, the therapist must first look at the methods being used. If all methods have been tried and the goal is still not met, limiting factors should be identified and a more realistic goal set.

This process of goal setting and re-evaluation ends when the therapist feels that the patient has reached his maximum level of functioning. Formal treatment is then discontinued. Further gains may be facilitated by issuing home programs or through family education. Both strategies help insure the carryover of new learning and facilitate continued independence after discharge.

Many variables influence the recovery process after HI. The degree to which a particular patient will benefit from therapy cannot be predicted with certainty. This, in turn, makes it difficult for the therapist to predict long-term outcomes and to set LTGs. In spite of these complicating variables, the therapist must combine existing information, knowledge gained through experience with other head-injured patients, and sound professional judgment to develop a treatment plan that will provide the patient with the opportunity to achieve his maximum level of independence.

Part II

Behavioral Components

Psychosocial Elements of Head Injury

Diane Bermann, OTR/L

Comprehensive management of the head-injured patient must address the psychosocial as well as the physical problems associated with trauma. While adjustments must be made by both the patient and his family to the various disabilities associated with head injury (HI), adjustments must also be made to roles in the family that often change as a result of disability. The head-injured individual may display changes in personality or exhibit behaviors that are no longer within the social and cultural norms of the family. This may impact on the family and their ability to interact with the patient. The family's ability to cope with these psychosocial changes ultimately affects successful discharge planning and may determine the need for continued long-term care.

Effective management of psychosocial issues requires a team effort. Each team member has a different perspective on the patient and family, as different demands are placed on the patient by each discipline. Therapists and nurses may have a clearer perspective on the patient's adjustment due to their daily contact, while the physician and social worker may be more aware of the family's coping skills. Nurses are best able to observe and provide information on patient and family interaction during nonstructured visiting hours and on weekends. The clinical psychologist can assist the team in formulating behavioral management strategies and, in conjunction with the social worker, can meet with the patient and family individually and help them verbalize and cope with their feelings. Periodic meetings are necessary to enable team members to share

information to insure the optimal management of the patient and to meet the family's needs. Plans and strategies to manage behavioral and other psychosocial issues must be shared with the family for consistency of approach and to prepare them for ongoing management of the patient.

Occupational therapists are trained in both physical disabilities and psychosocial dysfunction. Some of the behavioral manifestations of HI and psychosocial dysfunction are similar. They may include depression, passivity, aggressiveness, or loss of social inhibitions. Although the sources of these behaviors differ, some of the techniques used to manage them are similar. Occupational therapists can select activities appropriate to the physical, cognitive, and psychosocial needs of the patient. Activities can be used to channel aggressive behavior, increase self-esteem, and foster efforts to combat depression. The therapeutic use of groups can also be beneficial in the treatment of socially inappropriate behaviors. Occupational therapists should be prepared to draw on all of their resources to provide comprehensive treatment to the head-injured patient.

Studies have shown that psychosocial issues that impact on the patient and family most often include changes in affect and personality (Jellinek, Torkelson, & Harvey, 1982; Livingston, Brooks, & Bond, 1985a,b; McKinly, Brooks, Bond, Martinage, & Marshall, 1981). In follow-up studies done 3, 6, and 12 months post injury, loss of temper, irritability, mood swings, and depression were found to be the behaviors most distressing to the family. These changes were reported more frequently at 1 year post injury (McKinly et al., 1981). One may speculate that by then a routine is established and patterns of behavior are more apparent. The family's expectations for improved behavior may also change as the reality of chronic behavioral problems becomes evident. In the studies, disturbed social behavior was described as violent or inappropriate behaviors. While families reported fewer episodes of such behaviors as opposed to irritability or loss of temper, they were more upsetting to the family when they did occur and tended to fluctuate or increase over time (McKinly et al., 1981). This increase may indicate a learned response in dealing with situations that are difficult or frustrating or that the patient wishes to avoid. Overall, the family reported physical limitations to be less stressful than behavioral problems, while loss of independence more often affected the patient (Jellinek et al., 1982; Livingston et al., 1985a). This may indicate that the head-injured person is unaware of the behavioral manifestations of the disability and focuses more on physical limitations. Often, these inappropriate behaviors are noted while the patient is in the rehabilitation setting, and strategies must be developed to control them.

THE NEEDS OF THE FAMILY AND SIGNIFICANT OTHERS

Adjustment to a disability as devastating as HI can be a daily struggle for both the patient and family. Initially, family members must be accepted at whatever emotional state they present. The level and style of coping will vary for each family and family member. Periods of mourning, shock, anger, or denial are not unusual. Efforts should be made by the team to encourage appropriate displays of concern by the family and significant others and involve them as active members of the treatment team. The therapist's role as a team member is to offer support to the family members and provide them with basic information regarding OT as it relates to HI and the types of OT treatment being provided to the patient. Frequently, families cannot process specific information immediately after the patient's injury due to denial or inadequate coping mechanisms. Thus, information provided in general terms may be more effective. The process of meeting with the family and talking about the patient's premorbid life

style and interests serves as a means of establishing rapport. This is the first step in gaining the family's trust and acceptance of the therapist's professional judgment.

Because the general public's awareness of HI is often limited, and the family's expectation may be the patient's complete return to his premorbid state, they may ask similar questions of all professionals, waiting for someone to tell them what they want to hear. It is imperative that the interdisciplinary team communicate so that the family receives a consistent message from all professionals. Questions related to OT goals are answered in terms of specific skills the patient needs to develop to become independent. It is important to keep in mind the level of the family members' acceptance and their ability to understand and process what is being said. Questions regarding the long-term prognosis may be referred to the physician.

If one individual emerges as the potential caregiver or contact person, it is beneficial to have that person observe treatment whenever possible. This establishes an early basis for trust and understanding between the team and the caregiver. This individual can be gradually introduced to the patient's routine and guided to interact appropriately with the patient. It is important not to overwhelm the individual with information in the early stages and to encourage, but not force, participation. Some family members are eager to learn and become involved as soon as possible. Others are more reluctant. Each family member must be treated as an individual with differing abilities and needs.

The therapist should make a point of observing family members' abilities in learning simple aspects of the patient's care in order to determine or predict their comfort level and ability to learn routine care. Some people's strengths lie in the physical dimensions of care, such as ROM techniques and splint application, while others have strengths involving the psychosocial aspects of care, such as emotional support and interactions with the patient. The therapist can encourage the caregivers to gradually become involved in necessary tasks as their comfort level increases. Some family members are anxious to know what they can do to help when the patient is not in therapy. They can be observed interacting with the patient during treatment sessions and can be directed or reassured that they are helpful. Specific activities related to cognitive, perceptual, and motor goals can be outlined for the family to perform outside therapy. Early involvement with the patient and the team can assist family members in the daily coping with disabilities and form a basis for future interactions with the team.

In the early stages of recovery, family and significant others often require a great deal of support. Frequently, they are encouraged by the patient's increasing responsiveness, but their expectations may be disproportionate to the patient's abilities. Important aspects of psychosocial treatment with the family are problem identification and resolution, and providing information when it can be used by the individuals. The family must be informed of the patient's limited capacity for stimulation, be alert to signs of overstimulation, such as agitation or decreased levels of response, and be taught that frequent short periods of interaction may be more beneficial than prolonged sessions.

During the recovery process, many patients enter a phase of agitation. This is a difficult time for everyone involved with the patient, especially if it occurs after a period of increasing responsiveness. This confuses the family, and they may begin to question their previous enthusiasm and expectations.

Family members often cannot understand uncharacteristic verbal and/or physical aggressiveness by the patient. Specific methods used by the team of dealing with the agitation should be shared with the family. At this stage, family members are encouraged to be nonjudgmental and nonconfrontive with the patient. The team needs to stress the patient's inability to control such actions. The family needs to be assured that derogatory statements made by the patient should not be taken literally or personally. Families often feel helpless or hopeless during this stage. Sometimes asking them to be responsible for a particular task assists them in feeling useful and more in control. Information and support provided by the team can assist the family through this difficult period.

As discharge approaches, the team must prepare the family for any deficits the patient may retain and assist them in their adjustment. If the team has been communicating with the family on an ongoing basis, providing them with information and management strategies, gradual adjustment may have occurred. If communication has been limited, family adjustment may be more difficult, with much teaching being done by the therapists just before discharge. Even though there has been much communication between the team and the family, adjustment may be difficult due to their ineffective coping mechanisms or lack of adequate support

systems. All safety and judgment issues should be covered and concerns written as part of a home program. To ensure understanding, it is helpful to have family members describe the type of environment the patient will need for safe performance of daily living skills, those areas in which the patient will require supervision or assistance, and those activities that should not be attempted due to physical and/or cognitive limitations.

GOAL AREAS

Specific issues addressed by the therapist in the psychosocial treatment of the head-injured patient include participation in treatment, reflecting adjustment to disability; social interactions and behavior; and interest identification and role adjustment. Goals and treatment reflect the patient's level of recovery and continue to change as the patient progresses.

Participation in Treatment

Often the patient's adjustment to his disabilities is far more difficult than the family's or significant other's adjustment. He may acknowledge some obvious deficits, such as physical dysfunction or a memory problem, but continue to deny more subtle deficits. Frequently, this affects the patient's participation in therapy. Once the patient is in an alert state, specific abilities and deficits can be pointed out. Although some patients will still be unable to recognize their deficits, the therapist can provide them with specific reasons why they require therapy and why specific activities are therapeutic or dangerous to attempt alone. Some individuals who deny deficits and do not have the judgment necessary to be responsible for their safety may require more emphasis on their limitations to keep them involved in the therapy process. Patients who are overly aware of their deficits do better when their abilities are stressed. By emphasizing abilities, the patient may realize he is not helpless and that strengths do exist that can be built upon. The approach that is used will depend on the patient's response.

Many patients enter a period of transitional agitation, occurring before, after, or in conjunction with increasing periods of alertness. A small percentage of patients remain in this state for a prolonged time (Brooks, 1984; Wood, 1984). We refer to this population as chronically agitated.

Involving the patient in therapeutic activities can be difficult. Some patients demonstrate short periods of awareness of people and environment, but most have no or a very limited sense of their abilities and limitations. During this phase, few demands are placed on the patient that may trigger or increase the level of agitation. It is often helpful to limit the number of people working with the patient. Relaxation and inhibition techniques described in Unit 6 may reduce agitation, enabling active participation by the patient in a structured one-on-one session of limited duration. This usually involves use of automatic activities, such as overlearned self-care tasks that provide successful experiences.

The patient's limitations often need to be pointed out during orientation activities for safety purposes. This is done in a concrete manner, such as "Your leg does not move; you are not able to stand up by yourself." Points should not be argued nor confrontation used at this stage. If the patient denies his deficits and begins to become upset, changing the topic of the conversation or activity will often distract him and prevent an outburst. The issue can be approached again at the next treatment session. Increasing the patient's self-awareness is an important goal of therapy at this stage.

As agitation decreases, longer periods of alert attentiveness may be observed. Some patients may be confused and disoriented at first but gradually become oriented to the environment and their relation to it. The therapist assists the patient in adjusting to the disability by providing information to increase his awareness of his strengths and weaknesses. This is stated in concrete terms by primarily focusing on physical limitations that may be more obvious. Cognitive factors such as memory impairment may be addressed early on if the patient questions his performance. Information should be presented in clear and concise statements. Excessive descriptions are confusing. Many patients cannot follow logic, and arguing a point may lead to an agitated response.

The therapist should also point out the patient's strengths. It is important to emphasize patient achievement in the performance of selected activities. This is done verbally as well as nonverbally. Facial expressions and tactile contact can be reinforcing factors in treatment. As the patient improves, there may be an increase in his awareness of deficits. Awareness is a first step in achieving adjustment.

Patients who improve physically and cognitively often develop insight into their condition. This can have a dual effect: (1) It may enable the patient to recognize his deficits and encourage the use of compensatory strategies; and (2) The patient may experience overwhelming feelings of loss upon the realization that life may never be the same. Anger, denial, and depression may accompany this realization and need to be addressed by the therapist and the team.

At times, these feelings result in the patient's refusal to participate in treatment. It may be the occupational therapist who first encounters resistance or other behavioral problems. This is because most daily living skills are quite complex, requiring both physical and cognitive abilities. Memory, sequencing, spontaneous problem solving, and decision making are often affected by HI. Paresis, abnormal tone, incoordination, or ataxia may further complicate the patient's performance.

There is often a high level of frustration involved in completing daily living tasks that were once completed quickly, efficiently, and without much thought. These same tasks may now take maximum thought, effort, and time to complete. This becomes more obvious as the patient begins to develop insight into deficits and realizes the changes that have occurred in his life. Other patients with little insight may resist treatment because they see no need for it. They either do not recognize problems in their performance or deny the relevance of the problem, arguing that someone else will perform the task for them. The patient may demonstrate limited coping skills and may resort to avoidance or denial responses reflected by resistance or a refusal to participate in therapeutic activities. These issues must be dealt with by the family and the entire team. The approach developed, whether confrontive, supportive, or based on token reinforcement, requires consistency of application by all who interact with the patient.

Often the patient will require direction by the therapist to focus on task performance and outcome. In the early stages, it is important for the therapist to be concrete and specific in identifying deficit areas and related methods of treatment. Providing a reason for the difficulty the patient is experiencing and the relation to the therapeutic activity often facilitates participation. For example, the therapist may point out that the patient can put on a tee-shirt without help but cannot fasten the buttons on his outer shirt. If the patient cannot understand why buttoning is difficult, the therapist can provide possible reasons. They may include lack of fine motor coordination, inability to use one arm, or lack of sensation in the hands. The therapist can explain why certain remediation techniques are used. These may include repeating the task, performing fine motor activities using small pegs, or identifying small objects buried in a rice box to encourage attention to and use of the sense of touch. As the patient progresses, strengths and weaknesses in the less concrete aspects of function can be explored, such as problem solving and safety.

If the patient becomes aware of strengths and areas for growth, he should be encouraged to accept responsibility for selecting appropriate activities during OT sessions. The therapist should reinforce the selection based on the patient's identified priorities and insight into his disabilities. Initially, some structure is usually required. The patient may select the category, such as cooking skills, and the therapist provides choices, or vice versa, to ensure an appropriate level of difficulty.

Maintaining the patient's active participation in the therapeutic process necessitates changes in approach as he progresses in his psychosocial adjustment. His level of alertness, behavior, and insight indicate the type of interventions most appropriate. Initially, progress may be noted by the amount of time the patient can be engaged in activity. This can be qualified by the type of demands placed on him and the treatment situations tolerated. Finally, participation in treatment involves the patient taking responsibility for selecting goals and carrying out recommendations.

Social Interaction and Behavior

After an HI, the patient's ability to control his actions and conduct is often impaired. The behavioral disturbances may be transitional or may continue to be a disturbance for prolonged periods of time. The patient's level of cognitive functioning often affects his behavior and ability to interact with others in a socially acceptable fashion. Cognitive and psychosocial goals and treatment often overlap because both require complex interactions with a variety of people and situations. In OT, an important goal area is developing behaviors that promote effective social interactions and relationships. As the patient becomes more aware of others, treatment involves encouraging appropriate responses to others. Treatment progresses to facilitating the patient's abilities to initiate and maintain interactions with others in a socially and culturally acceptable manner. Some patients cannot regain sophisticated levels of these skills, including developing and sustaining relationships with others, due to residual cognitive and behavioral deficits.

In the early stages of recovery, a primary focus of treatment is establishing a method of consistent communication with the patient. This provides the patient with a means to respond to others and convey basic needs. Frequently, there is a joint effort with the speech and language pathologist in determining the most effective method for communication. A "yes" and "no" signal affords the individual some control over situations and allows at least a limited level of choice and communication with others.

Other factors include the effects of stress and the environment. Often a quiet, low-stimulus environment is best suited for the patient who cannot process large amounts of information. This allows the patient to focus on following single commands, which are often a primary focus of treatment at this stage. The therapist supplies a supportive atmosphere, providing the patient with orienting information and simple explanations of what is occurring during treatment. To prevent stress, demands should be minimal and within the patient's capabilities. This reduces the possibilities of adverse behavioral responses such as agitation or withdrawal. Integration of efforts with methods of treatment provided by other team members is crucial to reduce the patient's stress and confusion.

This is even more important when working with an agitated patient who is in a state of heightened excitability. It is important to provide a low-stimulus environment with a supportive atmosphere for patients in a state of transitional agitation. Information can be provided to the patient as to where he is and what is happening. The patient in this stage will often experience brief periods when attention to the therapist or to an activity is possible. Attempts are made to prolong these periods and allow for continued one-on-one interaction. During these periods, demands placed on the patient are limited, and appropriate social behaviors are reinforced by praise and attention.

Seemingly purposeless and sometimes aggressive movement is often associated with the agitated stage. The patient's heightened level of arousal may produce an over-reaction to stimuli. This may trigger a "fight or flight" response. Patients have been known to strike out, scratch, or bite in response to therapeutic intervention or stressful situations. Sometimes the aggressive movement can be channeled into purposeful behaviors. Hitting or catching a balloon or tossing bean bags are examples. During treatment, it is important for the therapist to avoid triggering violent responses. It is better to reduce expectations than to challenge or force an action on the patient. It is essential not to reinforce violent reactions that can be used by the patient to avoid difficult or unpleasant tasks later in the recovery sequence. As the patient progresses through this stage, periods of attention and appropriate interactions should increase as well as his tolerance to environmental stimulation and demands.

The patient in a chronic state of agitation is more difficult to manage. Behavior management is an ongoing concern for the team and long-term caregivers. This type of agitation is usually external or situation based and may result from learned behaviors (Wood, 1984). Responses range from irritability and low frustration tolerance to violent verbal and/or physical outbursts disproportionate to the situation. Often the outbursts erupt suddenly and without warning. These can be dangerous.

For patients who experience a gradual buildup of frustration, outbursts can be avoided by changing the activity or task structure. These outbursts necessitate a unified approach by all people interacting with the patient. Often, the clinical psychologist can assist the team in establishing a program to modify aggressive behaviors. Time-out periods, isolation, token systems, and positive reinforcement may be used. Certain behaviors may be targeted for modification, and a consistent response to those behaviors by all individuals working with the patient is necessary. It is often beneficial to have a private duty nurse or aide to assist in these patients' care and be responsible for the management program in the hours outside therapy.

The patient demonstrating agitated behaviors requires primarily one-on-one therapeutic intervention. Short-term goals for these patients involve task participation for progressively longer periods of time without agitated outbursts, the ability to communicate basic needs, and the gradual decrease in the structure required for task completion. An additional goal might be to identify specific factors or patterns contributing to agitation so that the team can manage outbursts better. For some patients, there are no observable patterns, and behavioral management is difficult.

Some patients become able to respond to others but have difficulty initiating appropriate interactions. They can usually convey basic needs but not always in a socially acceptable manner. Some have difficulty delaying gratification of their needs, and some may have little awareness of the needs or feelings of others. Nonthreatening correction of their behavior is the method used most often to promote appropriate social interactions. Examples of acceptable alternatives are

provided. Depending on the patient's skills and abilities, treatment may be expanded to include activities involving two patients in a structured activity. This might be a board game or a simple card game where the patients must relate by obeying rules, taking turns, responding to questions, and engaging in other interactions. Initially, the therapist may need to provide structure and guidance, but direction should gradually decrease.

Appropriate interactions are emphasized and praised, while socially inappropriate ones are corrected. During this stage, various behavioral characteristics may emerge. Behaviors exhibited may be exaggerations of premorbid characteristics or changes from the premorbid status. Some variation in appropriateness is based on the individual's social and cultural norms and should be considered in evaluating his interactions. If the demands placed on the patient become too great, the patient may revert to an agitated response.

As patients interact with greater numbers of people, behaviors affecting social interactions may become more evident. Some individuals lose their social inhibitions to various degrees. These may involve the type of questions asked of people or the type of approach used to gain another's attention. Inappropriate physical contact or social ineptness may also be evident. Some individuals become more aggressive after HI, others more passive.

Passive changes tend to include changes in or lack of affect, poor initiation of conversation and actions, and a generalized lack of interest in surroundings. This type of patient lacks motivation, and if left to his own resources could not plan his day. Often, introduction of previous interests will spark the patient's attention and provide a source of motivation. Structured small groups may also benefit this type of patient if the leader can draw out each participant in the activity, discussion, or planning of the event. Small groups provide the opportunity for patients to respond to the social initiative of others. Given the necessary structure, the passive individual may react in a more active manner in this type of environment.

Some individuals revert to an egocentric perspective. Their attention may be fleeting, and they may expound upon whatever catches their attention. There is little or no awareness of their effect on others or of the needs of others. During treatment, the fleeting attention and verbal monologues interfere with performance of therapeutic activities. Strict structure and limits must be set by those working with the patient for optimal patient performance. Structure is provided by redirecting the patient to the task and, at times, providing a low-stimulus environment. A structured group involving peer pressure and therapist role models can sometimes be effective. The group can be structured in such a way that time limits are set or turns taken to ensure equal participation. Depending on the individual, confrontation may reduce inappropriate behavior as long as it does not trigger other behavioral problems. A certain level of insight by the patient is necessary for confrontation to be effective. The specific inappropriate behavior is pointed out to the patient, and the reasons it is considered inappropriate are provided. The patient may be required to describe acceptable alternative behaviors, or if unable, they can be provided by the therapist or other group members.

For individuals to function within the social and cultural norms of society, they must be aware of behavioral norms and the needs and feelings of others. Loss of social inhibitions reflected by inappropriate verbalizations or behaviors can be very distressing to family members. This can be a transitional problem, or it can be chronic. A program of behavior modification may be useful if the problem involves one or two specific behaviors or actions found to be offensive, such as hand kissing. A behavior modification program may be less effective with a patient whose lack of insight allows for offensive statements to acquaintances or strangers. This type of behavior may be better dealt with by extinction techniques. The caregivers refuse to attend to inappropriate behaviors while giving positive attention for appropriate ones. This concept is important for all people working with or caring for the patient.

Family and staff can inadvertently reinforce inappropriate behaviors by providing excess attention to them. The patient can then learn to get attention by using the inappropriate behaviors. Videotapes may assist the individual in identifying the inappropriateness of an interaction. Token systems have been used to control behavior and to ensure participation in treatment. The patient accumulates tokens for specific tasks performed or for time spent in appropriate interactions. Tokens are lost when guidelines are broken.

The ability to interact with others in a variety of situations is an important aspect of daily living. Behaviors displayed can enhance or prevent effective social interactions. The occupational therapist, as part of the treatment team, can assist the patient in recognizing inappropriate behaviors and developing more effective means of interaction.

Interest Identification and Role Adjustments

Roles encompass a number of complex behaviors reflecting one's personal, sexual, familial-social, and occupational-vocational identity (Oakley, 1981). Roles and expectations associated with specific roles change throughout an individual's life depending on age, interests, goals, values, and circumstances. For example, the role of a son is very different at age 6 as compared with age 36. The role is maintained, but the expected behaviors associated with it change. Occupational roles typically change from student to worker to retiree or as one's vocational pursuits change. Over time, some roles are adjusted or deleted from an individual's repertoire as needs and skills change.

An HI can have a sudden, major impact on an individual's performance of life roles. Physical, cognitive, and behavioral limitations may affect the performance of the skills associated with them. Young adults, successful in their social and occupational roles, may lose that identity after an HI, producing a dependent role. This may result in a less mature parent-child relationship or may significantly affect husband-wife roles. To meet the psychosocial needs of the head-injured patient involving his self-concept and self-esteem, previous life roles and interests must be considered and addressed in the OT treatment process.

Interest identification and adjustment to life roles may have been addressed earlier in the recovery process with the family or significant others, but it is not usually addressed with the head-injured patient until he demonstrates awareness of his strengths and deficits. It is beneficial for the patient to display insight into his disability for successful adjustment. The first step in treatment of role adjustment is the patient's ability to define previous life roles and interests. Broad categories such as husband or father can usually be identified. The scope of these categories covers many skills and subroles, and the patient may require assistance in identifying them. For example, ''father'' may encompass such roles as full-time worker, groundskeeper, dishwasher, part-time child care provider, fix-it man, check book balancer, and disciplinarian. These subroles can be broken down into the specific skills necessary for adequate performance. Some skills are concrete, others more abstract. A skill list compiled by the patient and therapist may assist in assessing which roles will be possible to resume and which must be altered or assumed by others.

For some, new roles must be developed or old ones adapted to the patient's level of functioning. Even the most severely involved patients may be able to re-establish some aspects of previous roles. This is essential for the individual's self-concept and sense of worth. For example, a young woman suffered an HI that resulted in severe physical deficits and mild cognitive deficits. She was confined to a wheelchair and demonstrated very limited arm placement and hand function. She could feed herself with difficulty and perform limited oral facial hygiene tasks. She viewed her most significant role as that of mother to a 3-year-old girl. Although this woman could no longer provide total care for her child, the therapist helped her break down the role into subroles and skills. Together they identified several skills important to her and then developed those skills. Playing with the child had been a very rewarding part of her role as mother. Activities within the patient's capabilities were identified such as reading large-print storybooks to the child, blowing bubbles, and painting. This process allowed the patient to maintain an important aspect of her previous role.

Major role changes affect all family members. The social worker is best trained to assist the family in adjusting to role changes, while the therapist can focus attention on the patient's abilities and development of skills. If a patient realizes the potential loss or change in role, he may be able to identify alternatives or adaptations to previous roles. More often, it is the therapist who must recommend alternatives. The therapist, psychologist, and social worker must work together to help the family understand and accept the new roles and subroles the therapist and patient are developing.

Developing our roles in life occurs over many years. It may take many months or years for adjustment to the role changes in a family. Most often, it occurs gradually after the head-injured patient has left the rehabilitation setting and has encountered various successes and failures.

Treatment of the psychosocial issues associated with HI is complex and often frustrating. Ideally, treatment begins in the acute setting, but adjustments continue long after discharge. If the team can help the patient and family establish a foundation for the understanding of these issues, they may be better able to cope on a long-term basis with the many changes that will occur.

PROBLEM AREA: PSYCHOSOCIAL

Subcategory: Participation in Treatment

Long-term goals and indicators	Short-term goals	Treatment ideas
1. Patient will tolerate treatment for short periods of time. • unaware of effect on others • agitated, impulsive.	1. Patient will tolerate _____ minutes of structured treatment.	1. Use activities relevant to the patient.
2. Patient will actively participate in treatment. • agitation, impulsivity responds to redirection. • limited awareness of disability.	2. Patient will participate in (*1:1, group, or structured*) treatments for _____ amount of time with (*supervision, cues*).	2. • See above. • Provide information regarding reason for treatment activity in a manner appropriate to patient's recovery. • Use positive reinforcement. • Use token systems or contracts.
3. Patient will demonstrate carryover of treatment suggestions into daily activity. • incorporates compensation techniques with guidance from therapist • aware of deficits.	3. Patient will incorporate treatment suggestions (i.e., memory book, inhibition techniques) in the following ADL activity _____.	3. Provide patient with information regarding reason for treatment activity in a manner appropriate to his level of recovery.

Subcategory: Social Interaction

Long-term goals and indicators	Short-term goals	Treatment ideas
1. Patient will respond appropriately when interaction is initiated by others. • minimally aware of surroundings • may not respond consistently.	1. • Patient will demonstrate consistent (*yes/no response, use of communication device*). • Patient will respond to (*familiar other, therapist independently, when prompted*).	1. • Establish method of communication with speech therapist. • Use 1:1 treatment. • Reinforce appropriate interaction.
2. Patient will initiate appropriate social interactions. • initiates socialization • requires structure for complex social situations • egocentric, limited insight • limited impulse control.	2. Patient will initiate appropriate interaction with others in (*familiar, unfamiliar, group, 1:1*) settings. • Patient will identify (*one, two, three*) socially acceptable methods of interacting in a variety of simulated situations. • Patient will self-correct behavior in social situations in response to the reaction of others (*with, without*) cues. • Patient will (*occasionally, consistently*) identify the needs of others in social situations.	2. Use 1:1 and group situations. • Use role playing/simulated situations. • Reinforce appropriate interaction.

Subcategory: Interest Identification and/or Role Adjustment

Long-term goals and indicators	Short-term goals	Treatment ideas
1. Patient will be able to identify previous interests/roles. • limited insight concerning skills required for performance of roles/interests • limited awareness of abilities and limitations.	1. Patient will identify (1,2,3) previous (*interests, roles*). • Patient will identify skills necessary for performance of the following interest/role _____.	1. Identify roles/interests with patient and/or family. • Introduce activity relevant to interests/roles.
2. Patients will participate in _____ subroles/interests. • some awareness of abilities and limitations • physically/cognitively able to resume some portion of former role with modification/supervision.	2. Patient will describe realistic options for role or interest performance based on knowledge of abilities and limitations. • Patient will (*identify, demonstrate*) compensation techniques necessary for participation in _____ portions of former roles/interests.	2. See above. • Practice subroles of various roles. • Provide adaptive equipment.
3. Patient will perform one or more previous or new life roles. • good awareness of deficits and adaptations required • able to identify realistic alternate methods of reaching a goal.	3. Patient to perform _____ role (*with, without*) modification.	3. See above.

REFERENCES

Brooks, N. (1984). Head injury and family. In N. Brooks (Ed.), *Closed head injury: Psychological, social and family consequences*, Chap. 1. New York: Oxford University Press.

Jellinek, H.M., Torkelson, R.M., & Harvey, R.F. (1982). Functional abilities and distress levels in brain-injured patients at long-term follow-up. *Archives of Physical Medicine and Rehabilitation, 63*, 160–162.

Livingston, M.G., Brooks, D.N., & Bond, M.R. (1985a). Patient outcome in the year following severe head injury and relatives psychiatric functioning. *Journal of Neurology, Neurosurgery and Psychiatry, 48*, 876–881.

Livingston, M.G., Brooks, D.N., & Bond, M.R. (1985b). Three months after severe head injury: Psychiatric and social impact on relatives. *Journal of Neurology, Neurosurgery and Psychiatry, 48*, 870–875.

McKinly, W.W., Brooks, D.N., Bond, M.R., Martinage, D.P., & Marshall, M.M. (1981). Short-term outcome of severe blunt head injury as reported by relatives of the injured persons. *Journal of Neurology, Neurosurgery and Psychiatry, 44*, 527–533.

Oakley, F.M. (1981). The Role Checklist. Available from the author (9103 Autoville Dr. College Park, MD 20740).

Wood, R.L. (1984). Behavior disorders following severe brain injury. In N. Brooks (Ed.), *Closed head injury: Psychological, social and family consequences*, Chap. 10. New York: Oxford University Press.

Treatment of Sensory-Perceptual and Cognitive Deficits

Diane Bermann, OTR/L
Theresa Bush, OTR/L

The human brain functions as an integrated whole, sorting, selecting, and using numerous bits of information to allow the individual to function effectively. It is difficult to isolate the particular brain functions needed for efficient performance of daily living tasks. In the adult, processed sensory information from the environment, memory, and other cognitive skills overlap and build upon each other to allow the individual to produce effective responses. An individual adapts to his environment and learns either by recalling sensorimotor and perceptual experiences or, in more abstract ways, by reasoning and hypothesizing about things he has not experienced directly. An individual's ability to meet his physical and emotional needs, solve daily problems, and plan for the future is the result of the integration of these sensorimotor, perceptual, and cognitive processes.

Traumatic head injury (HI) often produces widespread, diffuse brain damage. HI often affects the brain's ability to integrate efficiently the processes necessary to meet the complex demands of daily living. Occupational therapy (OT) treatment of the head-injured patient is often aimed at optimizing his performance of daily living tasks. By using evaluation and observation, the occupational therapist, as a member of the treatment team, can identify cognitive and sensory-based perceptual deficits interfering with the patient's optimal performance of daily living tasks. In treatment, attempts are made to remediate the deficits or to assist the patient in developing effective compensation techniques.

The extent of the brain damage will ultimately affect the level of recovery. However, without challenging the patient both physically and cognitively by providing a stimulating environment and skill-appropriate activity, opportunities for adaptation and improvement would be very limited.

A developmental framework is the basis for the treatment of sensory-perceptual and cognitive deficits. We acknowledge the importance of early sensorimotor experiences in the development of perceptual and cognitive skills. This is reflected in the treatment provided in the very early stages of recovery, including controlled sensory stimulation.

As the patient progresses, we continue to appreciate the importance of the sensory components of perceptual skills. This includes the effective processing of tactile, vestibular, auditory, and visual information. There are five times as many afferent as efferent neurons that must be organized by the central nervous system (CNS). Under normal circumstances, the brain is self-organizing and can inhibit much of the input into its system. Inhibition is a major brain function. When the brain is injured, the capacity to inhibit extraneous sensory information and effectively organize meaningful information may be impaired.

If the patient is responding to all sensory information in a disorganized way, perceptual, cognitive, and functional skills will be affected. Judgment and reasoning skills may be impaired if decisions are based on faulty or insufficient information. Some individuals may be able to focus on only one aspect of a situation and make judgments accordingly. During evaluation, the therapist determines which sensory systems are most effective in processing information. She plans treatment involving learning strategies and compensatory cueing systems using the patient's strengths. For example, a patient with visual perceptual deficits would have a treatment program using tactile and auditory cueing to improve task performance.

THE TREATMENT ENVIRONMENT

The environment is important if the patient's capacity to process incoming sensory information adequately is deficient. An overstimulating environment combined with inadequate processing may trigger confusion or agitation in some patients and can produce avoidance responses in others. For these patients, the treatment environment needs to be controlled so the patient is better able to focus on the information necessary for participation in treatment. These patients tend to respond better when treated in their rooms or in a quiet area on the unit.

At the Rehabilitation Institute of Chicago (RIC), treatment areas on patient floors are used for this type of patient. Areas are staffed by occupational therapists, physical therapists, and speech and language pathologists. Three or four patients are scheduled simultaneously into a 3-hour block, which allows for interdisciplinary, comprehensive approaches and flexibility of treatment for each patient. The location and time frame provide opportunities for cotreatment among disciplines and shorter, more frequent periods of intervention for patients who require intermittent rest periods.

The environment can be upgraded as the patient is able to tolerate increased environmental stimuli. However, brain damage may continue to affect some patients' ability to process information and to function in an open environment. If the level of stress or environmental factors becomes too great, regression to a more primitive level of response can occur. This is true at any level of recovery and applies to patients with minimal deficits whose performance on complex tasks may deteriorate when under pressure.

For the patient to be functional in daily living situations, he must be able to perform activities in nonstructured settings. This is the ultimate goal of treatment for many patients. Performance on individual tasks may be improved by limiting environmental distractions. This is especially true as tasks become more complex. Even though the patient may be functioning independently, subtle problems with attention may continue to influence his performance long after injury, affecting memory, observation of detail, completion time of tasks, safety, and judgment.

CONSIDERATIONS FOR WORKING WITH AGITATED PATIENTS

Many patients pass through a transitional stage of agitation in their recovery process. This organic irritability rarely persists longer than 12 months (Wood, 1984). This may be a part of the CNS's attempts to reorganize after HI. This agitation can persist longer as a learned reaction to stress and may be maintained as a generalized response to difficult or unpleasant situations (Lishman, 1978). Agitation as a learned response, or prolonged agitation, is referred to as chronic agitation in this text.

The cognitive, behavioral, and sensory-perceptual responses of transitional and chronically agitated patients are related to their level of internal confusion or stress as well as to the degree of demands placed on them by the environment at any given time. The patient experiences a decreased ability to perceive stimuli due to a significantly reduced threshold to process both environmental and somatosensory information. This may result in quicker, more exaggerated responses to stimuli (Sinclair, 1967). Frontal lobe damage can also contribute to a state of disinhibition or loss of inhibitory control, producing impulsivity and decreased control over emotional tone. This may contribute to patients' angry or profane outbursts.

The transitionally agitated patient may be detached from the present and disoriented as to time, place, and sequence of events. If verbal, the patient may confabulate bizarre or paranoid events of others' attempts to cause him harm. Other episodes of confabulation may relate to the patient's recall of events out of sequence as he attempts to make sense of his disorganized processing and internal confusion. He may respond inappropriately to environmental stimuli by crying out or reacting physically to minimal levels of stimuli.

Overall attention to the environment or to a task is brief, with poor or no selective attention. The agitated patient's intense state of internal confusion makes it difficult for him to cooperate with treatment efforts or respond to attempts to reason.

The sometimes explosive nature of the agitated patient requires careful handling by the therapist. Clinical judgment must be used to develop a balanced plan of intervention. There can be a delicate line between involving the patient in a functional activity and triggering an agitated or violent reaction. There are times the therapist may feel ineffectual in treatment, but at this stage it is sometimes necessary to sacrifice patient involvement in activity for personal safety and control of agitated outbursts. Reinforcement of agitated behaviors is not desirable; therefore, it is important to be sensitive to the patient's emotional tone in order to end an activity or task before his limit has been reached.

Indicators of this limit vary with individuals, but some common signs include:

- attempts to remove himself from the task, such as pushing away from the table
- an increase in nonpurposeful body movements, fidgeting, or self-stimulating behavior, such as rocking
- loss of eye contact
- verbal comments indicating the task is too difficult or frustrating
- an increase in the rate of respiration, or flushing of the skin

Sensory-perceptual and cognitive goals of treatment for the agitated patient involve improved processing of sensory information to produce appropriate adaptive responses and improved orientation and selective attention for optimal participation in treatment. Highly structured treatment places specific demands on the patient and focuses on normalizing his response to environmental stimulation.

The agitated patient's CNS can be characterized as being in a constant state of hyperactivity. Some patients appear to respond to this internal distress by self-stimulating behaviors. Others use a "fight or flight" response. The type of stimulation the patient uses to calm himself may indicate effective treatment techniques. Self-produced vestibular stimulation, such as rocking or fidgeting, rolling back and forth when in bed or on a mat, or pacing, are commonly observed in agitated patients. This type of behavior might be an indicator to include meaningful vestibular input in the patient's treatment program. Movement has an organizing effect on sensory input, and it is often through movement that individuals produce adaptive responses. It is possible that through nonpurposeful movement the patient is demonstrating a need for vestibular input and is attempting to stimulate the CNS to better organize incoming information. The therapist may be able to structure activities to make the movement patterns more organized and meaningful to his system, allowing him to produce an adaptive response. It may be possible to channel the patient's spontaneous behaviors into more functional activities such as reaching and rolling or propelling a wheelchair.

General inhibitory techniques promoting relaxation can be an effective means of preparing some patients for task participation who may be responding to stimuli at the level of the autonomic nervous system (ANS). Theoretical principles of neurorehabilitation (Farber, 1982) and sensory integration (Ayres, 1972) refer to an optimal level of arousal necessary for effective task performance. Once this level is obtained, the therapist can introduce gross motor activities or simple self-care tasks as the focus of treatment. Techniques that have an inhibitory effect on the CNS include maintained deep pressure, neutral warmth, and slow vestibular input. The therapist is cautioned that these techniques are not appropriate for all agitated patients, and some individuals cannot tolerate the proximity of the therapist necessary to perform them.

Maintained deep pressure can have an inhibitory effect on the CNS (Geldard, 1972). Farber (1982) and Montgomery and Richter (1972) describe a technique consisting of supraoral pressure. The therapist applies deep pressure to the patient's upper lip and gradually decreases the pressure to a moderate touch. Maintained pressure using the palm and the flat surface of the fingers on the patient's stomach or cervical and lumbar spine areas and slow stroking of the spine can also prove inhibitory. The therapist provides firm pressure with the index and middle fingers on either side of the spine as it is stroked in a constant rhythmic pattern from the patient's neck to the small of the back (Frank, 1971; Rood, 1962).

Neutral warmth is another method of inhibition. The patient is wrapped in a light blanket. Tactile and proprioceptive input is provided by the pressure and tension of the blanket. The input can be varied by the therapist's control of the blanket. This technique can be combined with slow rocking, allowing the therapist to maintain distance from the patient if necessary. An alternate technique is to wrap the patient tightly in the blanket and allow him to lie prone for 10 to 15 minutes. Many agitated patients may find the restriction of the blanket distressing rather than comforting.

Vestibular input involving slow rocking can be provided by placing a large inflated ball in front of the patient while he is short-sitting. This provides support and pressure when the patient leans forward with his arms extended and attempts to rock himself or be gently rocked by the therapist. The same concept can be used with a tilt board or a rocking chair or during techniques used to inhibit abnormal muscle tone.

These techniques need to be monitored for effectiveness in readying the patient for activity. Prolonged inhibition may decrease the patient's level of arousal to below optimum for task performance. ANS functions can also be affected, including heart rate and respiration. These should be closely monitored when using inhibitory techniques with head-injured patients.

These inhibition techniques may be impractical for use with many agitated patients due to the degree of agitation. In these cases, allowing the patient a brief rest or walking break every few minutes may be an effective means of promoting participation while avoiding agitated responses.

Purposeful Activity

When the patient is in a calmed state, graded activities can be introduced. Frequently, automatic or overlearned self-care tasks such as combing the hair, shaving, or pouring and drinking from a cup are used. The patient is usually able to attend to these simple tasks at an automatic level because he has repeated them so many times in his life that they are overlearned and do not require sustained attention. Simple cognitive tasks such as orientation activities or naming objects and their uses, and gross motor activities involving reaching, tossing, or hitting a ball can be effective. The cognitive demands of these tasks are limited yet the activity provides sensory input and results in an adaptive response. At this level, the patient may require frequent breaks to prevent sensory overload of the CNS.

An agitated patient is often disoriented, and it is helpful for the therapist to provide orienting information and explain in a concrete manner where he is and what has happened to him. Interpretation of factual information may be distorted by the patient, and misperceptions of situations may occur. This can be especially difficult when the patient is ambulatory and attempts to leave the unit or resists safety measures. One way to deal with the situation is by redirecting the patient. The therapist may make a statement or ask a question far removed and unrelated to the situation or topic and draw the patient's attention away from the source of agitation. Involving the patient in a new activity may serve the same purpose.

Gradually, the patient's periods of agitation should decrease, with longer periods of attention to task. When this begins, activity-based treatment may be the most effective method of therapy. As the patient becomes involved, attention, memory, and sequencing skills can be addressed rather than his agitation. Depending on the patient's functional level, these tasks can begin with simple daily living tasks, such as oral facial hygiene and dressing, and progress to avocational or homemaking tasks based on premorbid or current interests. These activities are graded beginning with simple one- or two-step tasks such as sanding a piece of wood or glazing a ceramic mold with one color. By limiting the complexity of the task, there is less chance of producing frustration. As the patient tolerates it, the therapist can increase the complexity by increasing the number of steps, necessary directions, or pieces needed to complete the project.

It is usually best to change only one aspect of the activity at a time. Increasing the number of steps in a task or decreasing the amount of direction provided may be more effective than selecting a new activity where all three aspects would become more complex. For example, a patient's first project might be a one-piece wooden key holder that is sanded and painted. The next project might be a cutting board that is sanded, stained, and varnished. One extra step has been added. Activities continue to be graded until the patient is functioning at his maximum potential.

The Treatment Environment

Patients in an agitated state may benefit from a controlled environment. At times, specific environmental factors can be identified that produce or increase the patient's level of agitation. These may include auditory stimuli, such as loud talking, television or radio, or excessive visual stimuli. These may be produced by the patient's proximity to a high traffic hallway or an open treatment area with a high level of activity. Occasionally, proximity to another person will produce an adverse response. If the source of the agitation can be identified, the therapist can control the environment by removing the offensive stimulus or by moving the patient to a less-stimulating environment. Isolated treatment areas or private rooms are effective in decreasing auditory and visual stimuli. It is often easier for the therapist to provide structure for the patient in this type of closed environment.

SENSORY STIMULATION

In the early stages of recovery, when the patient is emerging from a comatose state, a primary focus of treatment is providing sensory stimulation. At this stage, it is difficult to separate evaluation and treatment. The goal of a stimulation program is to prolong the level of increased arousal by fostering the observable responses and building in higher levels of adaptation. This is done by changing the intensity of input while still producing an appropriate response. Controlled stimulation is provided to produce an adaptive response. The therapist evaluates the patient's response to various stimuli, often beginning with noxious input such as loud noises, a pinprick, or unpleasant odors. Input is refined as the patient responds to more subtle input such as voice, light touch, and familiar scents. The initial sensorimotor responses may develop into components of movement and cognitive schemes necessary for function.

Resources regarding the effectiveness of sensory stimulation of the minimally responsive patient theorize that the stimulation affects the reticular formation associated with arousal and attention and reduces the threshold necessary to perceive incoming sensory information (Farber, 1982; Moore, 1978). A stimulation program can be initiated as soon as possible post injury to:

- prevent sensory deprivation
- provide opportunities for the patient to respond to the environment in an adaptive way
- incorporate physical mobility that provides appropriate sensory input

Subtle variations in response to input, such as changes in speed, consistency, or flexibility of response to a higher level of adaptation, are recorded by the therapist. Responses to stimuli at this level of recovery can be divided into three categories.

1. *No response:* The patient does not react in any observable way to the sensory input provided.
2. *Generalized response:* The patient's response to sensory input is not specifically related to that input. Responses may include total body movements or ANS responses such as increased heart rate, changes in skin color or temperature, or diaphoresis. The reaction may be delayed, inconsistent, or the same for all sensory input.
3. *Localized response:* The patient's response to sensory input is specific to that input, such as withdrawing an extremity from painful stimuli or turning one's head to auditory input. Latency and some inconsistency of response may exist.

A patient may display a variety of responses depending on the type of input. Response to pain may be localized while response to auditory or vestibular input may be generalized. A list of possible stimulus items and examples of responses are given in Table 5-1. The generalized responses can relate to any of the stimuli and are not repeated in the chart for each type of sensory input.

A holistic stimulation program involves controlled input into all sensory systems. Some clinicians recommend a phylogenetic approach to stimulation beginning with tactile and vestibular, while vision and audition are emphasized later (Farber, 1982). When treating the head-injured adult, some systems may be more affected than others. Developmentally higher systems such as audition may work more effectively than lower-level systems. By using the higher-level processing, the therapist may be able to enhance the lower-level processing to produce a more adaptive response.

In these cases, the amount of stimulation may be more important than the order of stimulation. It is important not to overstimulate the patient and to allow enough time between stimuli for him to respond. One to two minutes between the administration of different stimuli can be used as an initial guideline until latency of response can be established. If the patient's CNS is unable to process the amount or intensity of stimulation, it may block out the input.

Sensory overload can also trigger hyperexcitement or agitation. Either consequence of overstimulation does not produce the desired adaptive response. Family members can be cautioned about sensory overload and taught warning signals appropriate to the particular patient. These may include:

- flushing
- perspiring
- prolonged increase in respiration rate
- agitation

TABLE 5-1   Sensory input and possible responses

Input	Generalized	Localized

Tactile
  Pinprick
  Ice
  Light touch
	Mass body flexion or extension patterns.
	  ANS changes, i.e.:
	
	  • Increased respiration
	  • Decreased respiration
	  • Increased muscle tone
	  • Perspiration
	  • Flushing or other skin changes
	
	Moaning
	Crying
	Any generalized responses below
		Movement of extremity away from stimulus
		Pushing stimulus away
		Turning toward stimulus.

Vestibular
  Rolling/rocking
 	
  Movement to sit
	Increased arousal
	Decreased arousal
	Increased muscle tone
	Extensor patterning
	Any generalized responses above or below
		Eye opening
		Head turning in direction of movement

Visual
  Light
  Mirror/face
	Change in pupil size
	Blink
	Any generalized responses above or below
		Turning head
		Closing eyes
		Focus, track

Auditory
  Clap, bell
  Voice, name
  1-Step command
	Blinking, startle
	Increased arousal
	Grimace
	Increased movement
	Calming effect
		Turning head to stimulus
		Opening eyes
		Attempt to follow command

Olfactory
  Vanilla, banana
  Familiar scent
  Mustard
	Increased arousal
	Decreased arousal
		Swallowing
		Lip-tongue movements
		Eye opening

Gustatory
  Sweet, salty, sour solution
  Lemon swab
	Whole body response
	Change in level of arousal
		Tongue movements
		Licking lips
		Swallowing
		Eyes open
		Head turning

- closing of eyes
- sudden decrease in level of arousal
- increase in muscle tone

Families can be reminded that patients benefit from periods of low or no stimulation periodically during the day and that constant stimulation is contraindicated.

Tactile Stimulation

Tactile input can be facilitory or inhibitory. Pain and light touch to the skin can produce a facilitory response, while maintained touch to the skin, pressure to the oral area, and slow stroking of the spine are generally inhibitory to the CNS. The face and, especially, the oral musculature area are the most sensitive. Noxious stimuli such as a pinprick and ice should be used with caution. Ice to the face or midline may trigger a sympathetic response and is usually avoided (Farber, 1982). Tactile input sources include such things as brushes, fabrics of differing textures, and lotions applied to the patient's skin. Vibration is sometimes used to stimulate proprioceptors. It may prove inhibitory when applied over a muscle on stretch, or excitatory, producing a protective response, when applied to contracting muscles (Farber, 1982). It is important to monitor the patient for increases in spasticity or other adverse responses during stimulation.

Vestibular Stimulation

Vestibular stimulation often produces dramatic changes in the patient's level of arousal. When providing vestibular input to an adult, it is important that it be meaningful and familiar. Such activities as rolling, rocking in a chair or on a mat, or coming to a sit from a supine position are appropriate. Mechanical input such as raising and lowering a hospital bed has little functional meaning for the patient and produces limited or no adaptive response. Spinning an adult patient is contraindicated due to his lack of active participation, the potential for triggering seizures, and the infrequent ability of the CNS to process such intense stimulation (Chapparo & Ranka, 1982).

Slow vestibular input tends to be inhibitory while faster movement patterns tend to facilitate arousal in the patient. Often, controlled vestibular input produces eye opening and increased alertness. The therapist can then introduce other visual or auditory input in an attempt to prolong the state of arousal or to produce a higher level of response. The increased level of response and arousal may be brief, but alternating between vestibular and other sensory input may help sustain it. The initial change in position from supine to sitting may increase the patient's alertness, but he may quickly accommodate to the position. By changing the position again to a sidesit or by leaning the patient down onto his elbow, he may again be able to attend to visual or other sensory input and produce the desired response.

Tonal changes in body musculature must be considered when providing vestibular stimulation. Increased muscle tone post HI is a frequent occurrence. While slow movement patterns can have an inhibitory effect, decreasing or even normalizing the muscle tone, they may also reduce the patient's level of arousal. Often, a combination of slow rhythmic movement to inhibit abnormal muscle tone followed by normal facilitory movement patterns such as rolling or coming to a sit from a supine position produces an adaptive response in the patient.

Visual Stimulation

When the patient exhibits eye opening, visual abilities can begin to be assessed and can provide another avenue for sensory input. Patients will often respond to and focus on a person, especially a friend or family member, before focusing on objects. Once visual focusing is established, attempts at tracking begin. Tracking usually begins in midline, and the patient can gradually follow the stimulus horizontally and vertically. A mirror, familiar face, or familiar object, such as a stuffed animal or a photograph, may hold the patient's attention and elicit a visual response. If tracking is limited to one plane of vision, such as from the midline to the right side, with no spontaneous tracking to the left, the patient's room may be arranged so that visual stimuli and activity occur primarily on the left. Staff and family members can be encouraged to approach the patient from the neglected side. Visual tracking provides input into the vestibular system via brainstem and cerebellar connections (Ayres, 1972). Visual focusing and tracking combine with motor responses to produce purposeful reaching when the patient can track consistently.

Auditory Stimulation

The first response of the patient emerging from coma to auditory input may be to loud noises such as clapping or ringing a bell. This stimulus requires little processing, triggering the patient to respond in a generalized or localized manner. Processing language is a more complex task and may be more difficult. However, they may respond to the sound of a voice even if they cannot comprehend the words. The human voice can have a calming or arousing effect, depending on the pitch, volume, and familiarity. It is important that requests of the patient be within his physical abilities. They may include opening or closing the eyes, turning the head, or producing movement patterns that have already been observed. Other effective means of auditory stimulation include music and tapes of family members' voices, especially if they cannot regularly visit the patient.

How much the patient is understanding at this level of recovery is difficult to ascertain. Some patients recall events or things heard, while others possess no recall. As with any patient, conversations in his presence should include only information one would want him to hear.

Olfactory and Gustatory Stimulation

Olfactory stimulation produces an arousal response by affecting the reticular formation (Ayres, 1972; Chusid, 1976). Familiar scents such as perfume, aftershave lotion, a favorite shampoo, lotions, or foods may produce increased arousal or eye opening. Olfactory and gustatory stimulation may be used in conjunction with prefeeding activities. Nutritive scents such as banana or vanilla may produce sucking or swallowing responses (Farber, 1982). A cotton ball saturated with the scent or a bottle of the scent can be placed under the patient's nostrils for about 10 seconds. Care should be taken not to touch the patient's skin with the scent as accommodation to the scent will occur with prolonged exposure. Damage to the olfactory nerve or a tracheostomy will affect the patient's response to the stimuli. Noxious odors such as vinegar and ammonia that irritate the trigeminal nerve are not recommended (Farber, 1982); garlic and mustard are often used as noxious stimuli.

Gustatory stimulation can be provided by placing one or two drops of sweet, salty, or sour solution on the patient's tongue with an eyedropper. Other methods include the use of a cotton swab dipped in the solution or a glycerine swab. The use of a swab provides tactile and gustatory input and may affect the patient's response. Sweet tastes tend to increase salivation, which may be contraindicated if the patient has difficulty with secretions. Tastes that are meaningful to the patient such as chocolate or even beer have been used to increase his level of arousal.

Multisensory Stimulation

Most activities are multisensory in nature. The CNS processes input from the various senses so that the information can be used by the individual. It is theorized that input from one sensory system validates another. Effective multisensory processing is necessary for an individual to obtain adequate information from and function in his environment. Multisensory input is often provided to the patient during routine daily activities. For example, daily hygiene tasks provide tactile input of various temperatures and textures as the patient is washed and dried. Vestibular input of normal movement patterns is provided as the extremities and body are moved for thorough cleansing. The procedure can be further enhanced by providing the auditory input of naming body parts as they are moved or cleansed.

Patterns of Arousal

It should be made clear to family members that the early stages of recovery are often characterized by inconsistency of response to stimulation, which may be affected by time of day, position, and type of input. The patient may produce localized responses to a variety of stimuli in the morning if his level of arousal is heightened and no response to the same stimuli in the afternoon or evening. Treatment programs can capitalize on periods of alertness and provide meaningful input in the hope of expanding this state. To help establish optimal treatment times, a program providing several sessions of graded sensory input for 15 to 30 minutes throughout the day can be initiated. Specific patient responses can be charted and posted so that all disciplines can document the type of stimulus provided, patient response, and time of day. Often with charts such as these, patterns may be determined indicating increased levels of arousal throughout the day.

Some patients do not progress out of the state of limited arousal. They may be classified as being in a persistent vegetative state. The physician has the medical information necessary to make the diagnosis, which is usually the result of massive cortical axonal damage. These patients may be admitted to rehabilitation centers for trial periods of therapy and to provide proper positioning equipment for the bed and wheelchair. Patients who continue to progress to a more consistent state of arousal have greater demands placed on them for active participation in activities and adaptation to the environment.

SENSORY-PERCEPTUAL AREAS OF TREATMENT

Treatment progresses from single-modality sensory stimulation to that of intersensory stimulation, requiring active patient participation and integration of more complex information. Treatment follows a developmental progression; the early stages of treatment may necessitate that the patient produce gross movement patterns such as assisting in rolling, coming to sitting, or following one- or two-step commands. For example, in reaching for and placing an object, tactile, vestibular, visual, and verbal information relating to the same goal are processed by the patient. This activity assists him in re-establishing a sense of body scheme by relearning where and how his body can move. Sensory-perceptual treatment at this stage may be incorporated into the physical handling techniques used to control abnormal tone, facilitate functional use of extremities, and improve balance and equilibrium responses. These techniques, described in Unit 6, incorporate meaningful proprioceptive, tactile, and vestibular input while challenging the individual to respond motorically in an adaptive way.

Simple gross motor activities such as hitting a balloon require limited physical skills but produce an adaptive motor response in relation to a visual stimulus. Simple visual perceptual tasks can also be attempted at this level of functioning, such as the use of a form board, puzzles, or sorting boxes. This serves the dual purpose of assessing basic visual form and space skills as well as sustained attention to a basic cognitive perceptual task. Stimulation of the primary senses continues, but the patient is now required to participate actively by identifying visual stimuli, naming a scent or flavor, or pointing to the location of a tactile stimulus.

Some patients may be characterized by their slowed processing of sensory information. Visual-perceptual or motor planning deficits may become more apparent as the patient attempts more functional activities. The patient may be unable to tolerate formalized testing to determine the basis of the motor planning deficits observed clinically, so treatment is more general. It continues to involve total body movements in an attempt to improve the patient's awareness of his body in space through meaningful tactile and vestibular input.

Movement sequences can be varied by repositioning the activity, thus requiring differing movement patterns. Observations can be made concerning the patient's:

- ability to cross the midline spontaneously
- bilateral integration skills
- awareness of affected extremities
- gross motor planning skills
- visual tracking skills

Cognitive tasks such as adding and subtracting can also be incorporated into the sequences by using number boards with Velcro targets. For example, the therapist

can give the patient a math problem and he can answer by reaching and placing the Velcro ball on the correct number.

As the patient becomes more functional in daily living tasks, sensory-perceptual dysfunction may be exhibited in many ways. Difficulties in coordination, motor planning, and task completion can be the results of poor or slowed processing of sensory information. Impulsivity and disinhibition can be the result of the patient's inability to filter out extraneous environmental information or his ability to focus on only one aspect of the environment.

For some patients, problems may be obvious when they attempt to perform even simple functional tasks. For others, problems may emerge only when unfamiliar tasks are attempted or when they must process several environmental or task factors simultaneously, such as a cooking activity or a community outing. A balance needs to be maintained between demands placed on the patient and his processing abilities. If demands exceed the patient's capabilities, signs of stress, such as confusion, agitation, immature motor response, or withdrawal from involvement in the task, may occur. The balance can be maintained by adjusting either the activity or the environment. For example, if the structure of the environment is reduced, providing increased auditory and visual stimuli, the patient must process more complex information. The demands of the task selected can be decreased until the patient adjusts to the increased environmental demands. In this situation, the therapist may select an activity previously mastered rather than combining a new activity with a new environment.

The basis of sensory-perceptual dysfunction must be determined in order to provide effective treatment and to use the patient's strengths for compensation of deficits. However, patients must reach a certain level of alertness and attention before they will be able to tolerate formalized testing.

A battery of tests evaluating tactile, motor, and visual skills can be used in conjunction with clinical observations to evaluate the patient's deficits. The test battery used at RIC includes several subtests in the areas of tactile processing, motor planning, visual perceptual, and visual motor processing (Chapparo & Ranka, 1980). Subtests vary in the components needed to complete the tasks accurately. For example, some tactile processing subtests have visual components, and others require a motoric response.

The patient's patterns of performance are assessed in an attempt to determine which primary processing systems are working effectively and which are impaired. For example, a patient performs well on tactile processing subtests in which vision is occluded but demonstrates difficulty performing tactile subtests where vision is required to select responses. If the patient also demonstrates difficulty performing visual processing subtests, his pattern of performance indicates visual processing deficits as the probable cause of dysfunction as opposed to tactile processing deficits. Systems working most effectively can be used to build skills and can be incorporated into the patient's cueing systems. Impaired systems can be the focus of treatment by attempting to enhance the processing of sensory information.

Through clinical observation, the therapist can often determine the patient's spontaneous compensation for processing deficits. Some patients may use vision to compensate for somatosensory deficits or touch to compensate for visual perceptual deficits. An example is a patient groping for the brake on his wheelchair. Some patients with adequate visual processing can quickly distinguish the brake from the other hardware. Patients whose visual processing is impaired may have to touch the wheel, the foot pedal release mechanism, or the wheelchair frame before discriminating the brake lever and using it. In an open environment with many external demands, the compensation may not be spontaneous enough to ensure a safe, efficient response.

Often, sensory-perceptual treatment is combined with cognitive tasks or physical handling techniques. This is accomplished by positioning the components of the activity to encourage total body movement patterns. If somatosensory processing is impaired, activities that emphasize tactile exploration and vestibular input can be incorporated into treatment. This is done by combining a simple cognitive task with normal movement patterns. For example, the patient is directed to find nuts, bolts, and screws buried in a rice box (enhanced tactile input) and sort them into containers (cognitive component). Positioning the rice box on the floor requires the patient to bend over to pick out the item while the sorting containers are placed high on the patient's opposite side (vestibular movement, crossing the midline). This activity can be further graded by using clear sorting boxes so the patient can see the contents. Color-coded or opaque containers encourage recall as to where each object should be placed in the absence of visual cues. Some patients can use their visual skills to compensate for tactile processing deficits, but this tends to slow task completion and may not

be totally effective in multistimulus environments. Fine motor coordination may also continue to be affected.

The relation among movement, motor learning, and visual perception has been established (Held, 1965). Treatment of visual processing deficits can be enhanced by positioning treatment media in such a way that the patient must use rotational movement patterns to cross the midline and visually scan the area in order to complete the task. When learning new tasks, manual cues may be more effective than visual or verbal direction for such patients. Patients who demonstrate only visual perceptual problems may benefit from computer programs designed to enhance visual processing. From clinical observation, it appears that patients whose good tactile processing skills are a basis for their perceptual skills are better able to benefit from visual perceptual training than those with deficits in both tactile and visual processing.

Form and space deficits may be based on poor visual processing, tactile processing, postural adjustment, or any combination. Form and space perception involves the individual's relationship to the environment and how objects relate to each other. Developmentally, we learn these concepts by performing postural adjustments and experiencing the effects of gravity on our body before learning how objects relate to each other. Along these lines, treatment can affect the patient's postural mechanism by combining gross motor activities and heavy proprioceptive input with visual or tactile processing tasks. This incorporates weight shift, rotation, and crossing the midline and is accomplished before progressing to finer visual or motor skills.

The basis for motor planning problems may be generalized form and space deficits, primarily somatosensory or visual processing deficits. Activities selected often reinforce the development of body scheme. Activities can be graded by changing the number of steps and the amount of sequencing required to complete the task. Depending on the cause of the motor planning deficit, activities selected can place more emphasis on tactile or visual skills.

COGNITIVE AREAS OF TREATMENT

Orientation

Often, head-injured patients require frequent orientation to person, place, and time. If verbal, the patient may confuse past and present events and people. It is helpful to have biographical information about the patient readily available to provide him with accurate information and to verify his statements. Pictures of family members are often useful. Information regarding what has happened to the patient and why he is in a hospital can be provided in a concrete or simplified fashion according to his responsiveness.

Some patients demonstrate episodes of confabulation where they compensate for memory and other deficits by inventing details to meet their needs. These episodes may increase in frequency or duration in some patients, while others encounter brief periods or none at all. Some patients may be aware enough of their disorientation and disorganized thought processes to attempt to make sense of their situation, resulting in confabulation. In this sense, the confabulation may be a positive sign that the patient is becoming more aware of his condition. Confabulation can have a negative impact when prolonged or used as part of a denial of deficits. It should be monitored, especially if it becomes hallucinatory or exaggerated. If this occurs, the physician should be contacted to assess the possibilities of hydrocephalus, a seizure-related disorder, or a toxic reaction to medication (Adams & Victor, 1981).

Basic orientation can be graded for individual skill levels as to person, place, and time by providing cues rather than information. For example, rather than informing the patient that it is Monday, the therapist might state that it is the first day of the work week and allow the patient to provide the day. In the early stages of treatment, it is important for activities, therapists, and daily schedules to be consistent. A daily familiar routine promotes orientation to the environment. It is helpful to structure treatment sessions and allow for intermittent reality orientation as necessary. This can be provided every 10 or 15 minutes or at the conclusion of each activity during the treatment session. Large calendars in the patient's room and in the treatment areas and reality-orientation boards with day, date, season, weather, and name of hospital listed can assist the patient in recalling basic orientation information.

Orientation questions are initially related to biographical information. This includes identification of family members, friends, pets, or places through pictures or visits. These tasks are concrete, require a single association, and are retrieved from long-term memory storage. Once achieved, questions can then progress to incorporate date, day of the week, present time, therapy, and city. Improvement is noted if the patient can provide the correct answers with more consistency, fewer cues, or in less time. Questions then become more abstract, requiring associations such as dates and holidays, current events, and a developing sense of time. Basic orientation concepts relating to the topography of the hospital environment can be introduced such as location of patient's room, physician's office, elevators, and therapy areas. The therapist can help orient the patient by cueing him to environmental landmarks such as the nurses' station, signs indicating room numbers, name plates, or color-coded treatment areas and units. Topographical orientation becomes even more important for patients with independent mobility. Care must be taken that they do not wander off, especially if other cognitive deficits in safety and judgment exist.

Memory and Attention

Memory is an integral part of daily living routines and is often affected after trauma to the brain. Memory impairments may affect a person's ability to carry out daily living tasks, hinder new learning, or cause difficulty in recall. There are various theories of the mechanisms of memory (Atkinson & Shiffrin, 1968; Baddeley, 1982; Craik, 1972; Wilson & Moffat, 1984), and certain general concepts are consistent. Effective memory requires adequate functioning of three processes: input, storage, and retrieval.

Input

Input can involve any combination of visual, auditory, verbal, tactile, motor, olfactory, or gustatory information that is coded or processed by the CNS. New information is coded by meaning, association, or phonemics. An adequate level of attention is required for information to be coded and stored. Attention can be divided into three processes that relate to all functional tasks as well as to memory:

1. *Sustained attention or vigilance* is the ability to maintain focus, or concentrate on a task.
2. *Selective attention* is the ability to discriminate between important and nonessential information in the environment. It enables an individual to read a book or perform a task with music playing in the background.
3. *Sequential attention* involves attending to a series of facts or events as well as to their order. It can also involve fixing those events in a time sequence. Recalling and following a series of directions is an example of this skill.

Storage

The framework of memory storage has been described as having three major systems (Atkinson & Shiffrin, 1968):

1. The *sensory register* refers to information entering the system by one or more primary senses. Information is stored in this system briefly until it can be given meaning based on previous experiences and is then stored, used, further processed, or disregarded.
2. *Short-term memories* are stored as long as they are needed for immediate use or task completion. Then, they are further assessed and a subcortical decision is made to disregard the information, for example, a telephone number after it is dialed, or to process it further into long-term storage. The storage of short-term memory is limited by its capacity both in the amount of information and length of time it can be held. The system quickly becomes overloaded, and information is lost. It is probable that brain damage resulting from HI reduces this capacity even further.
3. *Long-term memories* encompass vast amounts of information about ourselves and the world. Psychosocially, the stored information provides an individual with his sense of personal history and involvement within a social group. Information is coded and, when retrieved, appears to pass between long- and short-term stores to be used by the individual.

Retrieval

Retrieval is essential for functional memory. It would appear that individuals who can recall information in response to a cue or clue are having difficulty retrieving information that was properly encoded and stored. For patients unable to respond to cues, the problem may relate to encoding or improper storage. It is possible that the information never reached the long-term storage banks or that it was improperly stored due to poor organization or incorrect association.

A certain degree of memory is necessary for independent functioning. For example, one must remember to look at a list in order to benefit from its cues. After HI, memory deficits can range from mildly annoying forgetfulness to a debilitating problem affecting one's safety and preventing independent living.

Application of the Mechanics of Memory

Much of the research in the area of memory function and dysfunction is based on tests of word, letter, or digit recall (Gronwall & Wrightson, 1981; Lezak, 1979) and recall of biographical information (Levin et al., 1985). Follow-up studies on head-injured patients 1, 2, and 3 years post injury show gradual improvement in simple immediate recall, as evidenced by accurately repeating a series of numbers, but little or no improvement on more complex tasks, such as reversing a series of numbers. In a few cases, there is a general deterioration in memory function. Factors most apparent in affecting performance are timed aspects (Gronwall & Wrightson, 1981), task complexity, and severity of injury (Lezak, 1979). Performance on recall tests may not directly relate to functional performance in everyday routines where environmental cues and overlearning of tasks often assist the head-injured person in carrying out a task and where time restraints may not be an issue.

Memory impairments usually become evident once the patient can communicate. Patients who are alert and oriented may begin to recognize their memory deficits. Knowing whether the breakdown is occurring in input, storage, or retrieval and which sensory systems are working most effectively can help the therapist in formulating compensation strategies.

Compensation strategies for memory impairment can be internal or external. Both require at least some memory capacity. Mnemonics, a series of techniques to improve memory, require time and effort to learn. Examples of mnemonics include making up a story to remember a list of words, learning a rhyme such as "i before e," or making up phrases using the first letter of each word to remember an ordered sequence (as many of us did to learn the cranial nerves). Visual imagery is sometimes helpful in remembering people's names. The same cues used to store the information are used to retrieve it. With repetition, mnemonic cues can sometimes be reduced or discontinued. Because many of these internal strategies require so much effort to learn, external cues are often more practical.

General factors that may be effective in enhancing input are:

- organization and clarity of information presented
- elimination or reduction of distractions
- repetition

- associating new information with old
- use of mnemonic cues during input
- input through multiple sensory systems (auditory and written)
- input by meaning
- emphasizing pertinent factors

Retrieval of information may be enhanced by:

- using the same associations and cues as used during input
- written cues or references
- an environment similar to the one where the information or task was learned (Goddem & Baddeley, 1980)

External compensation strategies include:

- memory books
- timers or watches that beep
- lists or charts
- diagrams or maps

If memory dysfunction is a problem, compensatory measures are introduced. This usually incorporates the use of a memory book, which contains appointments, daily schedules, and lists of things the patient needs to do each day. It can also include a weekly planner, calendar, and significant people's names and telephone numbers. At the start of each treatment session, the patient's daily activities can be reviewed using the schedule or daily log. At the end of the session, results of treatment or the activities performed can be recorded. Gradually, the patient may be able to take more responsibility by recording the day's events with cueing, or independently. As the patient progresses, introduction of unfamiliar tasks with the expectations of next-day carryover can be a realistic goal. If there is good carryover, the therapist can encourage spontaneous use of the compensatory lists by decreasing or changing the cueing provided. Often, by helping the patient organize the information needed, it can be better retained and recalled.

In the early stages of recovery, attention may still be fleeting, and it is helpful if the therapist prepares several activities for a single treatment session. Being aware of the physical and cognitive demands of each activity allows for its modification to the skill level of the patient. This reduces stress responses or lower levels of adaptation. Some patients can attend to gross motor activities for longer periods than to table-top tasks. This is most likely because the former may require a more automatic and developmentally lower level of function, whereas the latter typically require sustained attention and cognitive processing. When monitoring the patient's level of attention, time estimates can be documented, but it is also important to note the type of activity performed based on the cognitive components of the task. The therapist may be able to introduce simple sequencing tasks of two or three steps and monitor the patient's ability to attend and remember the sequence. Memory tasks such as recalling the therapist's name or following two- or three-step directions can also be introduced.

Attention and memory are important components of task completion, new learning, and consistent daily functioning. The patient's level of attention will affect memory in that attention is necessary for information to be processed and stored. His attention may fluctuate depending on environmental stimuli and the complexity of the task. The therapist has some control over both. Initially, the therapist may choose a low-stimulus environment and upgrade it as the patient's attention to task improves so that the patient can eventually function in an open, unstructured environment. The complexity of the task can be graded as to the number of steps and the skills required.

Increased time spans involved in task performance without cueing or redirection are encouraged to the maximum of the individual's ability. Activities to promote attention at this stage are most effective if they are simple, familiar, interesting to the patient, and provide immediate gratification. An example is the card game "21." It is familiar to many people, requires the cognitive factors of addition, memory, and decision making, yet each round is completed quickly. The number of rounds can be increased based on the patient's performance.

As attention to task improves, the selection of activities can become more varied, increasing the complexity of the task and the number of steps. Cueing by the therapist should be decreased as indicated. Often, as the patient's processing of sensory information improves, his ability to attend to specific tasks for longer periods also improves. Some patients may benefit from computer-assisted therapy programs (see Unit 11, Appendix A). As improvements in the computer tasks are noted, the influence on functional tasks can be assessed.

The patient's potential for new learning can be affected by memory deficits. Many patients' severe memory deficits clear after coma, and they eventually recall ongoing events. A small percentage continue to experience severe memory dysfunction, but most will have residual memory disturbances as compared with their premorbid status. The severity of the disturbance and its impact on functioning vary.

Severe attention and memory problems will limit a patient's independence. However, for patients with minimal to moderate deficits who recognize their problem and are willing to accept and use compensatory techniques, the prognosis for independence in functional tasks is much greater.

Initiation and Sequencing

Frontal lobe damage often affects the patient's ability to initiate tasks and impairs their sustained attention skills (Chusid, 1976). In severe cases, even familiar tasks such as the patient's morning care routine may require one-on-one supervision with daily review and cueing. Cues can be verbal or manual. Manual cues can involve touching the patient's arm to encourage the start of the movement pattern and puts cueing on a less cortical level than verbal cues.

Structuring the environment and the activity may help some patients compensate for initiation and sequencing deficits. For example, all items necessary to complete a task, such as brushing the teeth, can be displayed in the order used, such as brush, paste, and cup of water to rinse. The visual set-up may be sufficient cueing. Verbal cues can be added if necessary. Some patients can follow a written list for memory or sequencing problems. Appropriate self-care lists can be posted in the patient's room. Repetition of specific daily living tasks performed the same way each day is often an effective means of helping the patient retain the sequence on a more automatic level. This is not a useful technique with complex or highly variable activities.

Sequencing of tasks can be graded by increasing the number of steps and complexity as the patient's abilities improve. For example, once a patient can safely and accurately pour a glass of juice, the next step may be preparing a sandwich and juice. The progression can be continued to the preparation of soup, a sandwich,

and a hot beverage and then to two hot items and a beverage. Simple unfamiliar tasks can be introduced and graded starting with two or three steps and carried out over a few days so that recall of new learning can be incorporated into the task. To use the example of a patient completing a series of ceramic pieces, the patient may initially glaze a piece that has been poured and cleaned by someone else. The next step might be to clean and glaze a piece, followed by pouring, cleaning,and glazing the third piece. As each new step is introduced, the patient may be able to recall the previous steps. Starting with a nearly completed project and working backward to include more steps is sometimes termed "backward chaining."

Initiation and sequencing are components of all daily living activities. Severe impairment of these component skills may require continued supervision and cueing for performance of functional tasks.

Problem Solving and Abstract Thought

Problem solving, organization, and abstract thought processes are the most complex cognitive functions. They are the endproduct of the integration of initiation, attention, sequencing, memory, and sensory processing affecting the individual's safety and judgment in the performance of functional tasks and, ultimately, his level of functional independence.

The therapist can assist the patient in developing problem-solving strategies by helping him organize his thought processes and by prompting him with questions. The process of problem solving can be outlined as follows.

1. Identify problem based on the situation.
2. Analyze specific conditions of the problem.
3. Formulate a strategy and plan of action, including alternatives and possible consequences.
4. Choose the relevant tactics based on the individual's skills, and prioritize.
5. Execute the plan and monitor the operations.
6. Compare or verify the solution with the problem.
7. Evaluate performance based on which aspects were successful and which could be improved (closure).
8. Integrate skills based on the individual's attitudes, skills, and personality (Ben-Yishay & Diller, 1983).

Table 5-2 applies these steps to a specific problem. Initially, the therapist may need to review each step and provide maximal cues for completing the sequence. With repetition, some patients may be able to learn to self-cue by using the outline. Most patients will require assistance for a prolonged period in formulating alternate solutions, monitoring their performance, and deciding how their performance could be improved.

Simple problem solving can be introduced early, based on familiar or routine self-care tasks, by introducing "what if" questions to spark the patient's thought process. Gradually, less structured activities with more variables can be introduced, such as avocational tasks or homemaking activities where the patient's actions will directly affect the outcome. His actions and responses to various situations can be analyzed and reviewed mutually with him.

The therapist discusses the patient's decision-making process, reviewing the step-by-step sequence and results. It is helpful if the therapist takes a non-threatening approach when providing feedback. Questions incorporate how the patient felt about the success of the activity, perceptions of difficulties encountered, and incorporation of this information into the planning of activities. Treatment progresses to group and community-oriented activities where the patient takes more responsibility for their planning and execution. Problem-solving abilities may improve to the point where the patient can identify and prioritize problems and choose appropriate channels for assistance with difficult situations.

Gradually, the patient is required to take more responsibility to plan and review his performance for thoroughness and timeliness. Maximum independent functioning requires appropriate coping mechanisms and use of compensatory techniques. The individual's ability to integrate sensory-perceptual, and cognitive skills minimizes his deficits and allows for a greater level of functioning. Breakdown in skills may occur with increased stress or time constraints. As the patient becomes more independent and can define his needs, it is important for him to deal with the issues he views as priorities. It may be helpful to devote the beginning of each treatment session to brainstorming effective ways to resolve problems. Individual and group treatment at this stage often emphasizes community interactions and coping strategies needed for effective functioning post discharge.

CONCLUSION

OT treatment of cognitive and perceptual deficits at RIC uses functional activity relevant to the patient's needs. Premorbid interests are considered when avocational and prevocational tasks are introduced in therapy. The tasks are adapted when necessary or broken down into subskills dependent on the patient's level of recovery and deficit areas. Community reintegration skills related to the individual's needs are introduced when appropriate, based on the patient's cognitive, behavioral, and physical skills. When possible, the specific tasks the patient will need to perform post discharge are practiced in therapy. This is helpful because many patients exhibit difficulty with generalization and application of skills.

In treating sensory-perceptual, and cognitive dysfunction, it is important for the therapist to allow time for the patient to process information and attempt a response before cueing. This is especially important

TABLE 5-2   Problem solving

1. Identify problem	Experience hunger	
2. Analyze conditions	It's noon, have not eaten since 8:00 at home.	
3. Formulate strategy	A. Go to restaurant (cost of food, transportation). B. Eat at home (food on hand for soup and sandwich). Must clean up.	
4. Choose tactics	Unable to drive, too far to walk, no public transportation, therefore must eat at home.	
5. Execute plan	Open can of soup and put on stove. Gather ingredients needed for sandwich and assemble. Set table, pour beverage, pour soup. Eat. Wash pot and dishes.	
6. Verify solution	No longer hungry.	
7. Closure/evaluation	Lunch adequate, but would have preferred restaurant. Next time plan ahead.	
8. Integration of skills	Call friend and arrange transportation.	

when attempts are being made by the patient to use compensatory techniques such as memory books, sequencing lists, problem-solving outlines, schedules, or written instructions spontaneously so they do not become dependent on the cueing. Some patients will remain limited in independence by their sensory-perceptual, cognitive, physical, or combined disabilities. These patients may continue to require a supervised living situation and assistance for community involvement. Other patients may achieve a level of abstract thought that will allow them to return to independent living. For these patients, it is important for the therapist to prepare them as much as possible for the challenges and frustrations they may encounter.

PROBLEM AREA: SENSORY-PERCEPTUAL MOTOR

Subcategory: Somatosensory

Long-term goals and indicators	Short-term goals	Treatment ideas
1. Family will show awareness of sensory deficits by safely positioning and handling affected upper extremities: • patient cognitively unable to compensate for sensory deficits • sensory deficits interfere with safe performance of daily living tasks.	1. • Patient/family will describe sensory deficits. • Patient/family will (*describe, demonstrate*) use of compensation techniques for sensory deficits.	1. • Show/describe area of sensory loss to caregiver. • Show/describe effects of these deficits on task performance. • Provide suggestions for positioning, handling, compensation. • Provide opportunities for caregiver to practice these techniques.
2. Patient will demonstrate somatosensory skills sufficient for safe and effective functioning in _____ daily living tasks. • shows tactile defensiveness • demonstrates decreased awareness of affected extremities • difficulty identifying objects by touch although sensation is adequate.	2. • Patient will demonstrate localized response to _____ stimuli (*consistently, inconsistently*). • Patient will demonstrate awareness of affected extremities by (*properly positioning upper extremities in wheelchair, bed, etc., compensating for sensory loss in daily tasks*) (*with, without*) cues. • Patient will demonstrate ability to discriminate (*shape, size, texture*) of objects through tactile exploration.	2. • Provide graded single-sensory input. • Record responses to stimuli and time of day. • Use stimuli that elicit most consistent response to increase arousal/alertness. • Alter environment to increase or decrease stimuli as needed. • Use movement to enhance response to sensory input. • Provide graded tactile activities requiring improved selectivity of response.
3. Patient will demonstrate body awareness skills sufficient for effective functioning in _____ daily living tasks. • unable to identify body parts • task performance affected by poor body concept • unable to identify right/left.	3. • Patient will demonstrate awareness of body scheme as evidenced by correct identification of body parts (*on self, others, picture*). • Patient will demonstrate improved right/left discrimination by correctly identifying right/left on (*self, others*) or by following instructions re direction in (*ADL therapeutic activities, community activities*).	3. • Improve awareness of body parts and body in space through movement and tactile stimulation. • Provide bilateral activities to encourage use of affected extremity. • Name body parts and use right/left directions. • Provide activities to enhance awareness of self before emphasizing body scheme of others or directionality.

Subcategory: Visual/Visual Motor

Long-term goals and indicators	Short-term goals	Treatment ideas
1. Patient will demonstrate consistent visual (*tracking, scanning*). • difficulty noted with visual fixation, tracking, scanning	1. • Patient will visually track a (*brightly colored object, familiar face, etc.*) through (*right, left, all*) visual fields. • Patient will scan the environment to locate (*brightly colored objects, familiar people, self-care items*) located in (*right, left*) visual field (*with, without*) cues.	1. • Use visual stimuli that elicit most consistent response. • Record responses to visual stimuli and time of day. • Alter environment to increase/decrease stimuli as needed. • Use movement to enhance response to visual motor activities.
2. Patient will demonstrate visual motor skills for safe and effective function in _____ daily living tasks. • difficulty in performing visual screening assessments during evaluation • difficulty attending to relevant visual stimuli • difficulty with eye-hand coordination.	2. • Patient will demonstrate (*visual discrimination, figure ground, visual closure, visual memory, visual integration*) skills sufficient for performance of (*functional tasks, specific activity, specific assessment*) (*with, without*) cues. • Patient/family will describe effect of visual motor deficits on (*safety, quality*) of performance of _____ tasks.	2. • Use movement to enhance response to visual motor activities. • Provide graded activities requiring improved visual selectivity. • Provide graded activities that require improved integration of sensory systems. • Describe visual motor problems and demonstrate effect on function. • Describe compensation techniques. • Provide opportunities for family to practice suggested methods.

Subcategory: Motor Planning

Long-term goals and indicators	Short-term goals	Treatment ideas
1. Patient will demonstrate motor planning and motor integration skills for safe and effective functioning in _____ daily living tasks. • unable to identify or demonstrate use of common objects • difficulty sequencing task, may perseverate on previous actions • understands concept of task, but has difficulty with execution (i.e., unrefined movement, errors in selection of movement) • difficulty shown in using two body sides together in coordinated tasks.	1. • Patient will demonstrate ability to conceptualize motor tasks as indicated by (*describing or performing*) _____ (*familiar, unfamiliar*) activity. • Patient will demonstrate ability to execute _____ (*familiar, unfamiliar, simple, complex*) motor tasks. • Patient will demonstrate bilateral integration skills sufficient for performing _____ (*self-care task, therapeutic activity, assessment*). • Patient/family will describe effect of motor planning deficits on (*safety, speed, accuracy*) of task performance.	1. • Begin by assisting patient in identifying use of objects. • Use simple, routine ADL tasks with hand-over-hand assistance as needed. • Use physical, verbal, or visual cues to help patient to the next step. • Minimize the need for patient to learn new techniques until adequate performance of routine tasks is shown. • Increase complexity of task to provide mild challenges. • Provide bilateral activities to improve gross and fine coordination/integration. • Incorporate appropriate tactile and vestibular input into gross motor activities.

PROBLEM AREA: COGNITIVE

Subcategory: Arousal/Attention

Long-term goals and indicators	Short-term goals	Treatment ideas
1. Patient will demonstrate optimal arousal during _____ activities. • difficult/unable to maintain level of arousal for participation in treatment • unaware of surroundings.	1. Patient will demonstrate eye opening for _____ periods of time following _____ stimulation.	1. • Initiate stimulation program. • Vary patient position and time of day of treatment.
2. Patient will demonstrate ability to attend to _____ task. • attention dependent on environmental factors, complexity of task • requires redirection.	2. • Patient will attend to _____ (*visual, auditory*) tasks for _____ minutes in (*distracting, nondistracting, home, community*) environment (*with, without*) (*cues, structure*). • Patient will refocus attention to _____ task independently.	2. • Use activities relevant to the patient. • Provide variety of tasks throughout treatment session. • Grade motoric and cognitive complexity of task to increase attentional demands. • Grade amount of time attention to task is required. • Use computer-assisted treatment.

Subcategory: Memory

Long-term goals and indicators	Short-term goals	Treatment ideas
1. Patient is able to retain information relevant to task at hand. • able to attend to environment • shows some recall for automatic repetitious activities.	1. • Patient is able to recall _____ (*visual, auditory*) information for _____ amount of time (not more than therapy session). • Patient can use memory book to assist in recalling _____ information.	1. • Repeat consistent technique and approach to task. • Use relevant information. • Use compensatory measures such as memory books, lists, tactile or visual cues. • Organize information for more effective input into storage (i.e., present information in short, logical steps, have patient repeat steps before and after completion).
2. Patient is able to retain information from one situation to another: • uses compensation techniques as needed, able to recall relevant or routine information • oriented to self, environment, and time.	2. • Patient will recall _____ information for _____ amount of elapsed time. • Patient will use (*memory book, environment cues*) to assist in recalling _____ information.	2. See above.

Subcategory: Orientation

Long-term goals and indicators	Short-term goals	Treatment ideas
1. Patient will demonstrate orientation to familiar others and environments. • disoriented X3 • memory deficits • aware of self, responds to name.	1. • Patient will demonstrate orientation to (*self, familiar others*). • Patient will demonstrate orientation to (*daily schedule, familiar surroundings*).	1. • Repeat information. • Use familiar surroundings. • Use compensation techniques such as memory book.
2. Patient will demonstrate full orientation. • able to identify familiar places, year, season, month • may have difficulty with specific time (i.e., time of day, date) • able to identify familiar others by name.	2. • Patient will demonstrate orientation to unfamiliar others (*independently, with cues*). • Patient will demonstrate orientation to (*date, time of day*). • Patient will demonstrate topographical orientation within community (*independently, with supervision*).	2. See above and use additional environmental cues (i.e., calendar, signs, watches).

Subcategory: Initiation

Long-term goals and indicators	Short-term goals	Treatment ideas
1. Patient will initiate participation in functional tasks in order to fulfill basic needs. • requires cues to initiate or continue all tasks	1. • Patient will initiate (*first, each subsequent*) step of (*feeding, dressing, toileting*) sequence (*with, without*) cues.	1. • Use most effective cueing method (*verbal, visual, tactile*). • Use routine activities appropriate to time of day. • Structure activity to elicit automatic response.
2. Patient will initiate participation in tasks pertinent to life roles and interests. • able to begin/follow through with activities that are personally meaningful • may require cues to initiate tasks not of interest.	2. • Patient will initiate action in order to (*interact socially, perform leisure skills, pursue vocational interests*) (*with cues, independently*). • Patient will plan and perform (*simple meal preparation, community outtrip*) (*with cues, independently*).	2. As above, use activities personally relevant to patient.

Subcategory: Sequencing

If the patient can sequence tasks but has memory problems that interfere with day-to-day carryover, refer to the Memory subcategory.

Long-term goals and indicators	Short-term goals	Treatment ideas
1. Patient will demonstrate sequencing skills sufficient for completion of _____ daily living task. • unable to complete multistep task.	1. • Patient will sequence simple (*2, 3*) step task. • Patient will sequence familiar self-care task (*with, without*) cues. • Patient will sequence complex multistep task (*following initial instruction; with, without cues*). • Patient will simultaneously sequence (*2, 3, 4*) tasks for completion of _____ daily living task (*i.e., meal preparation, home maintenance*).	1. • Have patient sequence verbally or in writing before performance and/or during task. • Grade complexity and number of steps of task. • Repeat specific tasks/routines. • Use compensation techniques (*lists, set-ups*).

Subcategory: Problem Solving

Long-term goals and indicators	Short-term goals	Treatment ideas
1. Patient will demonstrate problem-solving skills sufficient for completion of _____ daily living tasks. • may have difficulty identifying problems or solutions • may persist in using an approach to a problem without assessing effectiveness.	1. • Patient will identify problems interfering with performance of _____ task (*with, without*) cues. • Patient will identify (*1, 2, or more*) solutions to problems encountered in _____ task (*with, without*) cues. • Patient will implement identified solutions to problems encountered in _____ task (*with, without*) cues. • Patient will evaluate effectiveness of identified solutions to problems in _____ task (*with, without*) cues. • Patient will anticipate problems in _____ task and take effective measures to avoid them (*with, without*) cues.	1. • Use graded real and simulated problem-solving situations. • Use cueing/structure to have patient anticipate problems. • Use problem-solving outline to review performance.

Subcategory: Judgment and Safety

Long-term goals and indicators	Short-term goals	Treatment ideas
1. Patient will demonstrate judgment for safe completion of simple, familiar tasks. • poor attention to task • impulsive • difficulty determining consequences of behavior.	1. Patient will demonstrate safe completion of (*feeding, dressing, bathing, toileting*) in a (*structured, unstructured*) environment (*with, without*) cues.	1. • Structure environment to minimize distraction. • Use most effective cueing method to promote safe performance. • Discuss possible consequences before task and review performance after.
2. Patient will demonstrate judgment for safe completion of all daily living tasks. • determines consequences of action in routine tasks • may require assistance for unfamiliar tasks or in a multistimulus environment.	2. Patient will demonstrate safe completion of (*homemaking, community living*) task (*with, without*) cues.	2. • Use most effective cueing method to promote safe performance. • Discuss possible consequences before task and review performance after.

REFERENCES

Adams, R., & Victor, M. (1981). *Principles of neurology.* New York: McGraw-Hill.

Atkinson, R.C., & Shiffrin, R.M. (1968). Human memory: A proposed system and its control processes. In K.W. Spence (Ed.), *The psychology of learning and motivation: Advances in research and theory* (Vol. 2). New York: Academic Press.

Ayres, A.J. (1972). *Sensory integration and learning disorders.* Los Angeles: Western Psychological Services.

Baddeley, A. (1982). *Your memory: A users guide.* New York: Macmillan.

Ben-Yishay, Y., & Diller, L. (1983). Cognitive remediation. In M. Rosenthal (Ed.), *Rehabilitation of the head injured adult.* Philadelphia: F.A. Davis Company.

Chapparo, C., & Ranka, J. (1980). Patterns of sensory integrative dysfunction in adult hemiplegia. Research Project RT-20, Project R-112. Rehabilitation Institute of Chicago.

Chapparo, C., & Ranka, J. (1982). Coursework from application of sensory integrative principles to adult head trauma and CVA: Advanced theory. Rehabilitation Institute of Chicago.

Chusid, J.G. (1976). *Correlative neuroanatomy and functional neurology* (16th ed.). Los Altos, CA: Lange Medical Publications.

Craik, F.I.M., & Lockhart, R.S. (1972). Levels of processing: A framework for memory research. *Journal of Verbal Learning and Verbal Behavior, 11,* 671–684.

Farber, S. (1982). *Neurohabilitation: A multisensory approach.* Philadelphia: W.B. Saunders.

Frank, L.K. (1971). Tactile communication. In C.D. Kopp (Ed.), *Readings in early development for occupational and physical therapy students.* Springfield, IL: Charles C Thomas.

Geldard, E.A. (1972). *The human senses* (2nd ed.). New York: Wiley.

Goddem, D.R., & Baddeley, A.D. (1980). When does context influence recognition memory? *British Journal of Psychology, 71,* 99–104.

Gronwall, D., & Wrightson, P. (1981). Memory and information processing capacity after closed head injury. *Journal of Neurology, Neurosurgery and Psychiatry, 44,* 889–895.

Held, R. (1965, November). Plasticity in sensory-motor systems. *Scientific American, 213* (5), 84–94.

Levin, H.S., High, W., Meyers, C.A., Van Laufen, A., Hayden, M.E., & Eisenberg, H.M. (1985). Impairment of remote memory after closed head injury. *Journal of Neurology, Neurosurgery and Psychiatry, 48,* 556–563.

Lezak, M.D. (1979). Recovery of memory and learning functions following traumatic brain injury. *Cortex, 15,* 63–72.

Lishman, W.A. (1978). *Organic psychiatry* (pp. 191–261). Oxford: Blackwell Scientific Publications.

Montgomery, P., & Richter, E. (1972). *Sensorimotor integration for developmentally delayed children: A handbook.* Los Angeles: Western Psychological Services.

Moore, J. (1978). Neuroanatomical considerations relating to recovery following brain lesions. In P. Bach-y-Rita (Ed.), *Recovery of function: Theoretical considerations for brain injury.* Baltimore: University Park Press.

Rood, M. (1962). The use of sensory receptors to activate, facilitate and inhibit motor response. In M. Sattely (Ed.), *Approaches to the treatment of patients with neuromuscular dysfunction.* Dubuque, IA: William C. Brown.

Sinclair, D. (1967). *Cutaneous sensation.* London: Oxford University Press.

Wilson, B., & Moffat, N. (1984). *Clinical management of memory problems.* Rockville, MD: Aspen Publishers.

Wood, R.L. (1984). Behavior disorders following severe brain injury. In N. Brooks (Ed.), *Closed head injury.* London: Oxford University Press.

Part III

Sensorimotor Components

Handling and Facilitation of Functional Movement

Karen Kovich, OTR/L
Diane Bermann, OTR/L

Movement is the basis of our functional capabilities and, developmentally, is the basis of our learning. Movement allows us to interact with the environment and to learn from those interactions. Traumatic head injury (HI) can limit an individual's mobility to varying degrees. This unit addresses the issues of normal development, muscle tone, function and how they are affected by HI. General inhibitory techniques and specific techniques used to facilitate movement are also discussed. Techniques are divided into specific problem areas so that the therapist can find them more easily. However, abnormal tone is rarely isolated to one limb, and with severely physically involved patients, it may be widespread.

The techniques described reflect some of the interventions that occupational therapists at the Rehabilitation Institute of Chicago (RIC) have found successful when working with head-injured patients at various levels of recovery. Many of the techniques reflect a Neurodevelopmental Treatment (NDT) orientation developed by Karl and Berta Bobath. Although there is a strong NDT influence on the treatment provided, techniques from other theoretical approaches are also presented.

MUSCLE TONE AS THE BASIS OF NORMAL MOVEMENT

Muscle tone is the foundation of functional movement patterns. It must be high enough for the individual to resist gravity and low enough to allow for smooth, coordinated movement. The Bobaths use the term "postural tone," as it reflects the influence of muscle tone on the dynamic components of balance and equilibrium responses necessary for function in all planes. The Bobaths describe a normal postural reflex mechanism as consisting of a great number and variety of automatic movements that gradually develop as the individual matures (Bobath, 1978). These include righting reactions, equilibrium reactions, and automatic adaptation of muscle to changes in posture.

Righting reactions serve to restore and maintain the head in its normal position in space during movement. The normal position is with the head vertical, with the eyes maintaining a horizontal gaze. Righting reactions also help maintain the head in proper alignment with the trunk and assist in movement from position to position, such as getting up from the floor, getting out of bed, and sitting down. Righting reactions are very difficult to separate from equilibrium reactions in the adult.

Equilibrium reactions are automatic reactions that serve to maintain and restore balance during all activities. Changes in the individual's center of gravity, which occur almost constantly during any functional activity, necessitate continuous postural adjustments. These adjustments may involve subtle tonal changes or, if displacement is great, movements of the entire body to counteract the displacement. To be effective, these movements and tonal changes must be well coordinated, quick, adequate in range, and well timed (Bobath, 1978).

Automatic adaptation of muscles to changes in posture overlaps, to some extent, with equilibrium responses but can also be observed in the trunk and limbs. It allows for smooth, coordinated movements both with and against gravity. Automatic adaptation allows for the balance of proximal stability and distal mobility that is necessary for functioning. It also allows for the graded control of agonists, antagonists, and synergists for proper timing and direction of movement. The normal postural reflex mechanism reflects three prerequisites necessary for voluntary and functional activity: normal postural tone, normal reciprocal interaction of muscles, and automatic movement patterns of righting and equilibrium.

Related to the postural reflex mechanism is the term "postural set." People perform certain activities in the same way, based on similar motor patterns, such as standing up, rolling, or running. Automatic changes in postural tone, or postural sets, not only accompany these movement patterns but precede them. For example, in sitting, we first pull our feet under the chair and lean forward before standing up. In that spontaneous movement, the postural set, or readiness, is established, enabling the movement pattern necessary to stand. Extension is the readiness state, or postural set, as the body prepares to assume an upright position. Postural sets vary depending on the activity or motor pattern performed.

EFFECTS OF HEAD INJURY ON NORMAL POSTURAL TONE AND FUNCTION

The effects of traumatic HI may be widespread or localized depending on the cause, severity, and location of the injury. Diffuse brain damage associated with high-impact acceleration/deceleration injuries often produces widespread physical impairments. An injury caused by a blow to the head may produce a more localized impairment. Both types of injuries produce upper motor neuron lesions that affect the ability of the central nervous system (CNS) to control or inhibit the firing of muscles. This unrestricted firing produces increased muscle tone. Similarly, the release of inhibitory control over primitive reflexes may occur, causing them to emerge and affect motor control and, therefore, functional abilities. Primitive reflexes most often observed in head-injured patients are the asymmetrical tonic neck reflex, symmetrical tonic neck reflex, tonic labyrinthine, grasp reflex, and positive supporting reaction. Often, changes in muscle tone are noted in the patient, as opposed to the patient assuming the reflexive posture.

In extreme cases, damage to the brainstem can produce decerebrate rigidity. It is theorized that destruction of an inhibitory center in the reticular substance extending from the medulla to the midbrain produces hyperactive extension reflexes and spasticity (Chusid, 1973). Typical posturing caused by decerebrate rigidity is hyperextension of the neck, extension of the lower extremities, extension and internal rotation of the upper extremities, and flexion of the wrists and hands. The presence of decerebrate rigidity for an extended time would indicate limited functional goals. Decorticate rigidity may also occur in the patient with severe cortical damage. It produces extension of the lower extremities and flexion of the neck and upper extremities.

Damage to the cerebellar region or connections to it may produce ataxia. If the ataxia affects the trunk, the patient may show a wide-based, unsteady gait pattern, which may affect proximal control of the upper extremities. If the ataxia affects the limbs, voluntary movements will be jerky and uncontrolled. An intention tremor may be present, as well as problems in estimating ranges of movement. This is exhibited by over- or under-reaching by the patient. Techniques to inhibit cerebellar ataxia are limited, and compensation techniques are often necessary to allow the patient to achieve the highest level of function possible.

The effects of abnormal postural tone and primitive reflexes are inhibited before facilitating function by the use of relaxation techniques and reflex inhibiting patterns (RIPs). RIPs are positions or movement patterns that reverse or counteract the effects of abnormal postural tone and primitive reflexes. Often, they are used to prepare the patient for effective weight bearing through the trunk or extremities. This allows for more normal sensory input and is frequently effective in maintaining normalized muscle tone in the patient in preparation for function.

Movement into or through RIPs can be controlled by the therapist using key points of control. The therapist places her hands on the patient at those points most effective in influencing muscle tone throughout the body. Proximal key points of control are the shoulders and hips. Distal key points of control are the hand and foot. Key points of control are often used to facilitate normal movement patterns once abnormal postural tone is inhibited.

DEVELOPMENTAL PRINCIPLES

Principles of normal development of function are presented here to assist the therapist in treatment planning. General principles are more useful than specific milestones because function and skills in the adult are variable after injury. In general, it is most effective to gain motor control:

- proximal to distal
- gross to fine
- static to dynamic

This indicates that treatment should start at the head, neck, and trunk when attempting to normalize muscle tone because the trunk provides the balance of mobility and stability needed for both upper and lower extremity function.

Developmentally, a child learns to function in one static position and then another before being able to move between the two. The dynamic component that allows movement between positions requires refined movement patterns that incorporate righting and equilibrium reactions. Initially, distal support is required to move between positions, but with continued repetition, effective movement patterns are learned and integrated into the CNS, and distal support is no longer necessary.

As the individual is challenged by higher developmental positions, function and skill at lower levels become more refined. For example, working in a half-kneel position may be challenging for a patient in relation to balance and equilibrium responses. As the patient gains more control during activity in this position, it becomes easier for him to function in sitting and standing. He may also be able to perform more complex tasks in those positions with less effort.

When applying these principles to the treatment of adult head-injured patients, the therapist considers:

- influence of head and neck on movement patterns
- effects of proximal control on distal function
- development of gross motor control as a prerequisite for effective fine motor control
- control of movement patterns into and out of static postures
- necessity of repetition and variation for the integration of motor patterns
- importance of challenging the patient to achieve higher levels of function as lower levels of skill are perfected

The following chart represents a developmental framework relating to the development of function in the upright position.

Developmental task	Components	Functional implications
Head control	Balance of flexion and extension Rotation Symmetry	Midline orientation Righting reactions Influences movement from position to position
Gradual increase in extensor tone in trunk	Balance of flexion, extension, and lateral flexion Symmetric weight bearing	Maintain postures against gravity Trunk stability Symmetry
Weight shift and rotation within body axis	Balance of lateral flexion and extension Rotation of upper trunk on lower trunk Separation of shoulders Anterior and posterior pelvic tilt	Movement from one upright position to another Ability to cross midline
Equilibrium responses	Balanced postural and tonal adjustments Automatic adaptation of muscles	Maintain balance when center of gravity changes Integration of both sides of body Background for movement patterns Ambulation
Hands set free for skilled function	Balance of proximal stability/mobility Good balance and equilibrium during activity	Hands no longer needed for support Development of skilled manipulation Able to function in upright Easily moves from position to position while engaged in activity

GENERAL INHIBITORY TECHNIQUES

Normal movement, which is necessary for functioning, is impaired by patterns of increased muscle tone such as spasticity and rigidity. In the head-injured patient, abnormal muscle tone ranges from mild to severe. By normalizing muscle tone before functional activity, the therapist helps the patient avoid abnormal movement patterns. Abnormal patterns may be influenced by synergies, associated reactions, and stress, which is produced as the patient attempts to move normally despite the abnormal muscle tone. Techniques that can be effective in inhibiting abnormal postural tone are:

- rotation
- mobilization of proximal joints
- slow rocking
- neutral warmth
- weight bearing
- inversion

Rotation provides a slow passive stretch that elongates one set of muscles while putting the opposing group on slack. Rotary patterns tend to reverse the pull of spasticity and therefore allow relaxation of the trunk and limb musculature. Rotation also incorporates the normal movement patterns of the trunk that are necessary for both balance and equilibrium responses and functional movement patterns of the arms.

Mobilization of proximal joints affects both the trunk and limbs. Because many trunk muscles attach to either the scapula or pelvis, the shoulder and pelvic girdles must be considered as part of the trunk. Spasticity often produces retraction and depression of the scapula, internal rotation and adduction of the humerus, and contraction of the lateral flexors of the trunk. Rigidity in the trunk itself often prevents separation of the upper trunk from the lower trunk in movement patterns. This affects spontaneous balance and equilibrium responses, and distal control of the limbs. The pelvis is often retracted and may be fixed in a posterior tilt by spasticity or rigidity. This affects sitting balance and often increases extensor tone in the lower extremities. Mobilization of the shoulder girdle and pelvis is an important preliminary step that is necessary to help reduce abnormal muscle tone and allow for:

- separation of movement in the upper and lower trunk
- elongation of trunk musculature
- freedom of movement in the shoulder
- effective anterior pelvic tilt for symmetric weight bearing

Slow rocking alone or in combination with **neutral warmth** can be effective in producing a generalized inhibitory state. This involves total body relaxation and may decrease respiration and heart rate. These techniques can be combined by wrapping the patient in a sheet or light blanket while controlling the rocking motion with the sheet. Further relaxation of the trunk musculature can be obtained by increasing the amount of rotation used in the rocking motion.

Weight bearing through the extremities and pelvis can have an inhibitory effect on spastic muscles. In the upper extremities, the resulting cocontraction helps to re-establish a normal agonist/antagonist relationship of muscles and facilitates normalized muscle tone (Eggers, 1984). Weight bearing in a sidelying position on a properly positioned arm produces relaxation at the shoulder girdle and in the arm. Symmetric weight bearing through the pelvis in sitting often produces a decrease in extensor tone in the lower extremities as well as relaxation in the upper extremities. When the patient is weight bearing on the upper extremities, it is important to keep both proximal and distal joints properly aligned. Prolonged static weight bearing on the upper extremities should be avoided, as the muscles accommodate to the stimulus and the normal cocontraction of muscles decreases.

Inversion, like slow rocking, can have an inhibitory effect on the CNS. When the patient is inverted, the carotid sinus is activated, producing a generalized calming and inhibition of all stretch reflexes except those facilitated by the labyrinthine reflex (Farber, 1982). Total inversion is contraindicated for patients with shunts. Extra care should be used with patients having tracheostomies, making sure the airway is kept clear, and with patients with abdominal feeding tubes, making sure they are not causing discomfort, which may result in increased muscle tone.

INHIBITORY TECHNIQUES SPECIFIC TO THE TRUNK AND NECK

When abnormal muscle tone is evident in the head-injured patient, it is important to follow the developmental principle of working from proximal to distal. Beginning treatment by using inhibitory techniques for the trunk and neck positively affects distal muscle tone and provides the necessary base for functional movement and activity. Spasticity in the lower trunk, resulting in retraction of the pelvis and shortening of the trunk, makes rotation and weight shift difficult, and a posterior pelvic tilt posture may develop. Spasticity in the latissimus dorsi, rhomboids, and trapezius can cause the scapula to become fixed in a downwardly rotated and retracted position, reinforcing lateral trunk flexion. This makes shoulder movement difficult or, in some cases, impossible. Scapular mobilization is often done in conjunction with trunk rotation.

Trunk

If the abnormal tone is mild, self-produced trunk rotation in supine or sitting may be enough to normalize muscle tone. In supine, the patient moves his hips and legs to the right side, elongating the left side of his trunk, and then reverses. For maximum stretch, the patient can incorporate counter-rotation of the upper trunk, as seen in Figure 6–1.

If abnormal muscle tone in the trunk is moderate to severe, or if the patient cannot produce the movement sequence independently, the therapist can assist in producing the rotary movements. Assistance can be provided at the shoulder girdle or at the lower extremities (Figure 6–2). Symmetric trunk rotation facilitated from the lower extremities with the patient supine is done by flexing the patient's hips and knees and slowly rotating them from side to side. This can also be accomplished by flexing one of the patient's legs and extending the other (Figure 6–3). The flexed leg is then rotated over the extended one, and the process is then reversed. If the patient tends to roll, the shoulders may require stabilization.

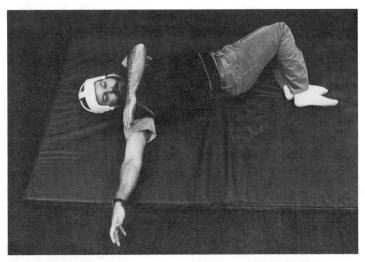

Figure 6–1 Self-produced rotation affects primarily the lower trunk.

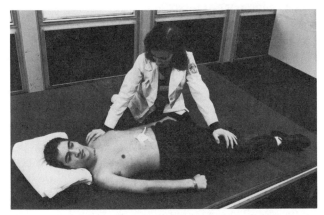

Figure 6–2 When the therapist assists in rotation, emphasis can be placed on either the upper or lower trunk.

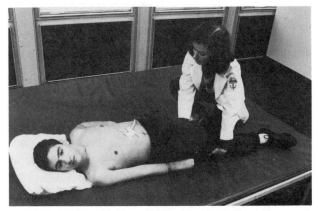

Figure 6–3 Rotation can also be facilitated from the lower extremities.

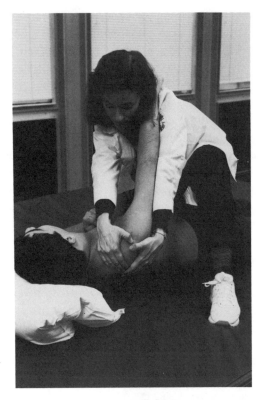

Figure 6–4 Rotation facilitated from the upper body can also incorporate scapular mobilization.

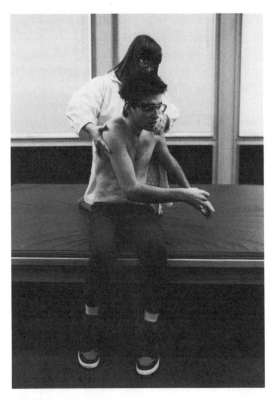

Figure 6–5 When the spine and pelvis can be properly aligned, trunk rotation can be facilitated in the more functional position of sitting.

An alternate method of trunk rotation in supine works well when the patient can actively participate in the movement sequence. To facilitate rotation of the right side, the therapist positions herself to the left of the patient and places her hands under the patient's right scapula. As the patient lifts his head, the therapist provides pressure and assistance from the scapula in an upward motion, while rotating the patient's upper body on the lower (Figure 6–4).

Trunk rotation can also be accomplished in the sidelying position. This position often serves to modify extensor tone in the trunk by reducing the extensor bias created by the supine position. When positioning the patient in sidelying, it is important to preposition the weight-bearing arm comfortably, attempting scapular protraction and external rotation of the humerus. The lower extremities should also be prepositioned, with the bottom leg extended. The top leg should be slightly flexed at the knee and hip to prevent total patterns of flexion or extension. A pillow can be placed between the patient's knees for comfort. The therapist then places one hand on the patient's scapula and the other on his hip and gently rotates the scapula forward while

either stabilizing the pelvis or rotating it backward. To reverse the motion, the therapist places one hand between the patient's clavicle and sternum to stabilize the shoulder girdle without causing scapular retraction and rotates the pelvis forward with her other hand. Movements should be slow and controlled, providing a constant amount of pressure.

Trunk rotation can also be accomplished with the patient in the sitting position if the therapist can maintain proper alignment of the patient's pelvis in a neutral or anterior tilt position. The therapist positions herself behind the seated patient and passively rotates the patient's upper trunk on the lower trunk (Figure 6–5). Weight bearing through the hips and lower extremities helps stabilize the lower trunk. This is not an effective technique if the patient's pelvis is fixed in a posterior tilt.

When trunk mobility is decreased because of rigidity or severe spasticity, it is useful to have two therapists to provide inhibition techniques. With the patient in supine, rotation is produced by moving the upper trunk on the stabilized pelvic girdle or by moving the pelvis on the stabilized shoulder girdle. Stabilization is necessary if there is no separation of upper and lower trunk mobility. Without separation, the patient rolls from side to side rather than achieving the desired alternating trunk elongation and shortening.

If the patient tolerates the technique, the therapists progress to counter-rotation, in which the patient's hips and lower extremities are rotated to the right while the shoulder girdle is rotated to the left. The movement pattern is then reversed. This produces an even greater stretch and elongation of the trunk. Movements should be slow and controlled, as abrupt or rapid movements can trigger stretch reflex responses. The patient should be encouraged to look in the direction in which his upper trunk is rotating. If this is not possible, one therapist should support the patient's head to prevent hyperextension of the neck. As the patterns are repeated, gradual increases in the trunk's range of movement should be noted.

When abnormal tone in the pelvic girdle is severe, or trunk shortening has occurred, passive mobilization may be necessary before implementing the rotation and weight-bearing techniques described. With the patient in a sidelying position, the therapist can stabilize the shoulder girdle with one hand while providing slow

rhythmic pressure to the pelvis. The pressure applied in a horizontal direction provides passive elongation of the trunk.

If the pelvis is fixed in a posterior tilt, the therapist can passively mobilize it into a more anterior position (Figures 6–6 and 6–7). This can be accomplished with the patient in a sitting position. The therapist provides pressure at the small of the back to move the pelvis forward into extension. Slow rhythmic movements can often increase the amount of passive motion available.

Neck

Increased tone in the neck flexors and sternocleidomastoid (SCM) muscle is common in severely physically involved head-injured patients. This makes head control against gravity difficult or impossible, and if uncorrected, can overstretch the neck extensors, preventing effective vertical head control. If the therapist attempts to push the flexed neck into extension, strong resistance will be encountered. However, by placing a palm on each of the patient's cheeks and incorporating slow rotational movements, the neck flexors will relax

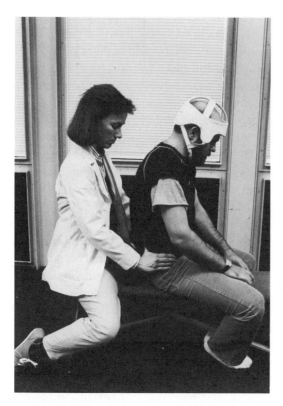

Figure 6–6 Patient sitting with a posteriorly tilted pelvis

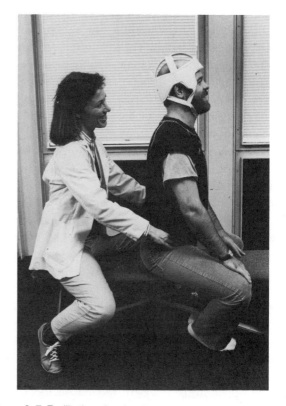

Figure 6–7 Facilitation of patient into an anterior pelvic tilt

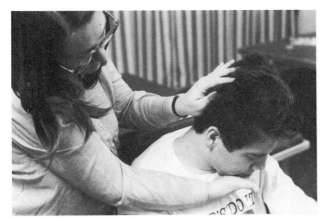

Figure 6–8 Tightness of the patient's SCM muscle causes his head to flex forward and rotate.

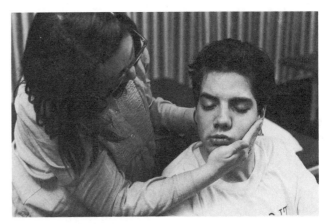

Figure 6–9 Tightness is often seen in the SCM muscle.

and the head can be positioned vertically (Figures 6–8 and 6–9). A similar technique is used if the patient's head is flexed and laterally rotated due to spasticity in the SCM muscle.

Scapula

Scapular mobilization involves passive movement of the scapula upward, forward, downward, and back to neutral. With the patient sidelying, the therapist supports the patient's arm on her shoulder and places one hand on the patient's scapula and the other on the anterior surface of the shoulder girdle. Pressure is directed between the hands. The therapist is careful not to dig her fingers into the patient. The therapist slowly moves the scapula and the supported humerus as a unit, elevating, depressing, upwardly rotating, retracting, and protracting. When this technique is performed with the patient in supine, the trunk will elongate as the scapula is upwardly rotated and the humerus flexed overhead. This technique can also be done with the patient in a sitting position.

Scapular mobilization may be combined with techniques designed to allow separation of movement between the patient's upper and lower trunk. This technique is performed with the patient in sitting, with arms supported on a table. The therapist places herself behind the patient and protracts and upwardly rotates one scapula, causing the humerus to flex slightly and elongate that side of the trunk. This technique encourages a separation of scapular movement as well as symmetric trunk elongation and extension. Because the pelvis is stabilized by the patient's weight-bearing position, the upper trunk is easily rotated on the lower trunk.

INHIBITORY TECHNIQUES FOR THE EXTREMITIES

After initial inhibition of abnormal tone in the trunk, the extremities may require additional inhibition to normalize their tone in order to allow active participation in functional tasks.

Inhibition of upper extremity flexor tone begins proximally. Flexor tone is usually dominant in the upper extremities. Thorough scapular mobilization is always a prerequisite to normalizing upper extremity tone, even if the trunk does not appear to be involved.

With the patient supine, the properly mobilized and positioned scapula can be held in place by the patient's weight against the mat. The therapist then begins to work more distally, slowly rotating the humerus into external rotation and back to neutral while applying gentle pressure into elbow extension (Figure 6–10). Moving further distally, the wrist is brought into neutral as the therapist continues the rotary movements. One hand is then placed on the patient's thenar eminence and the other at the ulnar ridge, and the hand is gently stretched as the wrist is extended further (Figure 6–11). The stretching of the hand usually produces relaxation of the fingers, and the thumb can be brought into abduction, which often produces continued relaxation of the hand and wrist, readying it for weight-bearing or voluntary movement patterns.

With the patient in sitting, the technique is similar, but extra care may need to be taken to ensure that continued scapular protraction and upward rotation remain when the patient's humerus is placed in flexion. The therapist guides the scapula in the proper movement pattern. It is also possible to extend and externally rotate the arm. This position has a continued inhibitory

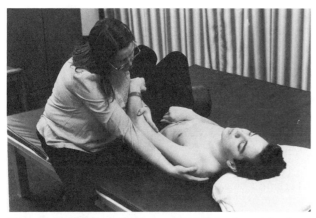

Figure 6–10 Inhibition of the upper extremity begins proximally.

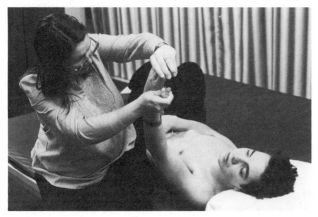

Figure 6–11 The therapist moves distally to achieve inhibition throughout the entire upper extremity.

effect on the extremity and adds to elongation of the trunk. It also puts the arm into a good position for upper extremity weight bearing. If controlled rotation and pressure into extension are not effective, gentle shaking of the extremity may offer momentary relaxation. The shoulder girdle is properly mobilized before working distally. To inhibit elbow flexor spasticity, the therapist grasps the patient's wrist and gently shakes the extremity while moving it into extension. Once relaxation begins, the therapist can maintain it by putting the patient's arm into external rotation and abducting the thumb.

Inhibition of the Tightly Flexed Wrist and Hand

Occasionally, the proximal parts of the arm can be inhibited while abnormal tone persists in the wrist and hand. With extra attention, relaxation may be produced in the hand as well. A flexed wrist and tightly fisted hand make it difficult for the therapist to reach the pa-

tient's thenar eminence and ulnar ridge in attempts to produce inhibition in the hand. In this case, further flexing of the wrist often allows the fingers to extend far enough for the therapist to position her hands in the patient's palm and begin mobilization techniques to inhibit the abnormal muscle tone.

Mobilization of the wrist may be necessary if the tone is severe, tendons are tight, or the wrist has been fixed in flexion for an extended period. In these cases, the therapist places her thumbs on the dorsal surface of the patient's wrist (Figure 6–12) and gently applies alternating pressure in all directions: forward and back, up and down, and finally in small rotary movements. This often permits extension of the wrist to neutral. Soft tissue contractures will not respond to these techniques, and casting may be a viable alternative for increasing range and providing inhibition (See Unit 7).

Inhibition of Extensor Tone in the Upper Extremities

Strong extensor tone in the upper extremities is occasionally encountered in the head-injured patient. This may be associated with overall decerebrate posturing,

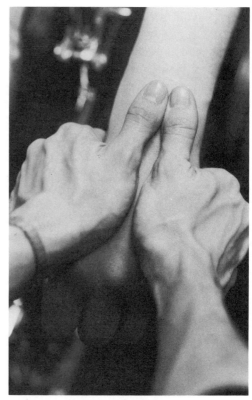

Figure 6–12 The therapist applies pressure to the patient's hand, using her fingers and thenar eminence.

which includes extension and internal rotation of the upper extremities, flexion of the wrist and hands, extension and internal rotation of the lower extremities, and strong extensor tone in the trunk. If this is the case, techniques to break up the extensor tone throughout the body are required before attempting upper extremity inhibition.

Supine and sidelying positions often reinforce the extensor posturing; sitting upright with hips flexed will help inhibit the posturing. The therapist works proximally to distally, but in this case, the scapula may be abnormally positioned in protraction, and the therapist may need to work for a more neutral position. Inhibition involves rotation and pressure into elbow flexion and then back to a neutral position, preventing the elbow from locking into extension. Use of the techniques described earlier to inhibit flexor tone in the wrist and hand can then be used.

Inhibition of Extensor Tone in the Lower Extremities

Extensor tone in the lower extremities is often seen alone or in conjunction with the positive supporting reaction. If the positive supporting reaction is triggering extensor spasms in the lower extremities, it is important to avoid pressure on the ball of the foot. Encouraging effective weight bearing through the heel is the best method of inhibiting the reaction. Flexion of the hips is effective in inhibiting generalized extensor tone in the lower extremities. This can be accomplished with the patient in supine by flexing his hips and knees with his feet flat on the mat. A small bolster placed under the knees may be effective in maintaining the

position, but if extensor tone is too strong, the therapist may need to provide downward pressure at the ankles. Properly positioning a patient in sitting will also serve to inhibit lower extremity extensor tone. Proper positioning includes hip flexion to at least 90°, a slight anterior pelvic tilt, equal weight bearing through both hips, and feet supported flat on the floor or a raised surface to provide weight bearing through the lower extremities.

Inversion Over a Ball

Inversion should produce a generalized relaxation of muscle tone, allowing for increased extension and external rotation of the upper extremities and passive elongation of the trunk. Active head control can sometimes be elicited in this position, and the use of a large mirror may facilitate the patient looking at himself. This position may be too stressful for some patients and may produce increased muscle tone throughout the body, in which case it should be discontinued. If the patient is alert, it may be helpful to explain or demonstrate the technique before attempting it.

For safety, two to three therapists should be available to control the inverted patient and monitor his responses. To invert a patient, it is best to start with the patient in short sitting on the edge of a mat. The ball is held in place while the patient is leaned forward and brought to the ball (Figure 6–13). The ball is then slowly rolled forward so that the patient achieves a prone position with one therapist supporting the patient under the axilla and another controlling the patient at the hips as his weight comes forward onto the ball (Figure 6–14). Because this technique can produce

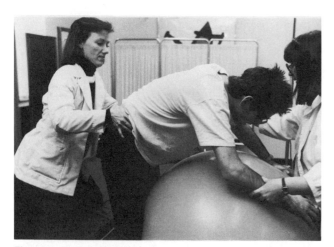

Figure 6–13 Two therapists are required to control the patient as he is placed over a ball.

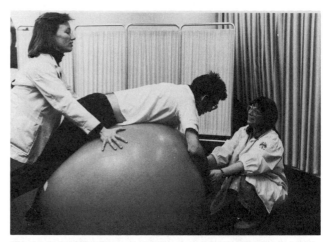

Figure 6–14 Note the patient's increased trunk extension and the beginning relaxation of his upper extremities.

generalized inhibition and is a dramatic postural change, blood pressure, pulse, and respiration should be monitored closely.

Partial inversion of the patient can produce some of the same effects as total inversion, is easier for one therapist to control, and can be used in preparation for total inversion. The patient assumes or is placed in short sitting with feet flat on the floor. He leans forward over a smaller ball with arms flexed or is draped over the ball. The therapist can slowly rock the ball from side to side, encouraging trunk elongation and further upper extremity relaxation.

GENERAL TECHNIQUES TO FACILITATE NORMAL MUSCLE TONE

While hypotonicity is less common than spasticity in the head-injured patient, it also prevents effective movement patterns. Facilitation techniques can be used to increase muscle tone. Since these techniques are similar to those used to facilitate functional use, they are first described generally and are then related to functional use.

Postural changes, which cause a spontaneous response to gravity, may normalize low muscle tone. Placing the patient with low postural tone in various developmental positions against gravity often increases muscle tone.

Joint approximation, or compressing a joint with more force than the body part itself can produce, tends to cause cocontraction of muscles and facilitates normal muscle tone (Farber, 1982).

Tapping individual muscle bellies is facilitory and can be used to normalize muscle tone. It is used to increase muscle tone steadily by making use of proprioceptive and tactile stimulation.

Weight bearing is both inhibitory and facilitory. It can be used to inhibit abnormal postural reflexes or to facilitate postural adaptation and muscle cocontraction. Intermittent weight bearing of properly aligned joints encourages spontaneous adjustments of postural tone (Eggers, 1984). Weight bearing is also a functional prerequisite for upper extremity use and is often used before eliciting voluntary upper extremity movement.

FACILITATION OF NORMAL MOVEMENT

As muscle tone approaches a more balanced state, the patient often demonstrates increased active movement throughout the body, which enables participation in functional activity. However, due to remaining influences of tone, movement often occurs in abnormal patterns rather than in an isolated manner. The patient may require hands-on assistance from the therapist to produce selective quality movements without excessive effort. To facilitate this quality movement, the therapist places her hands on the patient at those points at which they can influence tone throughout the body. These points of therapist/patient contact are referred to by the Bobaths as key points of control (Bobath, 1978).

Proximal key points of control, such as the pelvic and shoulder girdles, are used most frequently. Tone throughout both upper and lower extremities can often be influenced through these points. In addition, their use affords the therapist greater control. Distal points of control can be used with the higher-functioning patient who can independently produce proper movement components yet requires guidance to influence the quality of movement. The point of control used with each patient is determined by the specific amount and location of assistance needed and by the movement the therapist hopes to achieve.

Facilitation should be done from the point at which the patient requires the most control. The therapist, rather than the patient, controls movement at the point from which facilitation is provided. If a patient has fair upper extremity control, but a decreased ability to rotate the trunk actively, the hips may be used as a point of facilitation to encourage rotation yet allow independent control of the upper extremities. When assistance is needed to place the upper extremities, or when the therapist must assume much of the control, the shoulder girdle is often used as a point of facilitation.

The aim of treatment is to withdraw manual contact gradually as the patient gains the ability to produce quality selective movement. The therapist can then use intermittent rather than constant manual contact or can change the point of control from proximal to distal.

Before the awakening stage, handling and facilitation techniques are done solely by the therapist, with the patient a passive participant. The patient must be at least in the awakening stage to become an active participant in therapy. Active participation, even though it may be minimal, allows the therapist to introduce therapeutic activity into treatment. Through activity, desired movements are more easily obtained with less manual facilitation because demands are placed at a more automatic and less cortical level.

The ability to participate in therapeutic activity is dependent on the cognitive, sensory-perceptual, and behavioral status of the patient, as well as the physical demands of the task. When working with the patient in lower developmental positions that provide more external support, such as supine or sidelying, cognitively complex tasks or those requiring more selective distal movement may be used. When the patient is in positions that require postural adaptation, tasks that require less cognitive effort may be indicated. Therapeutic activities can be introduced to facilitate normal movement in and through the following positions, which are based on the normal developmental sequence.

Rolling and Reaching

When rolling from supine to sidelying, a normal increase in postural flexor tone automatically occurs. However, unless the individual can break up the total pattern of flexion, normal rolling cannot occur. Normal rolling is initiated by lateral rotation and slight flexion of the head toward the side to which the patient is moving. The shoulder girdle then rotates in the same direction to position the upper extremity, followed by the pelvis and the lower extremities.

The patient often cannot adapt postural tone before initiating movement. Rolling is often initiated by exaggerated head, neck, trunk, and lower extremity flexion, or by using the lower extremities to push off of the mat. Patients with increased tone in the trunk show little dissociation of the upper trunk from the lower trunk and roll as a unit. To assist the patient in developing a more normal rolling pattern, the therapist can use hands-on facilitation from the shoulder and pelvis, as well as activities positioned to encourage the proper movement components.

When the patient is rolling to an involved side or does not spontaneously position the upper extremities, the shoulder should be brought forward into protraction and abduction before the initiation of movement. As tone around the scapula relaxes, the arm is placed into increased abduction until a 90° angle is possible. Should retraction occur as the patient rolls onto the shoulder, the therapist can manually maintain protraction by placing her hand on the medial border of the scapula. When extensor tone dominates the lower extremities, or when the individual lacks the ability to flex the legs actively, his knees and hips may be placed in flexion to break up the abnormal tone and encourage segmental rolling.

When facilitating rolling from the shoulder girdle, the therapist places her hands on the patient's scapula

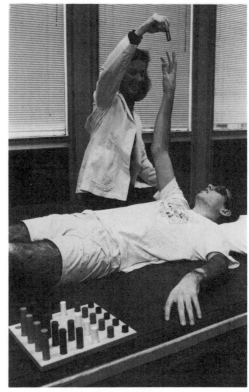

Figure 6–15 Use of an activity can facilitate active head and upper extremity movement during rolling.

from behind. Movement is then initiated by protraction and rotation of the leading shoulder girdle. The patient is simultaneously verbally cued to look in the direction toward which he is rolling to encourage lateral rotation and flexion of the head.

Asking the patient to reach for an object can be useful in facilitating the desired components of movement. An object held above the patient in supine encourages active extension through the leading upper extremity (Figure 6–15). Once the object is in the patient's hand, he is instructed to place it on the opposite side of the body. This requires active rolling to a sidelying position. Once in sidelying, the final placement of the object helps determine the amount of flexion or extension gained in the trunk. If the patient is asked to place the object at waist level, the head, neck, and trunk will remain in flexion (Figure 6–16). If the object is placed at 90° or more of shoulder flexion, extension of the head, neck, and upper trunk is encouraged (Figure 6–17).

Rolling facilitates trunk mobility while the patient is in a highly supported position. When combined with reaching, the patient can achieve greater separation of movement between the upper and lower body and may

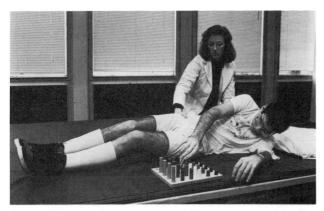

Figure 6–16 Stabilization at the hip encourages segmental rolling.

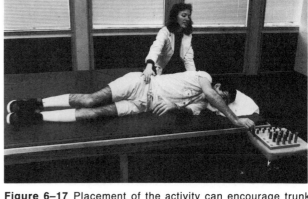

Figure 6–17 Placement of the activity can encourage trunk extension.

develop upper extremity control in and across midline in a gravity-reduced position. Functional implications include use of rolling to achieve greater bed mobility and in preparation for coming to a sitting position independently. Rolling is also used by the patient who dresses the lower extremities while in bed.

Prone

Due to increased tone in the abdominal muscles and lateral trunk flexors, many patients lack sufficient mobility to allow for trunk extension. The prone position is used to facilitate extension of the head, neck, and trunk. To assume prone, the patient rolls with the weight-bearing arm positioned in abduction over the head (Figure 6–18). A wedge is often used to support the patient in a weight-bearing position on the upper extremities, with the elbow flexed to 90° and aligned with the shoulder girdle (Figure 6–19). If the upper extremity cannot be positioned above the head, the patient can be gently lifted onto the wedge. Once in this position, he can accept joint approximation through the shoulder girdle. Symmetry and trunk alignment producing equal weight bearing should be maintained while completing all facilitation techniques (Figure 6–20). As the patient becomes able to shift weight from one side to the other, the scapula is mobilized on the thoracic wall, helping to achieve normalization of tone.

Joint approximation can also be applied to the head and neck in this position. After properly aligning the patient's head and neck, the therapist gently applies pressure to the rostral surface of the head in an attempt to normalize tone and facilitate head and neck extension (Figure 6–21). Tapping the trunk and neck mus-

culature can also be effective in facilitating active extension in the prone position.

The prone-on-elbows position is primarily used to work on head control and to achieve symmetric weight bearing and weight shifting in the upper extremities. The performance of functional activity is often difficult in this position due to the amount of body weight on the upper extremities. Because this can easily fatigue the musculature of the shoulder girdles, the patient should not be left in this position for prolonged periods.

Movement to Sitting

Assuming a sitting position from supine is an extension of rolling and requires further trunk rotation, hip flexion, lateral flexion of the head against gravity, and lateral flexion of the trunk on the leading side. Simultaneously, the weight bearing arm extends to assist in pushing up to a sitting position as the trunk, head, and neck actively extend to maintain the position against gravity.

Frequently, the patient does not have sufficient trunk control to alternate between active flexion and extension in coming to sitting. It is generally easier for him to sit up by moving toward the more involved side, allowing him to lead with the side over which he has greater control. However, moving in this way often makes it difficult to achieve enough elongation of the lateral trunk flexors and extension of the weight-bearing arm to enable him to sit with the trunk extended.

The therapist can facilitate movement to sitting from the shoulder girdle when behind the patient or by using both the shoulder and pelvis as points of control while standing in front of the patient. As with rolling, the arm on the weight-bearing side is placed in abduction with

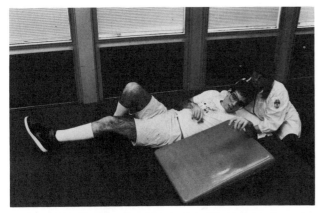

Figure 6-18 The upper extremity is prepositioned above the wedge in preparation for moving into the prone position.

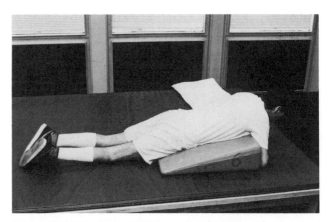

Figure 6-19 The prone position can facilitate extension throughout the neck, trunk, and lower extremities.

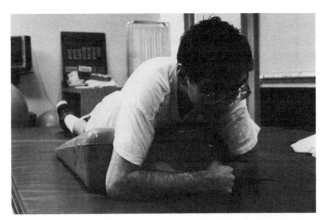

Figure 6-20 The upper extremities should be placed symmetrically for proper weight bearing, with the scapulae in protraction.

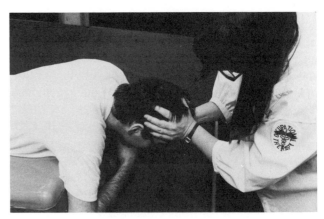

Figure 6-21 The hands are placed to preposition the patient's head in proper alignment before performing joint approximation.

the scapula in protraction. The movement is initiated with flexion and lateral rotation of the patient's head in combination with rotation of the upper body (Figure 6-22). The therapist can assist with protraction of the patient's leading upper extremity while simultaneously controlling the pelvis to encourage segmental rolling. Next, the lower extremities are flexed and brought down over the edge of the mat. Frequently, patients will attempt to hook the lower extremities under the mat and pull themselves to sitting from this point using only their legs and demonstrate increased extension throughout their trunk and lower extremities. The therapist can discourage this through proper placement of the feet as well as by facilitating the use of the trunk and upper extremity musculature to come to sitting.

The patient continues the movement to sitting by reaching across the body with the leading arm and placing it on the mat to push himself to a sitting position (Figure 6-23). As the patient sits up, the therapist can

facilitate weight bearing through the lower arm, first in flexion as the patient comes up onto the elbow, and then in extension as the patient sits up (Figure 6-24). Once the patient is sitting, neck and trunk extension are facilitated by the therapist through verbal cueing or by tapping the lumbar spine (Figure 6-25).

The short-sitting position facilitates postural stability in antigravity positions and encourages trunk extension. It also facilitates head and neck righting reactions and orientation of the body to the vertical midline. Functionally, the patient requires these skills to get out of bed and to attempt such tasks as upper extremity dressing in a sitting position.

When moving from supine to a side-sitting position, the components of normal movement are the same as those in coming to short sitting. The therapist usually facilitates from behind the patient, using the shoulder girdle as the point of control. Inhibitory techniques that normalize tone in the trunk and scapula in preparation

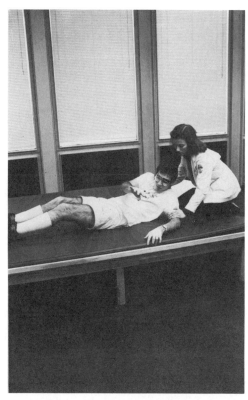

Figure 6–22 As the patient assumes sitting, the movement is initiated with the head and upper extremity while the weight-bearing side is stabilized.

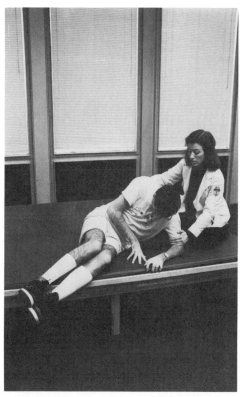

Figure 6–23 Once in a weight-bearing position, the patient is encouraged to use both upper extremities to assist in coming to sitting.

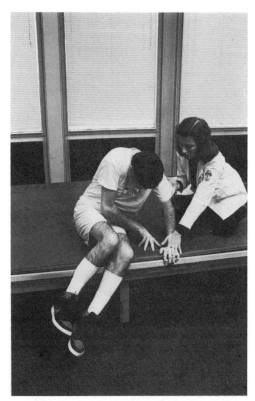

Figure 6–24 Extension of the weight-bearing arm can be facilitated by the therapist.

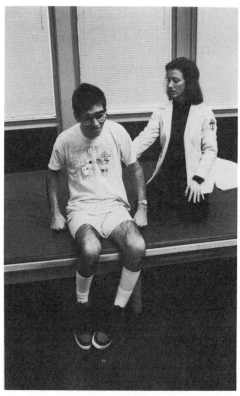

Figure 6–25 Once in sitting, extension of the lumbar spine often needs to be facilitated.

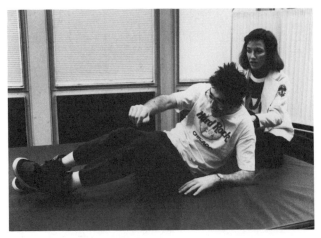

Figure 6–26 Facilitation may be needed to avoid excessive trunk flexion, as seen here.

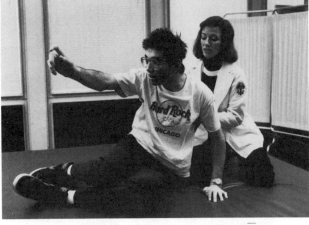

Figure 6–27 Once in side sitting, trunk flexion remains, and extension is facilitated.

for coming to short sitting also prepare the patient for side sitting.

Before moving to a side-sit position, the patient's arm is positioned in protraction, abduction, and internal rotation with the elbow flexed to 90°. The movement is initiated with lateral flexion and rotation of the upper trunk, followed by flexion of the lower extremities and segmental rotation of the trunk. Rather than rolling to a full sidelying position as one would when coming to short sitting, the patient is instructed or facilitated to reach with the leading arm diagonally across the body toward the feet (Figure 6–26). By doing this, the patient comes up onto the lower elbow in a weight-bearing position. As the patient further flexes the trunk, weight bearing in full extension occurs throughout the upper extremity with flexion of the lower extremities, followed by extension of the neck and trunk (Figure 6–27). Further rotation of the trunk throughout its vertical axis may be necessary for the individual to maintain a side-sitting position.

As the patient side sits, elongation of the lateral trunk flexors occurs on the weight-bearing side, with subsequent relaxation of the scapula. The side-sitting position may be painful or difficult for the patient with limited trunk mobility. Rather than achieving elongation, the weight-bearing side of the trunk may be shortened. By slowly guiding more weight over the weight-bearing hand in a gentle back-and-forth motion, elongation of the lateral trunk flexors can occur.

Once in this position, reaching activities that encourage movement toward the leading side and then across the body to the weight-bearing side can facilitate alternate shortening and lengthening of the lateral trunk

flexors (Figure 6–28). Further trunk rotation, as well as increased scapular mobility, may be achieved by having the patient reach for objects placed behind him with the non–weight-bearing arm (Figure 6–29).

Functionally, side sitting is a transitional position necessary to assume the upright position from the floor. It emphasizes the coordination of lateral trunk flexion and extension necessary for automatic postural responses that are then, in turn, necessary for effective balance and equilibrium reactions.

Function in Sitting

Sitting is one of the primary functional positions that we use throughout our lives. It enables us to observe the environment, eat, communicate, and participate in a variety of functional activities. For patients with increased tone, the force of gravity often places additional stress on postural muscles and increases tone, making it difficult to maintain the position or move the extremities. For patients with low tone, the gravitational demands of sitting upright can have a facilitory effect on muscle tone.

Maintaining the sitting position requires a bias toward extensor tone in the head, neck, and trunk. The patient's pelvis should be between a neutral and an anterior tilt with his hips and knees flexed to 90° and the feet supported. Initially, the hands may be fixed at the side to provide additional support.

To facilitate postural tone, tapping and joint approximation techniques described earlier can be used when the patient is properly aligned. Removing the external support of the therapist's hands momentarily to allow

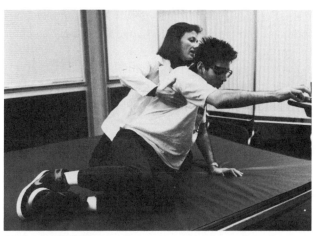

Figure 6–28 Placement of activity is used to encourage trunk extension.

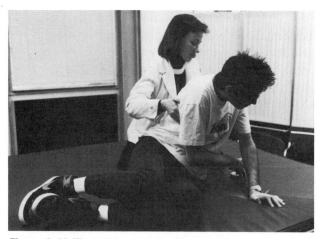

Figure 6–29 The activity can also be placed to encourage trunk flexion and scapula mobility.

for spontaneous postural responses will often increase tone in hypotonic muscles. The therapist facilitates this by placing herself in front of or behind the patient while providing trunk support with her hands. Support can be removed from one side first, and the response noted (Figure 6–30). Based on the level of response, support can be removed from the other side. Gentle tapping of the patient from one hand to the other 3 to 4 inches off

center may also produce a more normalized postural tone.

In sitting, patients with increased tone often exhibit flexion of the spine, due to the effects of gravity, and asymmetric weight bearing in the hips, making upper extremity function difficult (Figure 6–31). To be functional in sitting requires the ability to actively assume and maintain trunk extension and an anterior pelvic tilt.

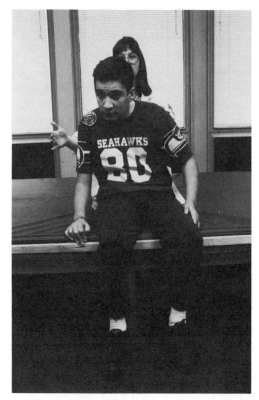

Figure 6–30 When support is removed, extension in head, neck, and upper trunk emerges.

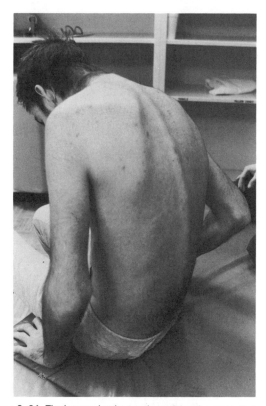

Figure 6–31 Flexion predominates throughout the patient's trunk.

This combination of movements is a postural set in preparation for participating in activity or standing and is difficult to maintain for extended periods even in individuals with normal muscle tone. To encourage this, the therapist places her hands on the iliac crests of the patient's pelvis and passively brings him into an anterior tilt. As the patient becomes able to maintain the position, manual contact is released.

The therapist can also facilitate trunk extension and anterior pelvic tilt when positioned in front of the patient by placing a rolled sheet around the patient's lumbar area. By pulling the sheet toward her, the therapist cues the patient to move into an anterior tilt and extend the spine. Tactile cues such as lightly tapping the small of the back may serve the same purpose.

The ability to move into and out of an anterior tilt assists in the development of static sitting balance. Many patients can maintain this balance for varying periods yet are unable to function in sitting due to poor righting and equilibrium reactions. To be functional in sitting, the patient must develop the ability to respond to changes in the center of gravity by transferring weight forward, backward, sideways, and diagonally and then reorienting the body toward midline. To assist the patient in developing this ability, the therapist facilitates movements that will change the patient's center of gravity.

It is often helpful to begin with the upper extremities supported on a bedside table (Figure 6–32). This increases the upper extremity support and reduces the patient's fear of falling while simultaneously encouraging upper extremity weight bearing. Using the shoulder as a point of control, the therapist guides the patient in shifting his weight forward and backward in small increments by moving the table first toward and then away from the patient. Facilitation of side-to-side weight shift can be done from the shoulder or pelvis by slowly guiding the patient in one direction and then the other. Proper weight shift in both directions encourages alternating lateral trunk elongation of the weight-bearing side with shortening of the opposite side.

As the patient develops the ability to shift his weight and is less fearful of falling, reaching activities can be incorporated to encourage the desired movement. The therapist can continue to use the table to maintain support of one upper extremity or may not. When working in sitting, reaching activities are initiated unilaterally with the least involved extremity. When activities are placed forward and upward, reaching encourages active weight shifting over the lower extremities and anterior pelvic tilting with extension of the trunk, head, and neck (Figure 6–33). Reaching to the side encourages lateral elongation of the trunk and weight shifting to that side (Figure 6–34). Bilateral reaching activities can also be used as the patient develops greater balance and no longer requires one upper extremity for support (Figure 6–35). Bilateral reaching facilitates many of the same movements as unilateral reaching, but does so symmetrically and uses the unaffected upper extremity to assist the affected one.

As the patient develops the ability to respond to changes in the center of gravity forward, backward, and sideways, the therapist facilitates movement in diagonal directions, which encourages greater trunk rotation. Reaching across midline encourages weight shifting to that side and trunk rotation (Figure 6–36). As rotational ability is developed around the body axis, the patient will be able to shift his weight and move from position to position more easily.

Activities are gradually placed farther away from midline to encourage reaching in all planes of movement. This may involve reaching to the floor for an object that is then placed over the head or moving objects from the far right to the far left.

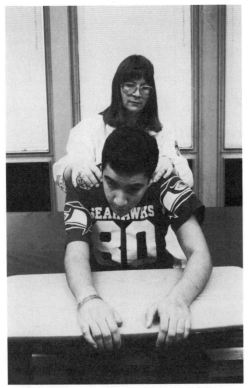

Figure 6-32 Facilitation of active movement in the trunk may be made less threatening when the upper extremities are supported.

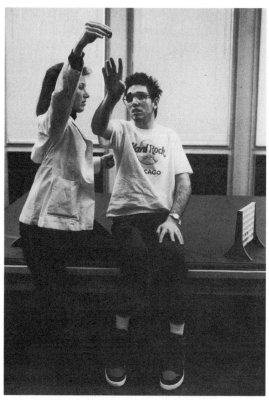

Figure 6–33 Forward reach can facilitate extension of the head, neck, and trunk.

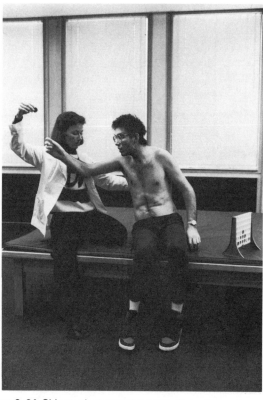

Figure 6–34 Side reach encourages trunk elongation on the weight-bearing side.

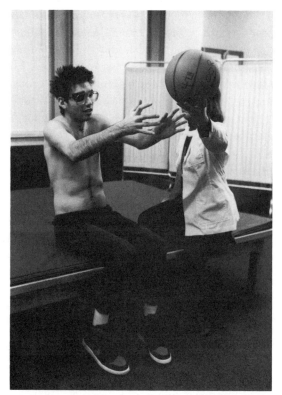

Figure 6–35 Bilateral reaching encourages symmetric weight bearing and extension through the trunk and upper extremities.

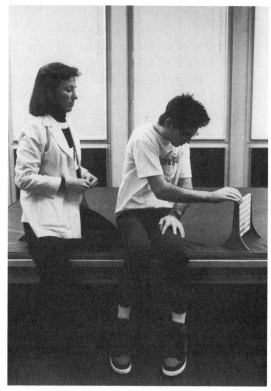

Figure 6–36 Initially, the object is placed close enough to achieve rotation without displacement of center of gravity.

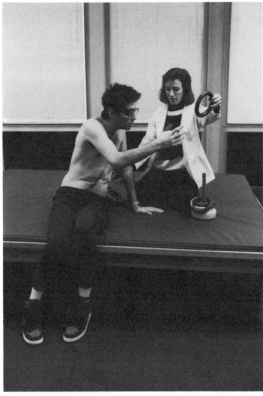

Figure 6–37 Displacement of the patient's center of gravity will produce greater trunk rotation.

Upper extremity weight bearing can be easily incorporated into dynamic sitting activities. When bearing weight on the flexed or extended upper extremity positioned at the patient's side, lateral elongation of that side is encouraged (Figure 6–37). Once in the weight-bearing position, movement of the body over a stable arm enables the center of gravity to be displaced farther from midline, provides proprioceptive input to the extremity, and encourages active use of the arm in maintaining or changing positions.

As dynamic sitting balance improves, the individual can automatically respond to changes in his center of gravity and no longer requires the use of upper extremities for support. This enables patients to perform a variety of functional activities in sitting, such as dressing, transfers, table-top and gross motor games, and the many other tasks performed in sitting throughout the day.

Movement to Standing

Developmentally, the ability to stand upright is not achieved by progressing from sitting. It is achieved through acquiring controlled movement in the transitional positions, such as quadruped and kneeling. The movement sequence most commonly used with patients to assume the upright positions from the floor is a progression through side sitting, quadruped, kneeling, half kneeling, and standing.

Quadruped

In side sitting, the hips and lower extremities are flexed and the trunk is extended and rotated toward the weight-bearing side. To help the patient assume a quadruped position, the shoulders are used as a point of control. Weight is taken off the upper extremities, and the trunk is counter-rotated away from the weight-bearing side (Figure 6–38). Forward weight shift is encouraged with the head and arms extended to assume the all-fours position (Figure 6–39). If control of the upper extremities is poor, the therapist can move her hands onto the humerus to guide placement of the arms. Once in the quadruped position, the arms should be in external rotation, with the elbows, wrists, and fingers fully extended. The hips and shoulders should both be in 90° flexion with the scapula protracted. The lumbar spine should be extended, and this can be facilitated by tapping upward on the abdomen. When the patient is in this position, the therapist should grade the amount of weight placed on involved upper extremities. Placing too much weight on the arms only serves to increase tone rather than facilitate a normalization of tone.

Activities can be used in this position to encourage forward and backward weight shifting and to improve proximal stability at the shoulders and hips. Activities placed to the patient's side encourages lateral weight shift, while reaching overhead facilitates extension of the head, neck, trunk, and upper extremity.

The ambulatory patient can be placed on a tilt board or Swiss ball in the quadruped position to facilitate more refined balance and equilibrium reactions (Figures 6–40 and 6–41). When the patient reaches for an object on the left side, the therapist should observe lateral flexion of the head and the trunk toward the right side.

The quadruped position is used primarily to develop proximal control and stability. Functionally, the position is used as a transitional position in standing up from the floor or in household activities, such as cleaning the floor.

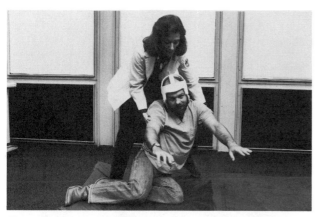

Figure 6–38 In moving from side sit to quadruped, the patient's weight is shifted forward over his knees.

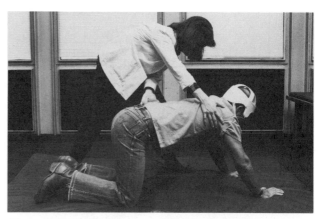

Figure 6–39 The upper extremities are guided so the patient may assume an effective weight-bearing position on all fours.

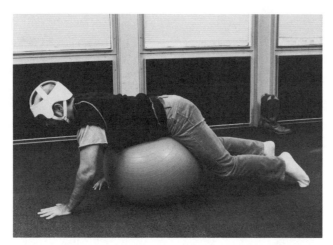

Figure 6–40 The patient must demonstrate a greater change in posture to accommodate to the moving surface beneath him.

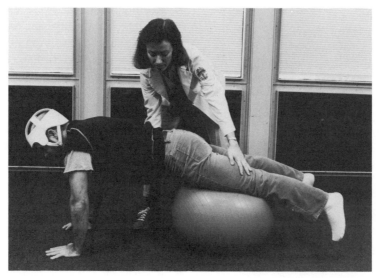

Figure 6–41 Postural challenge is greater as the ball is moved distally.

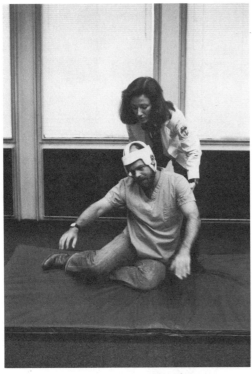

Figure 6–42 The patient's arms are rotated over his knees in preparation for weight shift forward.

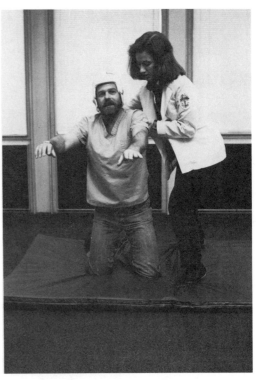

Figure 6–43 Weight is shifted forward to assume a kneeling position. Hips should be in an extended position.

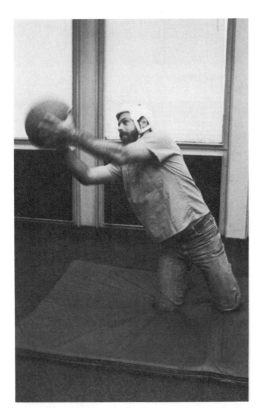

Figure 6–44 A gross motor activity in kneeling encourages spontaneous weight shift and equilibrium responses.

Kneeling

To assume the kneeling position from quadruped, one normally shifts his weight backward onto the lower extremities while extending the hips and trunk. Movement to kneeling from a side-sitting position can be facilitated using the pelvis or shoulder as a point of control. The weight is shifted off the upper extremities by rotating the trunk toward the leading side. The body is then flexed at the hips and the weight shifted forward to bring the center of gravity over the knees (Figure 6–42). The trunk is then counter-rotated while the hips and lower back extend simultaneously (Figure 6–43).

In kneeling, gross motor games and reaching activities facilitate automatic weight shift from side to side as well as trunk rotation (Figure 6–44). Kneeling on a floor mat in front of a bench provides the patient with an opportunity to work on trunk stability and control while moving in and out of upper extremity weight-bearing positions.

Equilibrium reactions can be facilitated by requiring the patient to reach away from midline to extreme ranges. When reaching to the right, lateral flexion of the head and trunk occur to the left, with extension of the left upper and lower extremities. Performing these

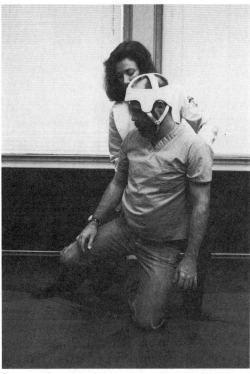

Figure 6–45 Weight shift must precede rotation of the hip to facilitate foot placement.

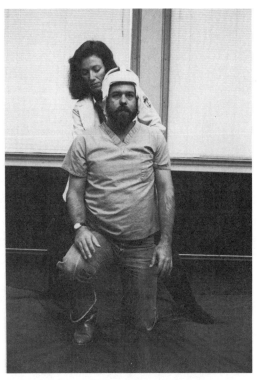

Figure 6–46 Once the foot is placed, weight is taken equally over both lower extremities.

activities on a tilt board is more challenging and will produce the same responses, but the patient will not have to reach so far to displace the center of gravity.

Functionally, for the adult, kneeling is a transitional position and is not used for static activity. Movement into kneeling from side sitting or out of kneeling to side sitting or half kneeling should be encouraged and practiced by the patient who requires development of effective weight shifting and rotation within these positions.

Half Kneeling

To assume half kneeling from a kneeling position, the patient shifts weight laterally with simultaneous rotation of the trunk toward the weight-bearing side. The therapist facilitates this from the shoulder girdle, pelvis, or a combination of the two. The weight must be shifted far enough to the side to allow the opposite leg to be brought up actively or to elicit an equilibrium response in which the movement is made automatically (Figure 6–45). Often, patients lack the ability to bring their lower extremity forward and up to assume half kneeling. The therapist can assist by moving the patient's foot forward with her own or by using her hand to place the lower extremity in the proper position for half kneeling. Once the leg is brought into the proper

position, either independently or with the assistance of the therapist, the trunk is counter-rotated to a neutral position (Figure 6–46).

Reaching activities in half kneeling can promote forward and backward weight shift on the lower extremities (Figures 6–47 to 6–49). This activity requires more than 90° of hip flexion and may be difficult for the patient with tight hip flexors. Refined balance and equilibrium reactions are encouraged by placing the patient's foot on a basketball and requiring him to move the ball from one side to the other, forward and backward (Figure 6–50). As with kneeling, half kneeling is a transitional position and should be used to encourage weight shift and trunk rotation as well as to improve balance and equilibrium reactions, rather than static positions.

To assume standing from a half-kneeling position, the therapist uses the scapula or hands as points of control. The patient's weight must be brought forward over the leading foot to enable him to stand by extending the lower extremity. When facilitating from the hands, patients who have not shifted their weight far enough forward or who lack sufficient strength in their lower extremities to push to standing may attempt to pull against the therapist to assist them in getting up. To

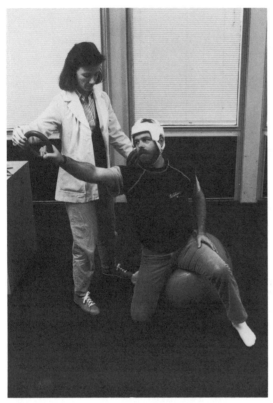

Figure 6–47 Treatment can be varied by using a ball.

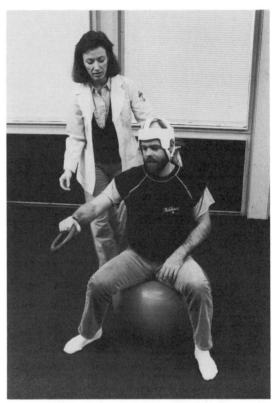

Figure 6–48 Greater trunk control is required during transition from one position to another.

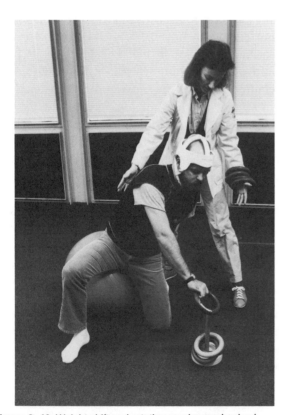

Figure 6–49 Weight shift and rotation can be emphasized.

avoid this, the therapist places her hands on top of the patient's hands rather than under them, allowing her enough control to guide the weight forward without giving the patient a surface to pull against (Figure 6–51).

Function in Standing

One's ability to function in standing depends on normal postural tone throughout the body, which enables selective movement, and balance and equilibrium reactions sufficient to free the upper extremities for use in functional tasks. When first working in standing, the patient may require the upper extremities to be fixed distally on a table or other surface for support. Because of this, reaching activities should first encourage the functional use of one upper extremity.

Patients may also be hesitant to bear weight equally on both lower extremities, placing the majority of their weight on the unaffected side. Activities can be placed on different surface heights to facilitate lateral weight shift in the standing position as well as flexion, extension, and rotation of the trunk (Figures 6–52 and 6–53). Once balance improves, bilateral reaching activities are encouraged. Gross motor games of catch

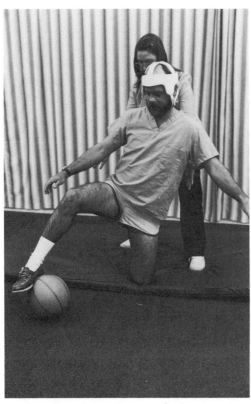

Figure 6–50 Greater challenges are provided as the patient progresses.

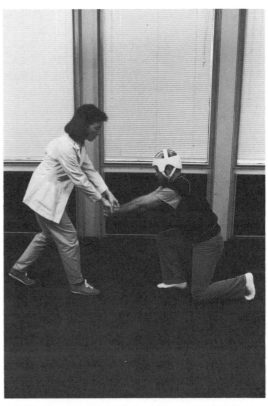

Figure 6–51 The patient's weight is guided forward as he extends to assume standing.

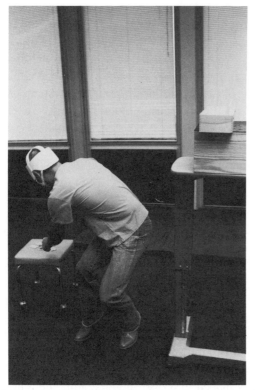

Figure 6–52 Weight shift and rotation allow for function in standing.

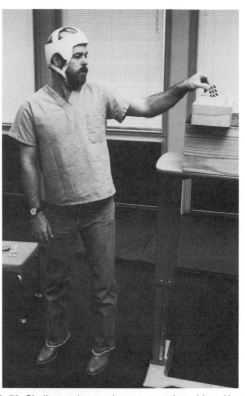

Figure 6–53 Challenges in arm placement can be achieved by placement of the activity.

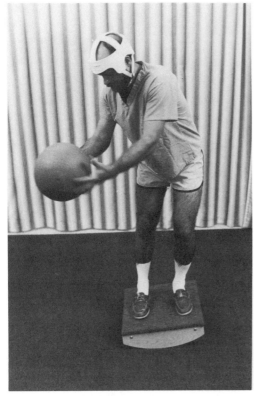

Figure 6–54 For the patient to gain full benefit from the use of moving surfaces, activities should produce equilibrium responses.

or bouncing a ball are useful in facilitating automatic weight shift as the therapist throws the ball to the patient in ranges that gradually work away from midline. Trunk rotation can be encouraged by the patient reaching across midline with one upper extremity or by reaching for objects at varying heights. Facilitation of balance and equilibrium reactions in standing can be achieved by requiring the patient to reach in ranges far enough from midline to displace the center of gravity. Moving surfaces can also be used, such as a small tilt board (Figure 6–54). These elicit the same response from the patient as reaching on a stable surface yet do not require movement in such extreme ranges.

The development of the components of weight shift and rotation in standing are prerequisites to the safe performance of functional activity in this position.

UPPER EXTREMITY FACILITATION

Supine

Although treatment of involved upper extremities is addressed when working in and through the develop-mental positions, patients frequently require treatment specifically focused on improving control, coordination, and the functional use of upper extremity musculature. When this is indicated, it is often beneficial for the patient to begin working in the supine position for several reasons:

- By placing the body in a supported position, abnormal postural tone may be decreased, which enables more selective use of the upper extremities.
- The therapist can evaluate tone and quality of movement in a position in which the resistance of gravity is reduced.
- In supine, upper extremity tone is biased toward extension due to the effects of the tonic labyrinthine supine reflex, which is often helpful in inhibiting the flexor pattern commonly seen in the upper extremity after HI.

Before facilitation of upper extremity movement, inhibition of abnormal tone in the trunk should be performed to enable the scapula to move more freely on the thoracic wall. Through the various techniques of range of motion (ROM) and scapular mobilization, inhibition of abnormal tone in and around the shoulder girdle can be achieved.

Facilitation of the upper extremity begins proximally, with the goal being to acquire stability at the shoulder girdle. This enables the patient to place the arm in various positions in space and is a prerequisite to both distal control and functional use. To facilitate stability, the therapist positions the patient's arms in 90° of shoulder flexion or perpendicular to the body. The arm should be in a position of external rotation, elbow extension, forearm supination, and wrist and finger extension with the thumb abducted and extended (Figure 6–55).

The patient is asked to hold the arm in this position while the therapist gradually withdraws manual contact. The therapist keeps her hands close by the patient for control as needed. If it is difficult for the patient to maintain this position, facilitation by joint compression can be used. By stimulating the joint receptors, a balanced contraction of agonist and antagonistic actions around a joint is elicited, thereby improving the ability to maintain the position. To apply compression, the joint is placed in proper alignment and held in a reflex inhibiting position. Gentle but firm intermittent pres-

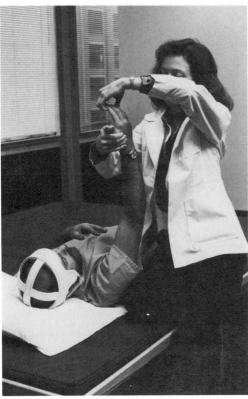

Figure 6–55 Inhibition techniques may be necessary before active control of the extremity.

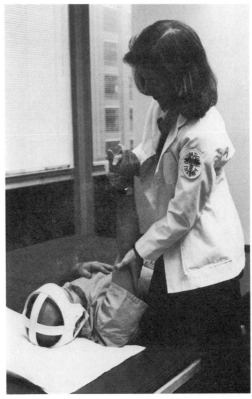

Figure 6–56 The shoulder girdle should be in proper alignment before performing joint approximation.

sure is exerted downward from the therapist's palm for 10 to 15 seconds (Figure 6–56). As the therapist releases control, the patient is asked to hold the position. Tapping the muscle belly of the biceps and triceps may increase their tone and assist in stability at the elbow. The tapping is done in an alternate sweeping motion.

As the patient becomes able to hold the arm proximally, the therapist may be able to release all manual contact or to provide only light distal contact to maintain the patient's digits in a relaxed position. The place and hold technique is attempted throughout all ranges of flexion, extension, abduction, and adduction.

Once the patient can actively hold a position, he is required to superimpose movement while maintaining shoulder stability. Starting with the arm placed perpendicular to the body, the patient is instructed to move in increments of 10° to 20° in one direction, hold the position, and reverse the movement. The therapist may place her hands at the end ranges of the desired movement, giving the patient a visual target as well as keeping the hands close by for support as needed.

Initially, movement is often quick and uncontrolled and responds to the force of gravity. Verbal cueing is used to instruct the patient to move as slowly as possible. As with the place and hold technique, the patient is required to move back and forth through small range increments, working his way through the entire range available at the shoulder girdle (Figure 6–57). Movements that are the components of the flexor synergy, such as flexion and adduction of the humerus, may be easier to perform initially in isolation than movements that deviate from the synergy pattern. Intermittent tactile and verbal cueing and distal facilitation are helpful in improving quality and control of movement.

As proximal control is achieved, the patient attempts to refine more distal movement. The patient places and holds the arm at the shoulder while performing activities that require active control of the elbow, forearm, wrist, and fingers. Beginning with improving control at the elbow, commands such as ''touch your mouth'' and ''reach toward the ceiling'' are often more successful and less cortically demanding than commands of ''bend or straighten your elbow.'' If hand function is present, activities such as placing light-weight objects on the mat over the opposite shoulder can be used to achieve the desired motion (Figures 6–58 and 6–59).

With the arm held at the shoulder, the patient is asked to bend the elbow to pick up an object and then extend the arm fully to hand the object to the therapist. As control develops, additional movements deviating from synergy are required, such as elbow flexion with supination and wrist and finger extension. As complexity of movement increases through the addition of various components, the therapist will often observe an increase in patterned movement that will initially require additional hands-on assistance or verbal cueing to correct. When working on distal control, slight assistance such as placement of the therapist's hand on the lateral humerus may assist in decreasing the effort the patient must exert.

Sitting and Standing

The majority of functional tasks are performed in sitting and standing positions. While the use of supine

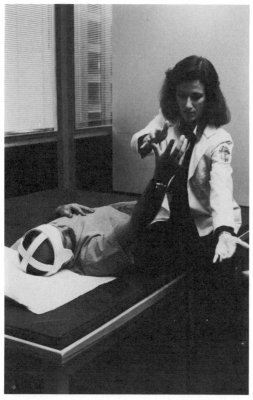

Figure 6–57 Extension and abduction are often more difficult to achieve than movement within a synergy pattern.

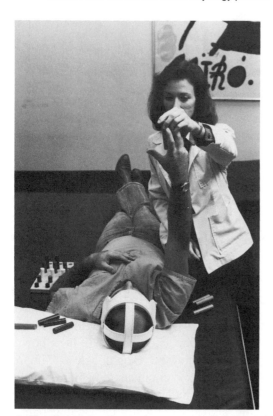

Figure 6–58 Movement patterns are put at a more automatic level through the use of activity.

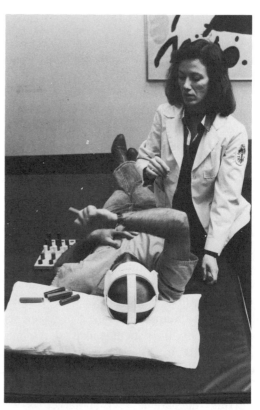

Figure 6–59 Various movement components can be added to increase the challenge.

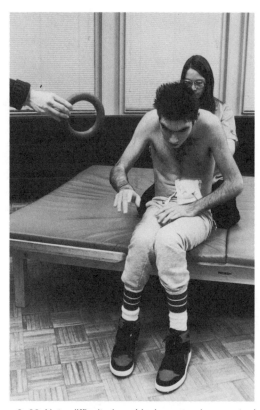

Figure 6–60 Note difficulty in achieving arm placement when the trunk is flexed and unsupported.

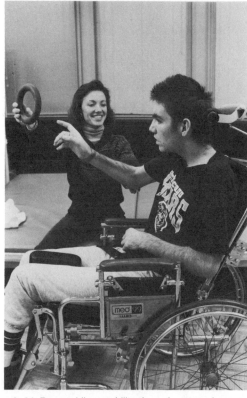

Figure 6–61 By providing stability through external support, trunk extension increases and greater arm placement is achieved.

is valuable in improving control, it is essential to progress the patient to development of control in antigravity positions and incorporate the use of the affected extremity in functional tasks.

When working with the patient in sitting, it is important that the body be positioned with lower extremity support sufficient to allow symmetric weight bearing at the hips. This encourages normal postural tone and allows for easier use of the extremities. When abnormal tone in the trunk is moderate to severe, it is often difficult to achieve sufficient trunk extension in sitting to enable use of the upper extremities (Figure 6–60). It is helpful to have two therapists position the trunk and facilitate upper extremity use simultaneously. Other options include working with the patient in a wheelchair with a solid back and seat to facilitate necessary trunk extension while freeing the therapist's hands for facilitation of upper extremity function (Figure 6–61).

Quite often with head-injured patients, the therapist will observe that movement that is isolated and controlled in supine may again appear patterned in sitting or standing. This is due to the increased resistance of

gravity and the change in demands of postural tone. When attempting to increase control in these positions, it is often beneficial for the therapist to sit next to the patient's affected side to enable her to provide hands-on assistance both proximally and distally.

The place and hold technique is used to gain stability in the shoulder girdle. The patient's arm is positioned in varying degrees of shoulder flexion and abduction (Figure 6–62). It is often most successful to place the arm in flexion and attempt to gain control of the arm downward. This allows gravity to assist the movement and may produce a less patterned response. As the therapist gradually releases manual contact, the patient is required to hold the position.

As the patient becomes able to hold a position, he is often able to begin actively moving into that position (Figure 6–63). An activity such as hitting a balloon encourages active movement against gravity while not increasing distal demands. When distal control is available, a patient may be asked to grab a ring or cone with the arm in a reflex inhibiting position and to place it at the end of the range desired. As proximal control

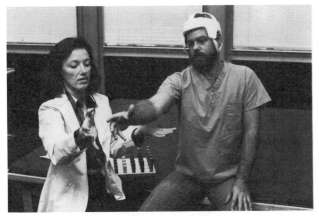

Figure 6–62 The postural demands of sitting often affect the quality of upper extremity function.

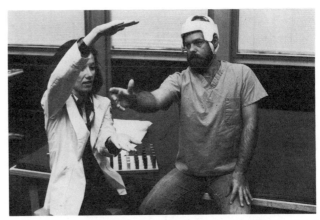

Figure 6–63 Quality of movement can be maintained when assisted by gravity.

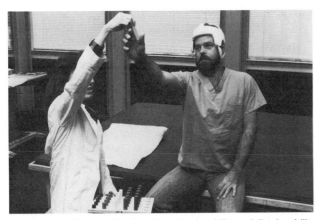

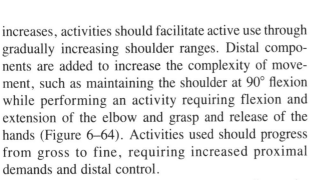

Figure 6–64 The coordination of proximal stability and distal mobility gives way to function.

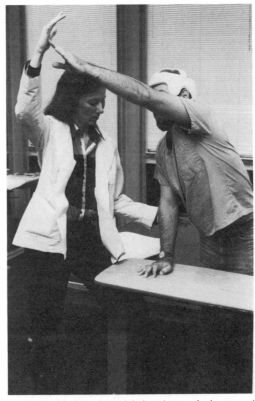

Figure 6–65 Upper extremity weight bearing can be incorporated into all developmental positions.

increases, activities should facilitate active use through gradually increasing shoulder ranges. Distal components are added to increase the complexity of movement, such as maintaining the shoulder at 90° flexion while performing an activity requiring flexion and extension of the elbow and grasp and release of the hands (Figure 6–64). Activities used should progress from gross to fine, requiring increased proximal demands and distal control.

Weight bearing through the upper extremity can be accomplished in sitting or standing by placing the arm on a mat or table in flexion or extension and using an activity to facilitate a weight shift onto and off of the extremity (Figure 6–65). If the arm is hypotonic, the therapist should be sure that all joints are aligned and may need to provide additional support at the shoulder or elbow.

Often, patients will compensate for poor proximal control by extending the upper trunk to achieve greater arm placement. The therapist should discourage this by placing the activity to require a slight forward flexion when reaching or by blocking trunk extension from behind the patient.

Hand Function

Increased flexor tone in the wrist and fingers is the most commonly seen pattern in the hand after HI. Early after injury, the patient frequently demonstrates a strong grasp reflex, causing flexion and adduction of the fingers when cutaneous stimulation is presented to the palmar surface. The grasp reflex can be inhibited by providing firm and maintained tactile input to the palm through weight bearing or work on grasp and release with solid objects such as cones or large pegs. As this reflex is integrated, patients commonly demonstrate gross active hook grasp, with little control of the amount of force and little active finger extension.

When attempting to facilitate active control of the hand, it is often beneficial to incorporate grasp and release activities with reaching, such as in a gross motor tossing game or placement of objects from one level to another. This may serve to encourage hand function on an automatic and less cortically demanding level. Other patients cannot combine hand function with arm placement without causing excessive patterned movement throughout the extremity. For these patients, it is beneficial to work on hand function alone, with the elbow supported, thereby decreasing the demands of proximal control. As distal function becomes more automatic, it can be incorporated into total arm movement.

When working on grasp activities, the patient actively holds the object and places the arm. Rather than instructing the patient to open his hand, the therapist can stimulate active release by a slight flexion of the patient's wrist (Figure 6–66). Active finger extension usually emerges in small ranges or in a mass reflex pattern. Use of varying-sized objects in the hand will determine the amount of finger flexion and extension required and will assist the patient in learning to vary the force of the grasp. Large objects, such as cones or balls, require small amounts of flexion and extension to control, while smaller objects, such as blocks or pegs, require greater degrees of finger control.

The first movement seen in the thumb is often flexion. This allows for a lateral prehension pattern. This prehension can be incorporated into activities such as writing, playing table-top games such as cards, or manipulation of small (1-inch) objects (Figure 6–67). As thumb control develops, the patient is required to combine finger and thumb flexion to produce a cylindrical or spherical grasp. This pattern can be incorporated into functional activities, such as drinking from a cup or using the hand to stabilize self-care items that require bilateral control, such as removing the tops from bottles. Isolated finger flexion and extension and palmar prehension patterns are encouraged through use of table-top activities that require manipulation of vary-

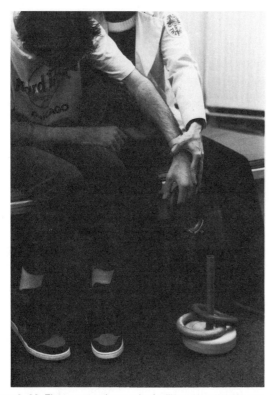

Figure 6–66 Finger extension can be facilitated by slight flexion of the wrist.

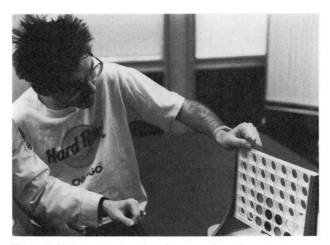

Figure 6–67 Lateral prehension often precedes palmar pinch.

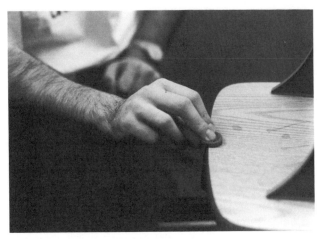

Figure 6–68 Palmar prehension can be encouraged by varying the placement of the checker.

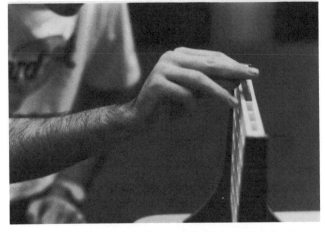

Figure 6–69 Palmar prehension can often be more functional than lateral prehension.

ing-sized objects (Figures 6–68 and 6–69). Items such as blocks, checkers, or pegs can be used to achieve greater manipulation skills. These patterns are then encouraged in self-care activities such as buttoning, shoelace tying, or utensil feeding.

MANAGEMENT OF CEREBELLAR ATAXIA

Ataxia in the head-injured patient presents as uncoordinated or uncontrolled motor patterns when attempts at movement and function are made. Ataxia affects postural stability and balance reactions as well as upper extremity function. Intention tremors and over- or underreaching contribute to the patient's difficulty with fine motor control. The trunk and proximal joints can be affected, as well as distal joints. Stabilization of proximal joints may improve distal function when distal joints are not involved.

We have observed several patients who initially demonstrate severe spasticity with emerging ataxia as their muscle tone was reduced. The spasticity may have masked the ataxia by producing abnormally high cocontraction of the musculature. When the muscle tone was reduced, so was the patient's ability to cocontract proximal joint muscles adequately for stability.

Ataxia can be frustrating for both the patient and therapist because it affects the patient's performance of most activities of daily living (ADL). Possible interventions are limited and are tailored to each patient. Some techniques may be successful initially but may lose their effectiveness over time.

Sensorimotor Approaches

The NDT approach emphasizes gaining control of movement patterns. This is achieved by improving the patient's postural tone, increasing proximal stabilization, and allowing the patient to experience controlled, purposeful movement sequences. Through handling techniques, the therapist attempts to:

- regulate abnormal tone, either decreasing or increasing, based on postural assessment
- increase postural control
- increase cocontraction of proximal musculature
- use static handling techniques, including weight bearing
- decrease or control movement in all ranges, but especially the mid-ranges

As with the handling techniques previously described, the therapist uses proximal key points to provide stability and gradually reduces assistance as the patient gains control.

The Proprioceptive Neuromuscular Facilitation (PNF) approach to the treatment of ataxia involves the use of specific manual techniques. The patient with severe ataxia may be unable to perform the isometric contractions necessary for rhythmic stabilization. In these cases, the therapist should use the slow reversal hold technique in smaller and smaller increments until the patient can hold the contraction (Voss, Ionta, & Myers, 1985).

Compensatory Techniques

Compensation techniques are used to improve the patient's functional performance when sensorimotor techniques do not prove effective or in conjunction with them. Specific suggestions for improving self-care performance are noted in Unit 9.

Weights (2 to 3 pounds) are sometimes placed proximally on the patient to provide extra proprioceptive input into the joints. This is thought to stimulate cocontraction and stability at the proximal joints. Weights are sometimes placed distally when ataxia affects those joints. With some patients, the effectiveness of weights seems to diminish. It is as if the CNS accommodates to the increased proprioceptive input.

External support often provides the necessary stability needed for function when ataxia affects the trunk. A head support may be useful as a distal point of contact to control ataxic movements even though it is not needed to maintain vertical head control. To improve distal upper extremity control, it is often useful to support the elbows on a stable surface. This proximal stability often allows for a functional hand-to-mouth pattern and improved control at the table-top level.

Severity of Ataxia

The severity of the patient's ataxia will ultimately affect the amount of control possible and the treatment positions used. The therapist working on functional activities will often choose positions that provide stability for the patient. When ataxia is severe, the choice may be for the patient to perform self-care activities from a wheelchair or semireclined in bed. When facilitating postural control, positions incorporating heavy weight bearing may be effective, such as four-point kneeling. In most cases of severe ataxia, positions that place the patient at high levels of challenge, such as the half kneel, are avoided. This is because the positions are unstable and further limit the patient's ability to participate in functional tasks. If ataxia is mild, these precautions may not be necessary. Depending on the patient's needs and goals, all developmental positions may be appropriate.

PRECAUTIONS

The head-injured patient often presents a complex medical picture, and the therapist must be aware of the precautions associated with various lifesaving medical interventions as well as common complications associated with HI. Common issues that may affect the therapist's handling of the patient are listed below.

- *Feeding tubes (nasogastric tubes, G-tubes, and J-tubes):*
  - Patients may pull and tug at tubes as they become more alert.
  - The therapist should be aware of tube placement during inhibition and facilitation techniques.
  - While the patient is ingesting tube feedings, he should be kept at a 30° angle to decrease the risk of regurgitation and/or aspiration.
  - Do not invert the patient within 1 hour of feeding.
  - Position tubes to avoid irritation if working with the patient in prone.
- *Tracheostomy:*
  - The airway must remain clear.
  - Care needs to be taken when working on head control if the patient tends to flex his head forward or is in prone.
  - The discharge from a tracheostomy should be disposed of properly.
  - If the patient is on oxygen or mist, be sure to keep tubing open and untwisted.
- *Infections requiring isolation:*
  - Wear appropriate protective devices (gloves, gowns, masks) as handling techniques necessitate proximity to the patient.
  - Gloves may decrease the therapist's sensation and affect handling, splinting, or casting, but must be worn according to isolation procedure.
  - Dispose of any discharge properly.
  - Disinfect any equipment and treatment areas that patients contact.
  - Use a sheet to protect the mat area and dispose of it according to isolation procedure.
- *Seizures:*
  - Avoid rapid rotary movements that may trigger a seizure.
  - Protect the patient if a seizure develops; follow the facility's policy and procedure.

- *Shunts:*
  - Avoid inversion.
  - Alert the physician to decreases in levels of arousal or drowsiness, and changes and functional performance that may indicate malfunction of shunt.
- *Unresolved fractures:* Follow or obtain the physician's recommendations for weight bearing and passive movement.
- *Pressure sores:*
  - Avoid pressure on area during handling techniques.

- Adhere to sitting tolerance restrictions.
- *Heterotopic ossification:*
  - Do not force joint motion.
  - Limit weight bearing if pain or swelling is present or if joint alignment is poor.
- *Osteoporosis:* Avoid aggressive ROM mobilization, or stressful weight bearing.
- *Autonomic nervous system responses to handling techniques:* Monitor heart rate, respiration, and blood pressure, especially when using inversion or when beginning facilitation techniques after prolonged bedrest.

PROBLEM AREA: MOTOR SKILLS

Subcategory: Range of Motion

Long-term goals and indicators	Short-term goals	Treatment ideas
1. Patient will maintain current (*active, passive*) ROM for prevention of further deformity in the following joints: _____. • severe limitations of motion • severe tone • long-standing contracture • heterotopic bone • pain that limits tolerance for Active/ Passive Range of Motion (A/ PROM) activities.	1. • Patient will tolerate (*orthosis, cast, ROM, tone management techniques*) _____ (*hours, minutes*) each day for maintenance of (*A/PROM*) in the following joints: _____. • Patient/caregiver will perform (*A/ PROM*) (*independently, with cues, with written instructions*). • Patient/caregiver will (*apply cast, orthosis*) correctly and follow recommended wearing schedule (*independently, with cues, with written instructions*).	1. • When casting, consult with the physician before casting to determine cause of limitations, i.e., ectopic bone, unresolved fracture. • Use orthotics. • Use positioning (bed and wheelchair). • Perform daily A/PROM and instruct caregiver as able. • Use of activity as possible to encourage ROM.
2. Patient will demonstrate functional (*A/PROM*) adequate for performance of ADLs (*by self, by caregiver*) in the following joints: _____. • moderate limitations of motion • moderate or mild spasticity that responds to tone management techniques • ectopic bone not present in joint(s) being addressed.	2. • Patient will increase (*right, left, both*) upper extremity (UE) (*A/ PROM*) by _____ degrees in (*the following joints: _____, in all limited joints*).	2. • See above; However, since the potential for upgrading function is better, the techniques may be used more aggressively.
3. Patient will demonstrate full (*right, left, both*) UE (*A/PROM*) for optimal function in ADLs. • mild limitations • zero to minimal spasticity.	3. • Patient will increase (*right, left, both*) UE (*A/PROM*) by _____ degrees (*in the following joints: _____, in all limited joints*).	3. • See above. Patient has potential to regain full ROM in specified joints.

Subcategory: Upper Extremity Muscle Tone

Long-term goals and indicators	*Short-term goals*	*Treatment ideas*

1. Patient will demonstrate improved muscle tone for optimal positioning of (*trunk, UE*).
• severe to moderate spasticity
• posturing
• little or no voluntary movement in extremity.
	1. • Patient/caregiver will demonstrate proper use of tone management techniques with (*cues, written instructions, independently*).	1. • Use inhibitory casting. (Do not cast if heterotopic bone is present.)
		• Use orthotics.
		• Use developmental positions to elicit more normal tonal bias.
		• Use positioning (bed and wheelchair).
		• Use inhibition techniques:
		  • neutral warmth
		  • slow rocking
		  • inversion
		  • ROM in RIP
		  • mobilization of proximal joints
		  • weight bearing
		  • rotation.

2. Patient will demonstrate control of muscle tone sufficient for beginning (*right, left, bilateral*) UE movement.
• moderate to minimal spasticity
• active patient participation
• active movement in joints being addressed.
	2. • Patient will demonstrate beginning movement at the following joints: _____, (*with, without*) (*facilitation, inhibition*).	2. • Use techniques listed above. Use facilitation techniques:
		  • weight bearing
		  • tapping
		  • vibration
		  • postural changes.

3. Patient will demonstrate control of muscle tone sufficient for isolated (*right, left, bilateral*) UE movement (*in the following joints* _____). • minimal spasticity • good sensation • limitations in ROM will not prevent UE movement.	3. • Patient will show beginning isolated control in the following joints: _____ while (*supine, sidelying, sitting, standing*) (*with, without*) (*facilitation, inhibition*). • Patient will show simultaneous control of (*shoulder and elbow, wrist and fingers, etc.*). • Patient will demonstrate control of muscle tone sufficient for full isolated (*right, left, bilateral*) UE movement. • Patient will control proximal UE muscle tone to allow performance of _____ repetitions of the task _____ in _____ (*minutes/seconds*). • Patient will compensate for ataxic movements through (*proximal stabilization techniques, adaptive equipment*). (This short-term goal is not part of the progression and is written to meet the needs of ataxic patients.)	3. • Use techniques listed above. • Facilitate UE movement in and through various developmental positions. • Provide graded gross motor activities to challenge speed and control. • Teach compensation techniques. • Instruct in use of adaptive equipment.

Subcategory: Upper Extremity Use

Long-term goals and indicators	Short-term goals	Treatment ideas
1. Patient will demonstrate beginning use of (*right, left, both*) UE(s) in _____ tasks. • inconsistent or no movement in UE • abnormal tone present • insufficient control for use as gross assist • poor sensation or UE awareness.	1. • Patient will use (*right/left*) UE as a (*passive, gross*) assist in _____ functional tasks (*with, without*) (*verbal, tactile*) cues.	1. • Use inhibition/facilitation to normalize tone and facilitate active movement. • Use activities to promote bilateral and unilateral use as gross or passive assist. • Use cueing.

2. Patient will demonstrate functional use of (*right, left, both*) UE(s) in _____ tasks.
• consistent synergistic or beginning isolated movement
• poor endurance
• limited strength
• good sensation or compensation for sensory loss.
	2. • Patient will spontaneously use (*right, left, both*) UE(s) as an active assist with (*fair, good, normal*) control.
	• Patient will spontaneously use (*right, left, both*) UE(s) as needed in any task.
		2. • See above; however, use activities to promote use of UE as active assist.
		• Activities to develop
		  • proximal stability (weight-bearing place and hold)
		  • bilateral use/control
		  • spontaneous use
		  • isolated movement at all joints.
		• As UE control develops, vary the physical complexity of activity and the position in which it is performed to grade influence on tone and movement.

Subcategory: Hand Function

Long-term goals and indicators	Short-term goals	Treatment ideas
1. Patient will demonstrate beginning use of (*right, left, both*) hands in _____ tasks. • abnormal tone, reflexes or synergistic movement noted • difficulty differentiating wrist/hand function • decreased muscle strength.	1. • Patient will demonstrate mass (*grasp, release*) of _____-sized object. • Patient will (*hold, pick up*) _____-sized object using (*lateral, palmar*) prehension. • Patient will oppose thumb to (*index, long, etc.*) finger.	1. • To optimize hand function, treatment should begin proximally to normalize tone and facilitate control as possible. • Use inhibition/facilitation to normalize distal tone as possible. • Use activities to develop grasp and release, lateral and palmar prehension. • Use casting and splinting to optimize ROM and to inhibit tone. • Use activities to develop isolated finger movement and manipulation of objects (gradually decrease size). • As control develops, vary the physical complexity of the task and the position in which it is performed to grade influence on distal tone and movement.
2. Patient will demonstrate functional use of (*right, left, both*) hand(s) in _____ fine motor tasks. • beginning isolated finger movement • minimal to no influence of abnormal tone • decreased strength • decreased coordination.	2. • Patient will demonstrate isolated finger movement. • Patient will improve score by _____ (*pounds, seconds*) in the following hand function tests: _____. • Patient will demonstrate increased fine motor control in _____ activities. • Patient will show (*fine motor coordination, hand strength*) within norms for use in _____ activities.	2. • See above • Emphasize manipulation of various sized objects. • Activities requiring speed and fine motor accuracy. • Resistive activities provided abnormal muscle tone is not elicited.

Subcategory: Head Control

Long-term goals and indicators	Short-term goals	Treatment ideas
1. Patient will maintain head in midline position with assistive device to maximize interaction with the environment. • zero to poor head control • severe to moderate abnormal tone.	1. • Caregiver will demonstrate correct use of head-positioning device.	1. • Provide external support. • Inhibit abnormal tone in neck. • Facilitate righting reactions of head/neck. • Use activities of interest to patient in planes requiring vertical head control. • Instruct caregiver in equipment use. • Use joint approximation through head and neck.
2. Patient will intermittently maintain head control. • poor endurance • decreased neck strength • beginning head control against gravity • poor awareness of head position in space • moderate to minimal abnormal tone	2. • Patient will demonstrate beginning head/neck control in (*prone, supine, sitting*). • Patient will maintain head control for _____ minutes (*with, without*) cueing.	2. • See above; however, gradually reduce use of head support as able. • Use developmental positions to optimize head control.
3. Patient will demonstrate independent head control for participation in functional tasks. • intermittent head control shown • aware of position of head in space.	3. • Patient will independently maintain head control for _____ minutes. • Patient will independently maintain head control during _____ dynamic activities in (*sitting, kneeling, standing*).	3. • See above; however, work toward removal of head support. • Challenge head control through use of developmental positions and dynamic activities.

Subcategory: Postural Adaptation

Long-term goals and indicators	Short-term goals	Treatment ideas
1. Patient will maintain proper postural alignment through positioning equipment to maximize interaction with the environment. • limited or no trunk control • poor awareness of body in space • severe spasticity or hypotonicity.	1. • Caregiver will demonstrate correct use of wheelchair-positioning equipment.	1. • Provide external support through positioning. • Instruct caregiver in use of equipment. • Inhibit abnormal tone in trunk, neck, and extremities.
2. Patient will demonstrate beginning adaptive postural responses in (*supine, prone, sidelying, sitting*). • may require cues and/or facilitation to initiate movement • poor protective and equilibrium responses seen in sitting • some awareness of body in space • moderate to minimal hyper/hypotonicity.	2. • Patient will demonstrate beginning adaptive postural responses in _____ position (*with, without*) facilitation. • Patient will demonstrate midline orientation, head righting, and weight shifting in supported sitting. • Patient will demonstrate adequate balance and equilibrium responses for unsuppported static sitting.	2. • Inhibit abnormal tone in trunk, neck, and extremities. • Facilitate adaptive postural responses (rotation, weight shift, righting, and equilibrium responses) in supine, prone, sidelying, and sitting. • Introduce activities incorporating movements above. • Provide activities that require use of transitional movements through sitting.

Subcategory: Postural Adaptation continued

Long-term goals and indicators	Short-term goals	Treatment ideas
3. Patient will demonstrate functional postural responses in (*sitting, standing, ambulation*). • protective and equilibrium response seen in sitting, standing and/or ambulating (delay may be noted) • good awareness of body in space • may be poor rotational components in trunk movement.	3. • Patient will demonstrate adequate balance and equilibrium responses for completion of functional tasks in dynamic sitting. • Patient will demonstrate adequate balance and equilibrium responses for completion of functional tasks in (*supported, unsupported, assisted, unassisted*) (*standing, ambulation*). • Patient will demonstrate adequate balance and equilibrium responses for completion of functional activity during (*standing, walking*).	3. • Facilitate adaptive postural response (rotation, weight shift, righting, and equilibrium responses) in standing and ambulation. • Introduce activities in standing position or activities that require transitional movements through developmental sequence. • Use moving surfaces (tilt board, ball). • Use activities that challenge gross motor skill and control (ball games, rhythm games).

Subcategory: Endurance

Long-term goals and indicators	Short-term goals	Treatment ideas
1. Patient will demonstrate endurance sufficient to participate in _____ daily living task(s). • requires frequent rest periods • impaired strength • medical complications may limit endurance • physical limitations may reduce efficiency of motion and thus decrease endurance in higher level tasks.	1. • Patient will participate in (*non, light, moderate*) resistive activity for _____ minutes during treatment session. • Patient will demonstrate endurance sufficient for participation in combined therapeutic and self-care activities for _____ hours with _____ rest periods. • Patient to demonstrate endurance for (*community, work simulation*) task _____ for _____ hours.	1. • Attempt to schedule treatment to accommodate endurance level. • Provide activities requiring participation of gradually increasing duration. • Provide activities requiring gradually increasing physical demands. • Provide activities that simulate work and community level endurance requirements. • Teach strategies for use at home/work to conserve energy.

REFERENCES

Bobath, B. (1978). *Adult hemiplegia: Evaluation and treatment.* London: William Heineman.

Chusid, J.G. (1973). *Correlative neuroanatomy and functional neurology.* Los Altos, CA: Large Medical Publications.

Eggers, O. (1984). *Occupational therapy in the treatment of adult hemiplegia.* Rockville, MD: Aspen Publishers.

Farber, S. (1982). *Neurorehabilitation: A multisensory approach.* Philadelphia: W.B. Saunders.

Voss, D., Ionta, M., & Myers, B. (1985). *Proprioceptive neuromuscular facilitation: Patterns and techniques.* Philadelphia: Harper & Row.

Management of Abnormal Tone Through Casting and Orthotics

Judy Hill, OTR/L

CLINICAL PROBLEMS AND TREATMENT OBJECTIVES

Muscle tone is characterized by subdued activity of a normal muscle at rest and an involuntary resistive reaction in opposition to mechanical stretch (Gatz, 1970). Abnormalities of muscle tonus include flaccidity, rigidity, and spasticity. Flaccidity is the lack of muscle tonus and tendon reflex elasticity. Rigidity is limb or joint and muscle stiffness and resistance to movement throughout the range of motion (ROM). The rigid extremity appears to be "stuck." Both agonist and antagonist are resistant to movement even when the velocity of the movement is low. For example, the elbow may remain positioned in 45° of flexion and may resist attempts at active or passive flexion and extension. Spasticity is increased tonus and is characterized by exaggerated resistance to passive motion, which is stronger at the beginning of motion and then gives way in the "clasp knife" phenomenon. Hyperactive tendon and stretch reflexes are also present. The hypertonicity in spasticity is not balanced between agonist and antagonist, as it is in rigidity, and is elicited by quick stretch or by any rapid movement.

Spasticity and rigidity, though caused by central nervous system (CNS) damage, appear to respond to external environmental stimuli, resulting in tonal fluctuations. These can be observed in normal and in CNS-damaged patients as a result of position change, sensory stimuli, such as noise or touch, and state of arousal.

Secondary problems that may occur with abnormal tone include:

- muscle and soft tissue contracture as a result of the muscle maintaining a shortened position
- joint stiffness due to lack of mobility
- edema resulting from constriction of vessels by tight muscles or from dependent positioning due to flaccidity
- joint damage as a result of spastic or rigid muscles exerting a prolonged and imbalanced pull on joint structures, as in subluxation of the wrist; joint damage can also occur when flaccid muscles fail to protect a joint, allowing it to be damaged by an external mechanical force, as in shoulder subluxation

Muscle and soft tissue contracture are treated with gentle and prolonged stretch. This allows for cell division (Brand, 1985), providing tissue expansion. When stretch is not gradual or prolonged enough, the tissues can tear, causing scarring, further shortening, and loss of elasticity.

Joint stiffness indicates a need for mobility. In severe cases, joints are sometimes mobilized or manipulated under anesthesia. After mobilization, attempts are made to maintain gains through passive ROM, splinting alternately in flexion and extension, and the use of continuous passive motion machines.

Edema secondary to constriction of vessels as a result of abnormal tone can be managed using treatment principles and techniques generally used with edema. These include mobilizing to loosen fluids, massaging to loosen and push fluids proximally, elevated positioning to allow fluids to flow proximally, and using pressurized garments and wraps to push fluid proximally and prevent fluid buildup. With edema due to vessel constriction resulting from joint malalignment, as can occur with spasticity or rigidity, attempts to obtain a more normal joint alignment may allow fluids to be mobilized and edema to be reduced.

When joint structures are damaged, joint mobilization may loosen and realign the boney components of the joint. Maintained spasticity and contracture of muscles may prevent manual mobilization and necessitate surgical intervention.

Before initiating a treatment program, it is necessary to evaluate the limb to ascertain the problems. Review of the medical record provides information on the history and etiology of the problem. Clinical observations and measurements are taken of edema, joint mobility,

alignment, and range. Response to rapid passive movement to elicit a stretch reflex and resistance to passive movement are assessed.

To discriminate between spasticity or rigidity and muscle contracture, both joint mobility and muscle length must be considered. For example, in assessing a hand, full finger joint ROM may be present with the wrist in neutral. Resistance to movement and/or a stretch reflex may be elicited at 45° of metacarpophalangeal (MP) flexion with the wrist in neutral and the interphalangeal joints (IPs) extended. However, if the wrist is brought to 60° of extension, it may no longer be possible to extend the fingers fully. This indicates a combination of spasticity and muscle contracture (Figure 7–1). If the IP joints cannot be fully extended, even with the wrist fully flexed and IP extension remaining the same when the wrist is brought into extension, joint stiffness and soft tissue contracture are present (Figure 7–2).

UPPER EXTREMITY CLINICAL PRESENTATION

A number of common clinical presentations are associated with abnormal tone in the upper extremities. Those frequently managed with orthotic devices and casting include:

- shoulder subluxation (Figure 7–3)
- elbow flexor spasticity or contracture (Figure 7–4)
- elbow extensor spasticity or contracture
- supinator spasticity or contracture
- pronator spasticity or contracture

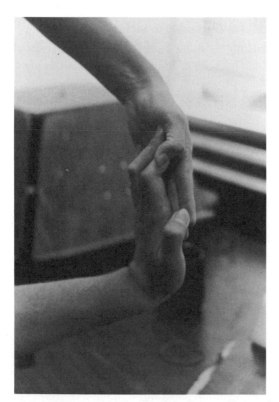

Figure 7–1 Inability to passively extend the fingers with the wrist in extension indicates finger flexor contracture.

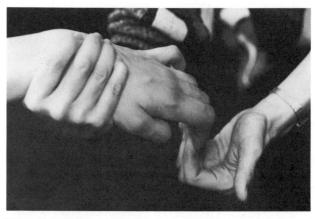

Figure 7–2 Inability to passively extend the fingers regardless of wrist position indicates contracture of joint structures.

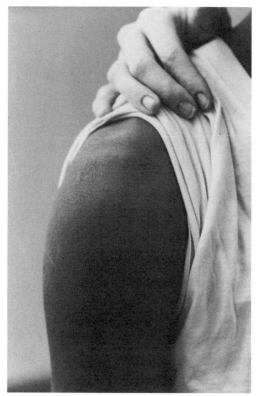

Figure 7–3 Shoulder subluxation can be observed as a space between the superior lip of the glenoid fossa and the head of the humerus.

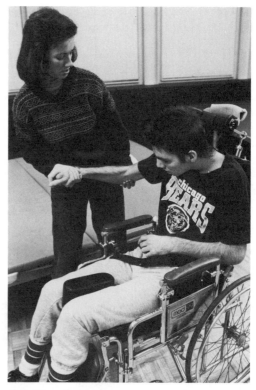

Figure 7–4 Elbow flexion contracture is common.

- wrist flexor spasticity or contracture
- wrist extensor spasticity or contracture
- wrist drop
- finger and thumb flexor spasticity or contracture (Figure 7–5)

- intrinsic hand musculature spasticity or contracture (Figure 7–6)
- intrinsic minus posturing or contracture (Figure 7–7)
- decerebrate rigidity or posturing (Figure 7–8)
- decorticate rigidity or posturing (Figure 7–9)
- synergistic, nonisolated, or patterned motion

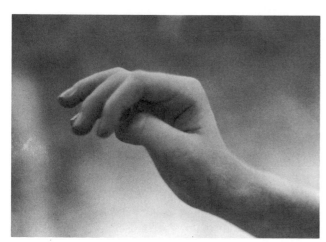

Figure 7–5 Finger and thumb flexor spasticity interfere with manipulation skills.

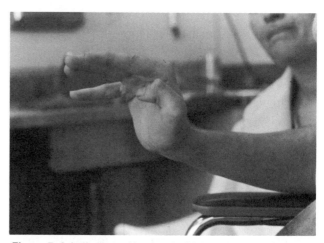

Figure 7–6 Intrinsic positive hand with spastic intrinsic hand musculature

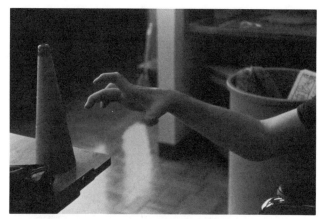

Figure 7–7 Intrinsic minus hand

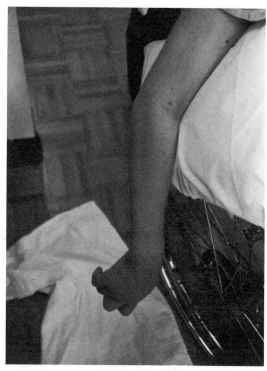

Figure 7–8 Decerebrate posture

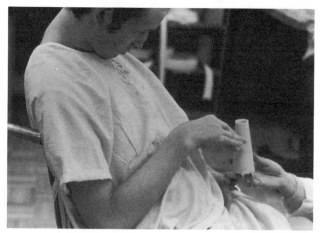

Figure 7–9 Decorticate posture

- prevent spastic muscles from assuming their most shortened position in an attempt to prevent increased abnormal tone
- provide positioning during nontreatment hours by incorporating into the orthosis positions of the joint and muscle that have an inhibitory effect on other muscles, such as thumb extension and abduction.

The Shoulder

At the shoulder, various types of slings can be used to support a flaccid or spastic subluxation by setting the head of the humerus in the glenoid fossa. Slings are also used to prevent further stretching of the rotator cuff muscles and traction on the brachial plexus. Elevation of the distal extremity for edema control and protection of a flail arm with patients who display disregard also may necessitate the use of a sling.

There is controversy over subluxation management, in particular the use of slings (Cailliet, 1980). Subluxation in the flaccid stage is believed to be caused by elongation of the rotator cuff muscles combined with downward rotation and depression of the scapula as a result of flaccid scapular stabilizers and the dependent

ORTHOTIC INTERVENTION

Orthotic devices are frequently used to manage flaccid, spastic, and rigid upper extremities and to prevent secondary problems. There is controversy over the effect of orthoses on abnormal tone (Carr & Shepherd, 1980; Farber & Huss, 1974; Logigian, 1982; McPherson, Dreimeyer, Aalderks, & Gallagher, 1982). Studies that have addressed the question of the effectiveness of orthotics in decreasing spasticity and rigidity have generally supported its effectiveness (Chariat, 1968; Long & Crochetiere, 1964; McPherson, 1981; Shah, 1982; Zablotny, Andric, & Gowland, 1987; Snook, 1979). At the Rehabilitation Institute of Chicago (RIC), orthotic devices are used with patients exhibiting abnormal tone to

- prevent secondary problems of contracture, edema, joint stiffness, and malalignment

weight of the upper extremity. This leaves the glenoid fossa oriented downward and the humerus in a relatively abducted position. When the humerus is in this position, capsular support is minimized.

Comprehensive intervention for the flaccid shoulder must realign the scapula, support the weight of the extremity, and support the humerus into the glenoid fossa. These factors are used to evaluate the effectiveness of slings. Spastic shoulder girdle musculature may contribute to subluxation by pulling the head of the humerus downward and out of the glenoid fossa. In these cases, the focus of treatment is to break up the strong pull of spastic adductors and depressors of the humerus by abducting the shoulder.

Slings may be categorized into six types.

- figure-of-8 sling (Figures 7–10 and 7–11)
- Kagle sling (Figures 7–12 and 7–13)
- vertical sling (Figure 7–14)
- clavicle strap (Figure 7–15)
- abductor rolls (Figure 7–16)
- slings suspended from an overhead bar attached to the patient's wheelchair.

Clinical observation suggests that slings are not effective in realigning the scapula except to the extent that they support the weight of the arm. An unpublished study at RIC by Ritt (1980) looked at the effectiveness of four slings in supporting the head of the humerus in the glenoid fossa. The results suggested that figure-of-8 slings are most effective. The Kagle sling was next, the shoulder saddle, a vertical type of sling third, and the clavicle strap last. There are disadvantages cited with sling use; the advantages and disadvantages are listed in Table 7–1.

Many clinicians discourage the use of slings because of their disadvantages; facilitation techniques and teaching the patient how to manage and protect the extremity are used instead. Wheelchair positioning devices such as armrests, lap trays, and overhead suspension slings are also used to support the upper extremities and to maintain the integrity of the shoulder joint (see Unit 8).

Questions to be asked when considering providing a sling include:

- Does the patient need the sling primarily for transfers and ambulation?

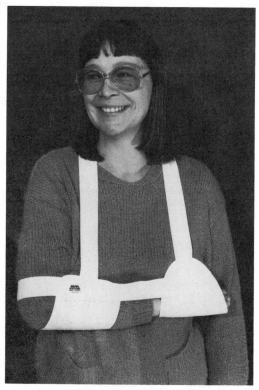

Figure 7–10. The "Universal Hemi-Sling" is a figure-of-8 type sling.

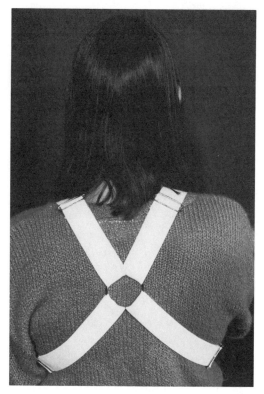

Figure 7–11. The figure-of-8 sling distributes weight evenly over both shoulders.

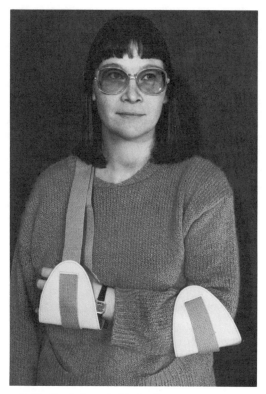

Figure 7–12 Front view of a Kagle sling

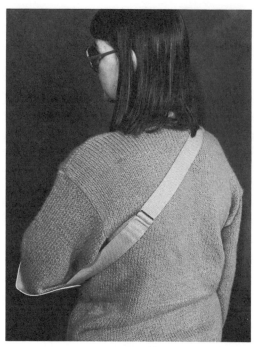

Figure 7–13 This sling provides less support than a figure-of-8 and distributes weight over one shoulder and the patient's back.

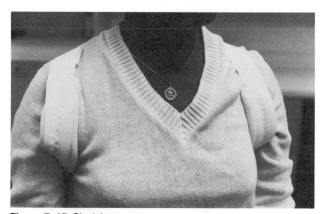

Figure 7–15 Clavicle strap

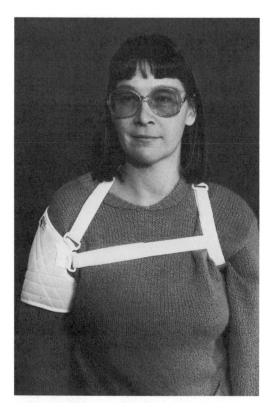

Figure 7-14 The "Hemi-arm Sling" is a vertical type sling. It allows the involved arm to extend at the elbow and distributes weight similar to the figure-of-8 sling.

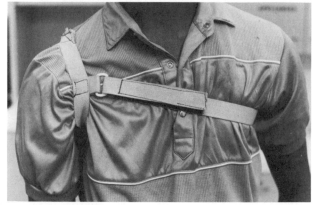

Figure 7–16 Abductor roll

TABLE 7-1   Comparison of shoulder slings

	Pros	*Cons*	*General guidelines for use*
Figure-of-8 sling	Can assist with edema control Protects flail extremity Provides maximum subluxation support	Difficult to don/doff independently Passively encourages flexion of elbow	Worn during ambulation but not in wheelchair where shoulder can be supported by wheelchair arm supports
Vertical sling	Allows arm to hang naturally at side Does not promote flexed positioning of elbow Can be worn in wheelchair and out	Difficult to don/doff independently Can contribute to edema through dependent positioning and constriction around the humerus Provides minimal subluxation support	Can be worn during ambulation or while in wheelchair; arm may or may not be supported on arm rest while in wheelchair
Kagle sling	Can assist with edema control Protects flail extremity Relatively easy to don/doff independently	Passively encourages flexion of elbow Provides moderate subluxation support	Worn during ambulation and removed when in wheelchair where shoulder can be supported by wheelchair arm supports
Clavicle strap	Allows arm to hang naturally at side Does not promote flexed positioning of elbow Can be worn in wheelchair and out Can be worn under clothing Relatively easy to don/doff independently	Can contribute to edema through positioning and constriction in the axilla if improperly fitted Provides minimal subluxation support	Same as for vertical sling
Abductor roll	Allows arm to hang naturally at side Does not promote flexed positioning of elbow Can be worn in wheelchair and out	Can contribute to edema through dependent positioning and constriction in the axilla if improperly fitted	Is used with spastic adductors, not with flaccid subluxation where abduction would decrease capsular support and contribute to glenohumeral instability

- If so, could the patient support his extremity without a sling during these tasks?
- Can the patient don and doff the sling independently so that it is not used continuously but only when needed for support?
- What happens to the subluxation when the patient stands or ambulates? Sometimes the more stressful bipedal position results in an increase in tone that reduces the subluxation without equipment.
- If the sling is needed primarily to protect the extremity, or when the patient finds the flail arm an irritant, could the extremity be supported in another manner, such as by putting the hand in a pocket?

The Elbow

When spasticity or rigidity causes flexion or extension posturing at the elbow, traditional elbow orthoses or bivalved casts can be used to prevent secondary complications. Bivalved casts are casts that have been cut in half and have finished edges and Velcro closures to allow removal and reapplication (Figure 7–17). Both bivalved casts and elbow extension orthoses may be used to maintain gains after an inhibitory casting program or independently of a casting program.

Bivalved casts are made from plaster or fiberglass. They offer full circumference contact throughout the upper extremity for maximum pressure distribution; skin tolerance for them is usually quite good. Thus,

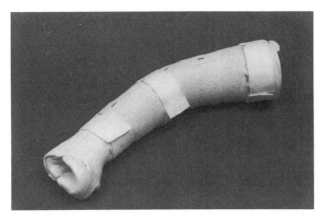

Figure 7–17 Bivalved casts offer good pressure distribution and removability for use as splints.

they can be left on the extremity for up to 5 days. The longer they are left on, the more they function like a cast in inhibiting spasticity and improving ROM. When removed more frequently, they function as orthoses by maintaining ROM and preventing secondary complications. Their durability varies from 4 weeks to 6 months for a plaster cast, to up to 1 year for a fiberglass cast. Fiberglass bivalves are lighter weight and, although more expensive than plaster, are also more breathable, which is an advantage for diaphoretic patients. Neither can be cleaned effectively, although the stockinette liner can be replaced.

There are a number of elbow orthoses, most of them fabricated by orthotists; some are commercially available (Figure 7–18). Some incorporate a turn buckle, spring, or ratcheting mechanism to allow gradual adjustment with changes in the patient's tone (Figure 7–19). Most are composed of humeral and forearm circumferential cuffs joined by metal slats with an axis

at the elbow. Some have a pad to provide counterpressure at the olecranon. Another type, the Yasukawa-Kozole (Kozole & Yasukawa, 1982), offers a full circumference pressure distribution. Pressure distribution and the prevention of skin breakdown are problems with traditional elbow orthoses (Atlas of Orthotics, 1975).

The Wrist and Hand

Orthotic intervention for the flaccid wrist and hand is focused on supporting the joints and arches of the hand, preventing wrist drop, and preventing overstretching and shortening of muscles by maintaining proper joint alignment. The functional position includes the following components.

- wrist positioned in 0° to 15° extension
- palmar arch curvature supported, allowing the 4th and 5th metacarpals to drop anterior to the 2nd and 3rd
- MP joints in 30° to 45° flexion
- IP joints slightly flexed to 10° to 30°
- thumb in opposition to index and middle fingers with MP and IP joints extended and metacarpals aligned with radius
- 30° to 45° of thumb abduction

There are various options for orthotic support.

- A wrist cockup splint is used to support the wrist in neutral and the curvature of the palmar arch (Figure 7–20).

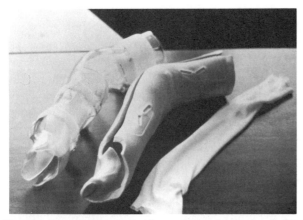

Figure 7–18 Definitive plastic elbow-wrist-hand orthosis with Plastizote liner

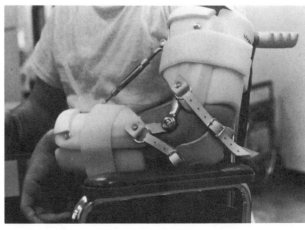

Figure 7–19 Turn buckle elbow extension orthosis

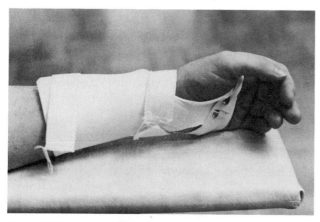

Figure 7–20 Wrist cockup splint

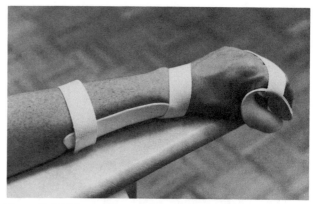

Figure 7–21 The resting hand splint offers full wrist and hand positioning.

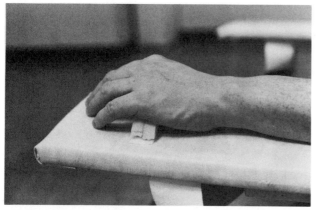

Figure 7–22 Hand support platform on wheelchair armrest

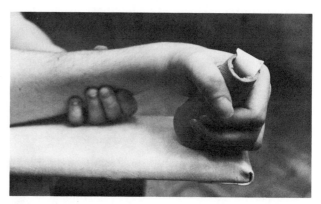

Figure 7–23 Cones can be used to manage severe wrist and hand spasticity or contracture.

- A resting hand orthosis is used, more frequently at night, to support the joints and musculature fully in a functional position (Figure 7–21).
- A simple wrist-hand or hand support can be added to an armrest or lap tray (Figure 7–22). This supports the palmar arch and allows the fingers to flex slightly and the thumb to drop into slight abduction while not being rigidly fixed to the patient's hand.

With the hypertonic wrist and hand, orthoses are used to maintain mobility, prevent increased hypertonicity, prevent secondary complications and skin breakdown, and maintain hand opening to allow for hygiene. Some investigators suggest that orthoses can help reduce spasticity (Chariat, 1968; Farber & Huss, 1974; Long & Crochetiere, 1964; McPherson, 1981; Shah, 1982; Snook, 1979; Zislis, 1964), while others maintain that orthoses interfere with recovery and increase hypertonicity or shift its effects to other joints (Carr & Shepherd, 1980; Neuhaus et al., 1981).

Clinical observation at RIC indicates that wrist-hand orthoses are useful in maintaining the patient's status but not in dramatically altering it. This may be because splints are removed and replaced a number of times during the day, thus eliciting stretch reflexes and interrupting gradual prolonged stretch. They help prevent contracture that would otherwise occur secondary to spastic or rigid posturing. There are a variety of wrist-hand orthoses used with patients at RIC.

- Cones or cone-shaped plastic hand orthoses are used when the totally flexed wrist and hand prevent fitting of wrist positioners (Figure 7–23). Cones are made of a hard plastic or dense foam (Plastizote) rather than soft materials, such as soft foams or washcloths, to prevent spastic muscles from pulling against the orthosis. In some cases, use of the cone results in enough finger relaxation to allow fitting a wrist-hand-finger orthosis, such as a modified resting hand splint, which places the wrist and fingers in a flexed position.

- Resting and modified resting hand orthoses are used to position all joints and muscles of the wrist and hand. A full resting orthosis is used most often with minimal hypertonicity. When abnormal tone is more exaggerated, modifications are made to prevent overstretch of muscles, which can promote deformity. The thumb may be positioned in extension or in combination with abduction, as opposed to direct abduction, if this has a relaxing effect on the rest of the hand. The finger platform may be rolled to prevent overstretching of the finger flexors (Figure 7–24). When the flexor digitorum superficialis is tighter than the profundus, the finger platform may be folded back severely or cut off proximal to the distal interphalangeal (DIP) joints to prevent the fingers from pulling against the platform and the DIP joints from hyperextending (Figures 7–25 and 7–26). Similarly, when the intrinsic hand musculature is relatively more hypertonic than the extrinsic, the finger platform is cut off just proximal to the proximal interphalangeal joints (PIPs) to prevent PIP hyperextension (Figure 7–27). In cases of intrinsic tightness with zero-to-minimal wrist and extrinsic tightness, a hand orthosis platform can be used to support the MPs in extension.

- Finger abduction orthoses are used to maintain finger abduction when this has an inhibitory effect. Simple foam finger abductors are advocated by some therapists using the Bobath approach to treatment. Snook's antispasticity splint (Snook, 1979) combines finger abduction on a volar finger platform, thumb extension, and a dorsal forearm trough. Precautions should be taken to avoid overstretching the finger flexors. Because these muscles are adductors as well as flexors, they are stretched when the fingers are abducted. If they are very spastic or contracted,

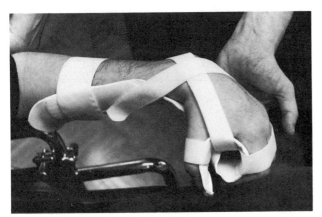

Figure 7–24 The rolled finger platform can provide a gentle stretch to the finger flexors.

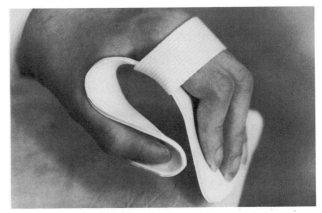

Figure 7–25 Overstretching the finger flexors can cause the DIPs to hyperextend against the splint as the PIPs pull into flexion.

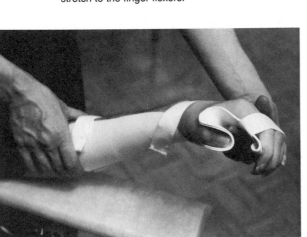

Figure 7–26 Cutting the finger platform off proximal to the DIPs relieves the hyperextension seen in Figure 7–25.

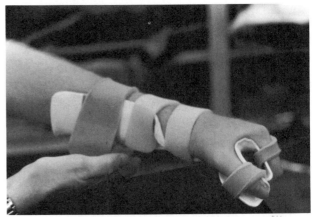

Figure 7–27 The finger platform cut off just proximal to the PIPs supports tight intrinsics.

they will exert an increased pull into finger flexion as the fingers are abducted. This will cause the hand to push against the splint platform.

- A simple dorsal plastic (Figure 7–28) or webbing (Figure 7–29) thumb extender can be effective for positioning for mild hypertonicity, especially with active finger motion and if thumb extension has a relaxing effect on the hand musculature.
- With more severe tone, where the wrist seems to "pull out" of an orthosis, a circumferential plaster or fiberglass bivalved cast can be used to position the wrist more securely.
- Dynamic orthoses are considered with minimal tone. The most commonly used at RIC is a finger extension assist outrigger.

Wrist-hand orthoses are fitted at or below the point of elicitation of the stretch reflex to avoid triggering abnormal responses. The wrist is positioned at a point where finger flexors are relaxed and not pulling into the orthosis. If it appears that the wrist or fingers are pulling strongly into the orthosis as the tone fluctuates, it is positioned in slightly more flexion until relaxation can be maintained.

To prevent contracture and stiffness, orthoses must be alternated with mobility and active and/or passive ROM. They should not interfere with available active motion and must be continuously monitored for fit and effect on the extremity. At the first sign of an increase in joint stiffness, a modification in the wearing schedule, an increase in mobility, or alternative orthoses should be considered. For example, if the MPs are becoming tight in extension, discontinuance of a resting hand orthosis should be considered, or it might be alternated

with a wrist cockup with flexion loops to pull the MPs into flexion gently. Edema should also be monitored because straps and immobility can contribute to its increase.

Orthoses must also be monitored for their effects on the skin. This is especially true when hypertonic muscles might pull the limb against the orthosis or fluctuating tone might cause shearing of the skin against the orthosis. The therapist must take additional responsibility for monitoring the orthosis when the patient's ability to monitor it is reduced secondary to decreased cognitive or sensory awareness. Other team and family members can be taught to monitor orthoses.

CAST INTERVENTION

Plaster casts are used in an attempt to reduce spasticity and to stretch contracted soft tissue and muscle. Clinical observation suggests casting is more effective than orthotic intervention in remediating contracture and the effects of spasticity. This may be due, in part, to the prolonged, gentle stretch that is provided when a cast is left in place for 5 to 7 days. Similarly, with muscles maintained in a relatively constant position, stretch reflexes are not elicited, and facilitory stimulation is minimized.

There is some indication (Hill, 1986) that the response to inhibitory casting and the maintenance of its results are most effective when volitional movement is present but limited by hypertonicity. Maintained improvement in limb position without the use of orthoses has been observed in some patients without volitional movement, but more often orthotic and sometimes surgical follow up is required.

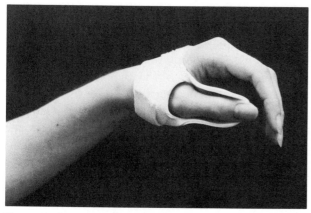

Figure 7–28 Dorsal thumb extender

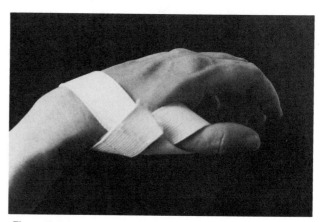

Figure 7–29 Webbing thumb extender

Considering these factors, the goals of casting should be defined before treatment is initiated. Casts should be applied by a therapist or cast technician who has received training in the techniques and precautions associated with casting the head-injured patient. Casts should be applied by occupational therapists only with a physician's order. It is desirable to have verification by an x-ray film that no boney malformation such as subluxation, fracture, or heterotopic ossification is limiting mobility. Casts are generally not applied over edematous areas or open wounds.

Serial casting is the use of a series of casts to stretch contractures gradually. Inhibitory casting is the use of a series of casts to influence spasticity and, in some cases, rigidity. The types of casts used are the same.

Serial cast type and position are based on biomechanical considerations. For example, with a severely contracted biceps, a drop-out cast may first be applied to gain elbow extension, followed by a long arm cast to pronate the forearm while extending the elbow. Another use for serial casting is for contracted finger flexors where applying a wrist cast in extension will result in the finger flexors pulling the fingers into tighter flexion. A finger shell might be added to stretch the finger flexors gently across the wrist, MPs, and IPs. Neurophysiological factors determine the choice of inhibitory cast and positioning of the arm. For example, if supinating the forearm relaxes the elbow flexors and makes elbow extension easier, a cast incorporating supination might be applied.

In head-injured patients, serial and inhibitory principles are usually combined to manage spasticity and contracture simultaneously. Where joint stiffness appears along with muscle contracture or hypertonicity, casting should be attempted only after other mobilizing techniques have failed and after a thorough discussion with the physician. Drop-out casts, allowing for mobility, or bivalved casts, which can be removed for daily mobility, are generally recommended in these circumstances.

Casts are left on the extremity for 5 to 7 days. When one cast in a series is removed, another is applied almost immediately after skin checking, cleansing, measuring ROM, and, in spastic patients, measuring the point at which the stretch reflex is elicited. Passive ROM is performed between casts to counteract stiffness. Usually no more than five casts are included in a series to avoid excess joint stiffness from prolonged immobility.

Goals of Cast Intervention

In the case of severe tone in the absence of volitional movement, casting might be used to evaluate the presence of volitional motion masked by spasticity or to improve limb position for hygiene, comfort, and ease in self-management of the extremity.

In patients with some volitional movement, the goal might be to facilitate greater ranges of active motion and to improve speed and coordination of motion by facilitating a balance of musculature around a joint. Improvements in these areas can be evaluated using ROM measurements, coordination tests, and comparison of performance on functional tasks.

An ROM gain of 10° to 20° per cast and a gain in angle at which the stretch reflex is elicited of 10° to 20° per cast are considered successful results. Slightly less gain might be considered successful in a patient longer post onset. Improved ability in arm placement and hand function tasks should be noted in patients exhibiting active motion after each cast. Examples of positive changes that can be quickly evaluated when casts are removed are the ability to reach forward with elbow extended and with forearm supinated or the wrist and finger position while picking up an object. If no improvement in these areas is noted after two casts, the series is usually discontinued. A different type of cast might be tried.

Even while setting less ambitious goals for patients with severe tone, the therapist must consider that long-term maintenance of any gains made with casting will be more difficult. Other methods, such as surgery or nerve blocks (Braun, Hoffer, & Mooney, 1973), may need to be considered. Cast application is also more difficult with severe tone. Temporary nerve blocking agents such as Xylocaine are sometimes used just before casting to enable the therapist to position the extremity. There is a danger with this technique that the cast will be applied in a position placing too much stretch on the muscles as they are relaxed by the Xylocaine. As its effects wear off, the cast may be painful, and tendonitis may occur from the pull on the muscle.

If goals have not been achieved after five casts, the casting program is temporarily discontinued. Gains are maintained through orthotics and bivalved casts and facilitation of functional movement. Reinitiation of the casting program is considered in 3 to 4 weeks or when joint stiffness has subsided and the patient can incorporate the gains made through casting into function. If gains are not significant after two casts, orthoses or bivalved casts are used to maintain the extremity, and the patient is reconsidered for casting in the future if changes in tone or volitional motion occur. Setting realistic and achievable goals is important in assessing the effectiveness of the technique and in giving the patient and family a realistic outcome expectation.

Types of Casts: Serial and Inhibitory

Many types of casts are used to decrease hypertonicity and its effects on the upper extremities. General guidelines can assist the therapist in deciding which cast to use with a particular patient. These guidelines, combined with a knowledge of anatomy, neurophysiologic treatment principles, and critical observation of the effects of casting, provide the therapist with a basis for deciding when to cast, what type of cast to use, and how to assess the results. There is often more than one acceptable option for a particular patient.

All casts are fabricated with a layer of stockinette smoothly covering the arm. Felt strips are placed on the stockinette over boney prominences for extra protection followed by four or five layers of cotton cast padding. This is covered with five or six layers of plaster gauze. The edges of the plaster are flared back to make a well-padded soft surface where they border the skin. Plaster is used rather than fiberglass for serial casts because it is less expensive, and its weight is thought to offer additional proprioceptive input of joint position. Fiberglass may be used in special cases, for example, when the patient is very diaphoretic or when a lighter-weight cast might be easier to manage.

Elbow and Forearm Casts

Three types of casts are used with hypertonicity affecting elbow motion. A fourth type is used when elbow flexion or extension hypertonicity is combined with pronation or supination limitations or in the unusual case where the primary problem is one of pronation or supination.

Drop-Out Casts. These casts incorporate a full circumference cast for part of the upper extremity and a half circumference shell for the other part. They get their name from the tendency of the partially enclosed portion of the arm to drop away from the cast as range increases. Drop-out casts allow the therapist and patient to observe range increasing as the extremity drops away from the shell. Skin condition on the partially enclosed portion of the extremity can be observed. Some joint mobility is also possible. This may be desirable where mobilization is the recommended treatment, such as in heterotopic ossification or with a secondary diagnosis of arthritis. Drop-out casts are generally used when spasticity is combined with contracture and when contracture is moderate to severe or represents a greater than 45° limitation of motion. When contracture is less than 45°, the drop-out cast may slip, decreasing its effectiveness and causing skin problems. Severe spasticity or widely fluctuating tone can also result in cast slippage. Drop-out casts are frequently used initially and replaced later with another type of cast when elbow limitations have been partly remediated. Two types of drop-out casts are used for flexor spasticity and contracture: (1) with humeral portion enclosed (Figure 7–30), and (2) with forearm portion enclosed (Figure 7–31).

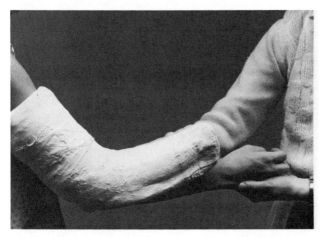

Figure 7–30 Drop-out cast with humeral portion enclosed

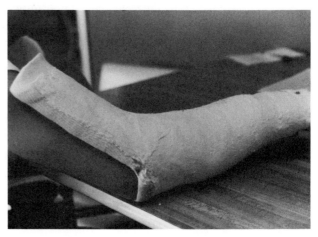

Figure 7–31 Drop-out cast with forearm portion enclosed

These casts are most effective when the patient is in an upright position, allowing gravity to pull the extremity away from the cast. Having the forearm portion enclosed adds more weight for gravity-assisted extension of the elbow, but the humeral shell may get bound by clothing or be cumbersome as it wedges away from the humerus as the elbow extends. Slippage is minimized with the forearm enclosed because the wrist provides a mechanical stop for the cast.

Reverse Drop-Out Cast. The reverse drop-out cast (Figure 7–32) is used to manage elbow extension spasticity and contracture as well as to put a weak biceps at a mechanical advantage in a shortened position. It is made with the humeral portion enclosed. Mechanically, it is most effective with the patient in a supine or sidelying position, allowing gravity to assist the forearm into elbow flexion.

None of the drop-out casts can control supination or pronation unless combined with a wrist cast, so the extremity must be allowed to assume the forearm rotation position it rests in. The forearm enclosed cast can be combined with a wrist cast, which allows managing wrist deformity simultaneously with the elbow.

Rigid Circular Elbow Cast. This cast is a full circumference enclosure of the forearm and humerus (Figure 7–33). It can be used with any degree of contracture and with hypertonicity in the absence of contracture. It is used for patients with severe or fluctuating hypertonus, when the patient is not positioned to allow the drop-out cast to work, and when minimal (less than 45°) limitations prevent the use of a drop-out cast. These casts are generally not used when mobility is required at the elbow joint because of severe rigidity or heterotopic ossification. If there is skin breakdown on any area to be covered by the cast, special precautions will need to be taken. A window is cut in the cast over any area of pink or delicate skin and the padding and stockinette pulled away to allow monitoring of the skin.

Long Arm Cast. The long arm cast (Figure 7–34) is the only type of cast effective in managing hypertonicity affecting supination or pronation. This is accomplished by using the hand as a lever to control the forearm position. They are also used to manage wrist and elbow problems simultaneously; when using the cast for this purpose, care is taken not to overstretch the spastic or tight muscles. Long arm casts are generally not used when there is skin breakdown in areas to be covered by the cast or with severe rigidity or other problems requiring mobility. With severe spasticity or

contractures at both the wrist and elbow, each joint is usually casted individually before applying the long arm cast. This approach facilitates application and minimizes the danger of overstretching the muscles. The area that has a greater inhibitory effect on the extremity is managed first. Often, elbow tone is managed first, followed by management of the wrist and hand.

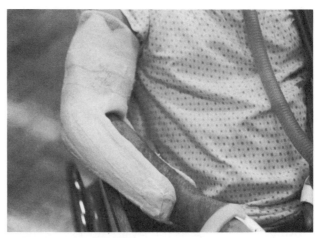

Figure 7–32 Reverse drop-out cast

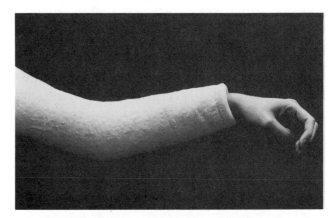

Figure 7–33 Rigid circular elbow cast

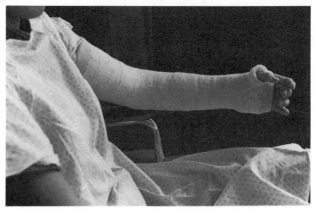

Figure 7–34 Long arm cast

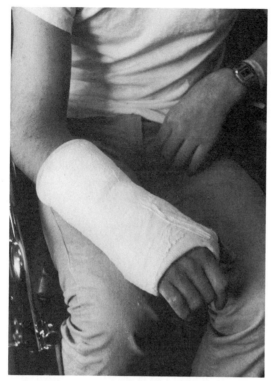

Figure 7–35 Rigid circular wrist cast

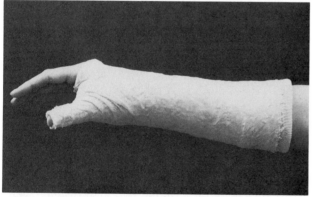

Figure 7–36 Rigid circular wrist cast with thumb post

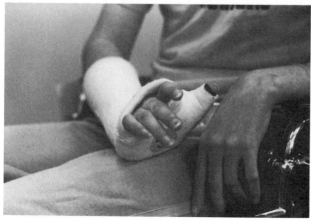

Figure 7–37 Rigid circular wrist and MP cast

Wrist and Hand Casts

One type of wrist cast is used with head-injured patients at RIC to manage hypertonicity. Modifications are made to this cast to manage different clinical problems.

Rigid Circular Wrist Cast. This full circumference cast (Figure 7–35) encloses the wrist and metacarpal areas and extends over the distal two-thirds of the forearm. It is used to control the wrist position while leaving the finger joints unaffected. It can be used to control wrist flexion, extension, or deviation. They seem most effective in influencing distal hand function when there is active finger motion. Goals of casting include achieving finger function in varying degrees of wrist extension and isolating wrist from hand function. The modifications made to the wrist cast enhance achievement of these goals based on different clinical presentations of wrist and hand function.

Rigid Circular Wrist Cast with Thumb Enclosed. The thumb portion is included on the rigid circular wrist cast (Figure 7–36) when pinch, grasp, and release are impaired by thumb flexor spasticity. This modification is also used when positioning the thumb relaxes the fingers.

Rigid Circular Wrist and MP Cast. When intrinsic, particularly lumbrical, spasticity is present, preventing full MP extension for function in picking up objects and manipulation, an MP platform is incorporated into the cast (Figure 7–37). The MPs are brought gradually into increased extension, while the IPs are allowed to flex and extend freely. With severe intrinsic contracture, the PIPs may hyperextend as the MPs are brought into extension, necessitating the addition of PIP flexion assist loops. Generally, a platform extending over the volar surface of the MPs and proximal phalanges is adequate to maintain MP extension, but a full circumference extension can also be used.

Rigid Circular Wrist Cast with Finger Shell. At times, the wrist cast alone is not effective in fostering active finger extension or remediating finger flexion contractures. In these cases, a full circumference finger shell that encloses the IP joints, middle phalanges, and part of the proximal and distal phalanges is fabricated (Figure 7–38). This shell is attached with Velcro to the cast to allow adjustability of the amount of stretch placed on the fingers. The primary indication for use of a finger shell is when the fingers remain flexed while in

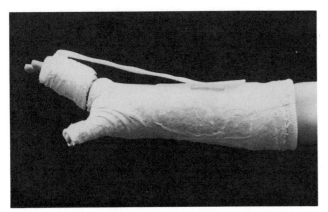

Figure 7–38 Finger shell attached to rigid circular wrist cast

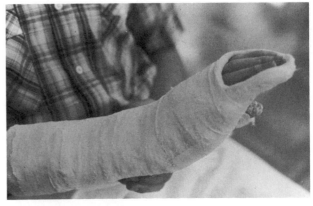

Figure 7–39 Finger platform cast

the cast, given that the wrist is not positioned in too much extension. Finger shells are removable to allow close monitoring of the fingers for stiffness and skin condition. Overstretch of finger musculature is a danger with the finger shell. Finger shells can be made to enclose all four fingers or only one or two fingers.

Rigid Circular Wrist Cast with Finger Platform. The finger platform is added to a wrist cast in cases of mild spasticity to achieve full simultaneous extension of the wrist and fingers (Figure 7–39). The patient is encouraged to try to lift his fingers off the platform with the cast in place. With moderate to severe spasticity, the patient's fingers tend to pull against a platform, causing a boutinerre effect. Platform casts are used only with minimal spasticity

Elbow and wrist casts can be combined. Any of the hand modifications can be added to a long arm cast, or a wrist cast can be combined with the forearm enclosed drop-out cast. Hand modifications, except enclosing the thumb, are seldom added to the long arm cast because this so completely immobilizes the patient, allowing little chance for work on improving control with the cast in place.

Determining the Position in Which to Cast

Casts are applied over a joint positioned 5° to 10° less than the range that is achieved with maximal traction. Consideration is also given to the point of stretch reflex, with initial casts positioning the upper extremity at or slightly less than that point. If the point of stretch reflex remains unchanged after the first cast, a second may be applied beyond that point and the results monitored. Inhibitory positions such as supination, thumb exten-

sion, and radial deviation can be incorporated into the position of the upper extremity to be casted. These are evaluated and determined for each patient. The amount of stress on tight muscles and soft tissues is minimized.

With fluctuating tone, the position in which to cast the patient varies greatly with total body position and amount of stimulation. It is determined by submaximal range, the point the stretch reflex is elicited, and the common resting position of the limb. Primary consideration is given to the latter. For example, if a patient usually rests with his elbow at 90° of flexion, if passive range at the joint is limited by only 30° when very relaxed but increases to 105° when very stressed, and if a stretch reflex is elicited at 90° of flexion, the initial cast would be placed at 80° to 90° of flexion. A rigid circular cast would be used.

Casts and other techniques incorporating a period of immobility are used only with extreme caution in cases of rigidity where increased mobility is needed. Where the rigidity is in an extreme of range, as in severe extension at the elbow in decerebrate rigidity, casting is often used to achieve motion in the opposite direction. In these cases, casting often results in an increase in passive or active motion, as movement away from the extreme range is gained. If this does not occur, and the cast leaves the limb rigid in a new position, casting is discontinued and mobilizing techniques attempted.

Often, with head injury, all four extremities show spasticity and contracture, and a team decision must be made on where to use cast intervention first. Generally, casting more than two extremities at once is not advised, as this limits the patient's ability to interact with the environment. The number of joints to be included is also an important consideration. While a rigid circular elbow cast, wrist cast, and ankle cast may not excessively inhibit the patient's interactions, two long arm casts probably would. The goal is to preserve the patient's ability to have motor interaction with the environment with his extremities while enhancing motor function through casting. When both upper extremities display volitional movement, but one is more functional than the other, casting the more functional one first may encourage use of the other. When one upper extremity is nonfunctional, casting several joints on the functional upper extremity may interfere with activity. Function and interaction with the environment should always be considered in deciding on the type and location of casts (Zablotny et al., 1987).

Cast Monitoring

Casts are monitored for the following complications.

- skin breakdown
- circulation compromise
- changes in sensation proximal or distal to the cast
- patient pain or discomfort
- an increase in restlessness or agitation

Casts are monitored until they are set for approximately 20 minutes, hourly for 2 hours after setting, and then daily until they are removed. Monitoring is increased if complications develop. The date of application and projected date of cast removal are written on the cast. Outpatients are candidates for casting only when they are dependable in keeping appointments and have someone to assist them in monitoring the cast if they cannot do so themselves.

Considerations in Casting Agitated and Confused Patients

Agitated and confused patients may be frightened and unable to understand why a cast is being applied. If a patient resists the cast application, it will be difficult to hold the extremity in the desired position. Often, it is the application process that elicits the most agitation, and the cast is no longer irritating after a couple of hours. If the cast continues to be an irritant, and increased agitation is noted, the casting program may need to be postponed until agitation decreases to prevent the possibility of harm to the patient or others. Occasionally, patients are sedated during cast application. If the cast continues to be an irritant after the sedative wears off, it will have to be removed.

TREATMENT USED IN CONJUNCTION WITH CASTING

Casts are used in conjunction with positioning, inhibition, and facilitation of normal movement. Using the casted limb in functional tasks and motor activities is encouraged. For example, a patient with a wrist cast might engage in a table-top game or pick up and place various-sized blocks. Active grasp and release is encouraged in this manner, with the cast holding the patient's wrist in a more normal position. Scapular stability, arm placement, and wrist-hand function might be facilitated while reaching for an object or playing catch with a rigid circular elbow cast. Neurophysiologic treatment techniques may also be used. These techniques are continued after the cast is removed to maintain and incorporate gains into functional motor activities. Bivalved casts or other orthoses may also be used to maintain gains while attempting to facilitate normal motor function.

Casting and orthotics can be important techniques in facilitating motor function in patients displaying abnormal tone and contracture. To achieve their maximum effectiveness, both orthoses and casts should be combined with treatment techniques that more actively engage the patient in functional motor activities. Casts, orthotic intervention, and other treatment of motor disorders associated with abnormal tone are based on a sound understanding of the problems and what is needed to remediate them.

REFERENCES

Brand, P. W. (1985). *Clinical mechanisms of the hand.* St. Louis: C. V. Mosby.

Braun, R. M., Hoffer, M. M., & Mooney, V. (1973). Phenol nerve block in the treatment of acquired spastic hemiplegia in the upper limb. *Journal of Bone and Joint Surgery, 55A,* 580–585.

Cailliet, R. (1980). *The shoulder in hemiplegia.* Philadelphia: F. A. Davis.

Carr, J. H., & Shepherd, R. B. (1980). *Physiotherapy in disorders of the brain.* Rockville, MD: Aspen Publishers.

Chariat, S. E. (1968). A comparison of volar and dorsal splinting of the hemiplegic hand. *American Journal of Occupational Therapy, 22,* 319–321.

Farber, S. E., & Huss, J.A. (1974). *Sensorimotor evaluation and treatment procedures for allied health personnel.* Indianapolis, IN: Indiana University, Purdue University, Indianapolis Medical Center.

Gatz, A. J. (1970). *Manter's essentials of clinical neuroanatomy and neurophysiology* (4th ed.). Philadelphia: F. A. Davis.

Hill, J. (1986). *The effects of casting on motor disorders associated with spasticity.* Unpublished manuscript (No. RT 20-PR 149A).

Rehabilitation Institute of Chicago, Research Dissemination RIC-RT 20.

Hunter, J., Sneider, L., Mackin, E., & Bell, J. (1978). *The rehabilitation of the hand*. St. Louis: C. V. Mosby.

Kozole, K., & Yasukawa, A. (1982). Elbow extension orthosis. *Journal of Orthotics and Prosthetics, 36*(1), 50–62.

Logigian, M. (1982). *Adult rehabilitation: A team approach for therapists*. Boston: Little Brown.

Long, T. D., & Crochetiere, W. (1964). Objective measurement of muscle tone in the hand. *Clinical Pharmacology Therapy, 5*, 909–917.

McPherson, J. (1981). Objective evaluation of a splint to reduce hypertonicity. *American Journal of Occupational Therapy, 35*, 189–194.

McPherson, J., Dreimeyer, D., Aalderks, M., & Gallagher, T. (1982). A comparison of dorsal and volar resting hand splints in the reduction of hypertonus. *American Journal of Occupational Therapy, 36*, 664–670.

Neuhaus, B., Ascher, E., Coullon, D., Einbond, A., Glover, J., Goldberg, S., & Takai, V. (1981). A survey of rationales for and against hand splinting in hemiplegia. *American Journal of Occupational Therapy, 35*, 83–90.

Ritt, B. (1980). *Comparative study of sling supports for the subluxed hemiplegic shoulder*. Unpublished manuscript (No. RT20-PR109 4/80). Rehabilitation Institute of Chicago, Research Dissemination RIC-RT-20.

Shah, S. K. (1982). Hand orthosis for upper motor neuron paralysis. *Australian Journal of Occupational Therapy, 29*(3), 97–101.

Snook, J. H. (1979). Spasticity reduction splint. *American Journal of Occupational Therapy, 33*, 648–651.

The atlas of orthotics. (1975). St. Louis: C. V. Mosby, p. 121.

Zablotny, C., Andric, M. F., & Gowland, C. (1987). Serial casting: Clinical implications for the head injured patient. *Journal of Head Trauma Rehabilitation, 2*(2), 46–52.

Zislis, J. M. (1964). Splinting of the hand in the spastic hemiplegic patient. *Archives of Physical Medicine and Rehabilitation, 45*(1), 41–43.

Positioning: An Adjunct to Therapy

Jessica Presperin, OTR/L

A large percentage of head-injured individuals use wheelchairs as the primary means of mobility, either temporarily or permanently. The procedure of ordering a wheelchair and prescribing interventions for positioning is an integral part of the rehabilitation process. In most cases, proper positioning is a viable adjunct to therapy and, occasionally, is a primary goal of the patient's admission.

Wheelchair seating and positioning is a specialty in its own right. This unit attempts to cover the basic information needed to position the head-injured child or adult. Positioning is defined in this unit as the provision of external intervention used to assist with the static positioning of the body as it relates to space. This unit focuses on linear seating for wheeled mobility. A linear system is based on straight planes of surface contact and is used for the majority of patients at the Rehabilitation Institute of Chicago (RIC). Customized contoured systems are discussed briefly and are more appropriate for patients with a fixed deformity. Alternative methods of positioning, such as sidelyers and bed positioning, are also discussed.

The goals of providing positioning equipment in a rehabilitation setting are to improve function, enable participation in therapy and nursing programs, and prevent the formation of contractures or pressure sores. A patient may progress through several stages during rehabilitation, requiring frequent changes in positioning intervention. Positioning systems must allow for adjustment as the individual changes physically and cognitively, grows, or becomes able to perform new functional tasks. Purchase of definitive positioning equipment or a wheelchair may not be necessary, as the goal may be ambulation.

At RIC, positioning is provided by a fleet of wheelchairs owned by the Institute that have interchangeable and adjustable positioning inserts. These systems can be used either as temporary supportive devices or in a trial to determine the definitive equipment to be ordered. The benefits of positioning are:

- aligns the body to provide symmetry and to prevent or control deformity caused by an abnormal neurologic influence on the body
- enhances the performance of the autonomic nervous system
- prevents decubitus ulcers
- provides stability to enhance distal mobility and function
- facilitates interaction with the environment

Abnormal tone and movement patterns often cause the patient to assume abnormal positions while sitting in a wheelchair or lying in bed. Without intervention, these positions may become habitual, leading to the possibility of structural deformity or muscle shortening. By providing external support to align the body symmetrically, the potential for deformity is decreased

(Bergen & Colangelo, 1985; Bergman, 1986; Hill & Presperin, 1986; Taylor, 1986; Trombley & Scott, 1977; Ward, 1983).

Respiration, swallowing, and cardiac performance may be enhanced by proper positioning. When the trunk is supported to allow increased diaphragmatic excursion, the effort necessary for the individual to breathe may decrease. This decreases demands on the heart, therefore increasing cardiac performance. The head and neck can be positioned to promote swallowing, decreasing the potential for aspiration of food or saliva (Bergen & Colangelo, 1985; Bergman, 1986; Brunswic, 1984; Hill & Presperin, 1986; Nwaobi & Smith, 1986; Trefler, 1984).

Independent pressure relief may be difficult due to the cognitive or physical involvement of the patient. A symmetric base of support and, in some cases, a special cushion may distribute pressure and assist in the prevention of decubitus ulcers (Anderson, 1979; Bergen, 1986b; Bergen & Colangelo, 1985; Bergman, 1986; Hage, 1985; Hill & Presperin, 1986; Trefler, 1984; Ward, 1983; Zacharkow, 1984).

Increased proximal stability often allows for increased distal mobility and function. When trunk supports are provided, an individual may be able to use the upper extremities for function rather than support. This allows him to participate in a broader range of activities of daily living or self-propulsion of his wheelchair (Bergen, 1986a,b; Bergen & Colangelo, 1985; Bergman, 1986; Trefler, 1984; Ward, 1983).

Vertical head positioning allows for eye contact and increases the patient's potential for social interaction. Once the head and trunk are positioned properly, he may be better able to participate with others in the environment. This may help increase attention span, visual tracking, visual orientation to the environment, and communication skills.

PRACTICAL CONSIDERATIONS AND EVALUATION

Before the therapist takes measurements or determines the equipment to be ordered, many factors must be considered. To obtain the necessary information, data can be collected from the primary caregiver, family, and team professionals. For example, the speech and language pathologist can contribute information pertaining to communication abilities, and the psychologist may assist with behavioral status.

Considerations such as funding, nursing, and follow through are more applicable to discharge and the ordering of definitive equipment. The following considerations are important when determining the patient's positioning needs.

- tonal characteristics
- orthopedic involvement
- functional capabilities
- level of cognitive functioning and behavioral status
- rehabilitation goals
- potential for follow through of program
- funding

Tonal Characteristics

Changes in muscle tone as the body is placed in different positions should be noted. Some positions may be stressful and increase abnormal tone, while others may be inhibitory. These inhibitory positions, as determined by the therapist, may be incorporated into the design of the seating system. For example, a patient with strong pelvic extension may have difficulty maintaining the sitting position. By fabricating a system to maintain hip flexion and stabilize the pelvis, extensor thrusting may be decreased. Provision of symmetric stabilization may inhibit the influence of asymmetric tone. A description of abnormal tone and how it affects seating should be included on the evaluation form.

Orthopedic Involvement

A range of motion (ROM) evaluation is needed to measure orthopedic limitations. ROM limitations from muscle contracture, fractures sustained at the time of injury, or ectopic bone formation are measured. Scoliosis, kyphosis, lordosis, leg length discrepancy, windswept legs, and boney prominences are also noted. Before a definitive system is decided upon, medical or surgical interventions planned to correct ROM limitations should be considered.

Functional Capabilities

The level of volitional movement and control will help determine the amount of definitive intervention needed. Head and trunk supports may stabilize the body to enable an individual to participate in a functional activity yet allow him to develop the agonist/antagonist muscle components needed for head or trunk control. The ideal positioning system allows functional volitional movement and encourages increased independence. Specific pieces of equipment, such as trunk supports and headrests, may vary, depending on the task being performed.

Cognitive and Behavioral Level

Deficits in cognition and perception often influence the type of wheeled mobility base ordered. Although a patient may be able to use an electric wheelchair base, unilateral neglect, apraxia, and poor problem-solving skills or judgment may put him or others in danger of getting hurt.

The mechanics of propelling a wheelchair may be difficult for the patient to understand. A therapist determining the type of wheelchair to order for the individual with unilateral involvement may find that a lever arm wheelchair is easier for him to propel than a one-armed drive wheelchair. This may be because the former correlates better to the direction the wheelchair is going than the latter.

As noted in Unit 5, many individuals experience an agitated state during recovery. With these individuals, positioning intervention includes safety modifications that may prevent them from injuring themselves or others. Antitippers can be attached to the chair to prevent patients from tipping over when they purposely push themselves backward. Parts of the wheelchair frame may need to be padded to prevent self-injury from kicking, hitting, or self-stimulation.

An individual may become increasingly agitated due to the frustrations of being unable to remove a piece of equipment or the feeling of entrapment. A compromise may have to be made if the agitation becomes uncontrollable or increases abnormal posturing. However, a seatbelt is a mandatory part of the system, despite agitation.

Rehabilitation Goals

Communication among professionals, family, and the patient concerning the goals of rehabilitation is essential before definitive equipment is ordered. Nursing issues include skin integrity, respiratory needs, feeding status, sleeping patterns, and medications. Vinyl coverings, nylon zippers, closed cell foam, or plastic may be incorporated into the seating system for patients with incontinence problems. Commercially available and custom-made trays to hold a respirator allow for easier mobility. Carriers to hold feeding bags are available for attachment to a chair. The patient's angle in space is a factor to consider for optimal food exchange.

Patients may have communication deficits or require specific body positioning to enhance voice output. If augmentative communication equipment is recommended by the speech and language pathologist, it should be accommodated as possible by the seating system. This may range from desk-type armrests allowing greater access to a computer terminal to a team discussion to determine placement of switches and communication systems. Positioning systems should also accommodate orthotic needs such as a body jacket, cast, or orthoses.

Potential for Follow Through of Positioning Program

Follow through with the use of equipment in the discharge environment depends on several factors, including acceptance of equipment, comprehension of its purpose, knowledge of its use, and provision of a maintenance system. The use of a wheelchair for mobility may be difficult for the patient or family to accept. Involvement in equipment selection may help them feel a part of the decision-making process and may help with acceptance and caretaking. The team should feel confident that the individual will consistently be positioned appropriately in the equipment in the discharge environment and that a positioning schedule will be followed. If the individual is not positioned correctly in the equipment or is left in it too long, the results may be detrimental, producing skin breakdown. It may be the decision of the team not to order equipment for the patient if they feel the follow through by the family or caregiver will be poor.

Funding

Purchase of equipment involves communication among the doctor, therapist, social worker, durable medical equipment (DME) dealer, third party payer, and family. Most DME dealers require prior financial approval from the third party payer before processing an order. A prescription and a letter of justification are often needed from the patient's physician. Documentation to assist in obtaining prior approval should be provided by the therapist. This may include goals and objectives of equipment, before and after pictures, and statements justifying the need for specific pieces of equipment. If reimbursement is not available through third party sources, charities, clubs, organizations, and churches are other possible sources of funding.

DETERMINING OPTIMAL POSITIONING AND INTERVENTION

Once preliminary data concerning functional needs are collected, the optimal positions for the individual and the means of intervention must be determined. General concepts of positioning have been developed by professionals studying the normal body and positions that provide optimal alignment, function, and comfort. Conceptualizing the normal biomechanical and neurodevelopmental components of sitting and formulating goals and objectives justifying the intervention used lead to optimal positioning (Midwest Regional RESNA/AART, 1986).

There is no "cookbook" method to proper seating, but a systematic approach following a developmental progression of proximal to distal can be applied. The pelvis is the first area of focus. Once the pelvis is stabilized, the therapist proceeds distally to the lower extremities, trunk, upper extremities, and head to assess positioning needs. With each intervention, note if the changes have affected positioning elsewhere in the body.

The majority of the equipment discussed and pictured in this unit describes systems used at RIC. Centers throughout the country use different types of equipment to produce the same effect. Technologic advances in the field of seating and positioning continuously change the materials and methods of fabrication used for seating systems. It is not the intent of the author to suggest or endorse specific equipment but to focus on how the equipment can assist in solving positioning problems. DME dealers, rehabilitation engineers, and seating specialists can be contacted to determine which materials and equipment sources will best fulfill the individual's needs.

HIPS AND LOWER EXTREMITIES

Tonal increases and tight hamstrings frequently found in patients pull the pelvis into a posterior tilt causing a rounded back and poor head alignment. If the pelvis is positioned on a level plane with a slight anterior tilt, the vertebrae align, allowing the facets to assist in providing trunk support. This position also provides greater weight distribution through the ischial tuberosities and femurs, decreasing the potential for pressure sores (Brunswic, 1984; Hage, 1985; Zacharkow, 1984). The neutral or slightly anteriorly tilted pelvis assists in inhibiting abnormal tone by preventing extension of the hips and encouraging cocontraction of the trunk muscles for assumption of active control (Saftler, Vaugn, & Hart, 1986).

The angle of the hip joint has an effect on pelvic alignment, weight distribution, and tonal influences. In this text, "hip angle" refers to the angle of measurement from the thigh to the anterior trunk. The optimal hip angle varies with the individual's needs and preferences and the therapist's theoretical philosophy. Optimally, the hip angle should support the desired pelvic position, and should range from 85° to 110° (Bergen & Colangelo, 1985; Payette, Albanese, & Carlson, 1985; Trefler, 1984; Ward, 1983).

The lower extremities should be in a neutral position, extending from the hip with the knees and ankles flexed to 90°. Feet are supported if they are not used to propel the wheelchair. Limitations at hips, knees, and ankles must be accommodated to provide maximal support.

Angle in Space

Angle in space refers to the patient's position in relation to the vertical plane. Changing angle in space refers to the procedure of tilting an entire seating system backward from an upright to a reclining position while maintaining the hip angle. The individual seated in the upright position may flop forward or demonstrate increased tone due to gravitational pull. By tilting the system backward, he may be able to demonstrate increased head and trunk control. Wheelchair bases providing a tilting mechanism are available, and travel wheelchairs have this component built in. Reclining wheelchairs may be used for this purpose if the seat is angled to maintain the desired hip angle. Function may be compromised when the individual is tilted back, as the effects of gravity are greater on the upper extremities during reaching activities. Feeding, swallowing, and visual orientation may also be compromised. For these reasons, an individual may require his position in space to be changed throughout the day to allow for participation in therapy and functional activities. For frequent changes, a travel chair or E & J Postura tilt hardware is recommended.

Firm Seat

With the introduction of the Everest and Jennings (E & J) folding wheelchair, the traditional wooden chair was replaced by a metallic frame with vinyl upholstery. Professionals and wheelchair users have noted that the vinyl tends to sag or "hammock" between the bars of the frame. For most individuals, this leads to a posterior pelvic tilt and adduction with internal rotation of the lower extremities. This promotes poor posture, decreased stability, and unequal weight bearing (Bergen & Colangelo, 1985; Trefler, 1984). A solution to this problem is to provide a firm base of support. This can be done by (1) purchasing a commercially available wheelchair with a folding firm seat, (2) inserting a firm board between the cushion and upholstery, or (3) mounting a solid seat board onto the frame.

When using a firm board between the cushion and the upholstery, the board may be covered with upholstery to prevent splintering. When using the mounted version, the board is modified for increased comfort. This is done by padding the board with pressure-distributing foam and then covering it with upholstery. A commercially available cushion can also be used on top of the board.

The mounted version, widely used at RIC, allows for stability of the seat board as well as adjustability in seat angle and height through the use of drop hook hardware (Figure 8-1).

Wedged Seat

A wedged seat decreases the patient's hip angle when seated in the wheelchair. Wedging the seat may be necessary for two reasons: (1) to increase the amount of hip flexion to counteract extensor tone and forward thrust of the hips, and (2) to maintain the desired hip angle when the individual requires a reclined position.

Wedging can be done by using a commercially available foam wedge, mounting the seat higher in front with adjustable drop hooks (Figure 8–2), or mounting E & J Postura tilt seat hardware onto a wheelchair frame. The knob in front of the Postura tilt seat allows for easy access to change the seat angle (Bergen, 1986b). If the wedged seat does not provide enough inhibition to control the extensor tone in the trunk and hips, an antithrust seat may be indicated.

Antithrust Seat

The theory behind the antithrust seat is to "form a soft tissue block which controls the inferior boney prominences of the pelvis in conjunction with a lap belt used to control the superior iliac crest" (Siekman & Flanigan, 1983). As the individual extends, the pelvis slides into the anterior roll, which prevents further extension. Eventually, the thrusting may decrease with resulting relaxation into the pelvic cutout. Siekman and Flanigan (1983) illustrate various shapes of the antithrust block to accommodate desired hip flexion and pelvic tilt. The shape and size of the antithrust block are determined by the amount of hip flexion needed to decrease the patient's extensor tone. Disadvantages of an antithrust seat are that the normal lordodic curve is de-

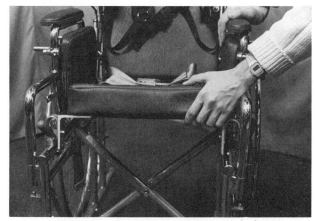

Figure 8–1 Drop hook hardware allows some adjustability in seat height and angle. The seat and back can be easily removed to fold the wheelchair.

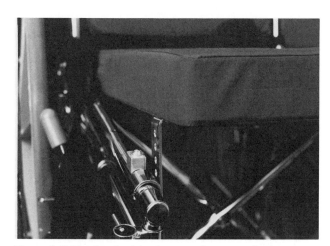

Figure 8–2 The drop hook hardware produces a wedged seat.

creased, the pelvis is slightly posteriorly tilted, and weight bearing may be increased at the ischial tuberosities.

Split Hip Angle Seat

Proper positioning accommodates hip angle discrepancies in individuals with ectopic bone or hip contractures. A split seat, allowing for varying hip angles, can be fabricated and antithrust features incorporated into the seat if necessary.

Seat Depth

Seat depth is measured from the buttocks to 1 inch to 1½ inches behind the popliteal fossa. It is necessary for the seat to extend this far to provide adequate stability for the distal femur and to decrease the chance of pressure where the seat rubs against the thigh. A seat extending farther cuts into the popliteal fossa, promoting extension of the lower extremities and a compensatory posterior pelvic tilt. Leg length discrepancy greater than 2 inches must be accommodated by fabricating one side of the seat deeper than the other. If the seat is fabricated to the measurements of the shorter leg, the longer leg will adduct and internally rotate, pulling the pelvis obliquely and posteriorly in an attempt to gain greater surface area support. If the seat is fabricated to the longer measurement, the seat will touch the shorter leg in the popliteal fossa or below, causing the leg to be pulled into extension with an oblique posteriorly tilted pelvis.

Seatbelts

In most cases, the pelvis must be stabilized to maintain the desired hip angle and pelvic tilt. The seatbelt is one of the primary stabilizers in maintaining optimal pelvic tilt. It should cross the pelvis at a 45° angle to the superior iliac crest (Bergen & Colangelo, 1985; Trefler, 1984).

The seatbelt can be attached at the bottom upholstery hole on the vertical upright bars of the wheelchair or at the second hole on the horizontal seat bars, depending on where the belt best stabilizes the pelvis. Auto-buckle and D-ring seatbelts are suggested, as they allow tightening once fastened and may help keep the hips positioned correctly in the wheelchair. Function and safety must be considered when determining the type of fastener. A cognitively aware individual may be inde-

pendent with transfers if able to don and doff the seatbelt. Agitated, impulsive, or unsafe individuals may have to be fitted with seatbelts that fasten behind or under the wheelchair to prevent independent seatbelt release.

Hip Blocks

Hip blocks center the pelvis in the seating system and prevent abduction of the femur. Hip blocks extending from the buttocks to the proximal femur are used to guide the pelvis, whereas those extending to the mid femur or knee assist in preventing abduction (Bergen, 1986b; Bergen & Colangelo, 1985) (Figure 8–3). With increased tone, hip blocks extending from the hip to the knee provide greater pressure distribution. However, small pads can be attached at the knee for localized support if distal pressure is enough to position the legs comfortably. Hip blocks are attached to the armrest to allow for ease in lateral transfers.

Pommel

A pommel, or adduction block, is used to prevent adduction and internal rotation of the lower extremi-

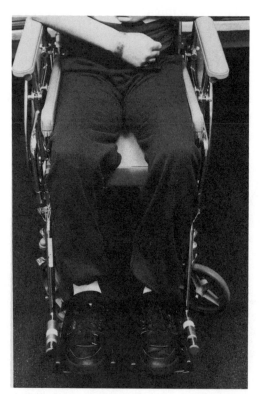

Figure 8–3 Hip blocks extending from hips to mid-femur guide hips and limit abduction.

ties. A pommel should not be used to hold an individual in the wheelchair or to stabilize the pelvis. A pommel placed from mid-thigh to the knees assists in reducing tone in the legs (Bergen & Colangelo, 1985). The width of the pommel should place the legs in a neutral position or in slight abduction. Surgical intervention, such as adductor releases, or a therapist's request for greater abduction to promote optimal seating may call for a wider pommel (Bergen, 1986b). A removable or flip down pommel allows for transfers, ease in catheter care, or use of a urinal (Figures 8–4 and 8–5).

Leg Rests

Elevating leg rests are generally adequate for positioning the lower extremities with greater than 90° of extension in the knee. To accommodate knees with less than 90° of extension, foot plates or a foot board may be placed behind the caster (Bergen & Colangelo, 1985; Butcher, 1985). Casters may have to be moved forward or changed in size from 8 inches to 5 inches to accommodate the foot board. The vertical bar of the leg rest may require bending to the desired angle. Commercially available adjustable angle foot plates (Pin Dot

Products) can also be used. For an individual with intermittent extension of the lower extremities, an elevating leg rest may be modified by removing the ratchet mechanism. This will allow the leg to swing up during extension but return to an optimal flexed position during relaxation.

Calf pads are used to prevent the lower extremities from slipping behind the foot plates. Webbing, latex material, or contoured Ethafoam may be incorporated if the commercially available pads are not effective or put too much pressure on the calves.

Foot Plates

The length of the leg rest affects the ankle, knee, and hip position. The feet should be supported to keep the knees in the optimal position with the femur parallel with the floor. The foot should be supported to achieve weight bearing through the heel and contact with the sole of the foot (Bergen & Colangelo, 1985; Trefler, 1984). Foot plates are available in several sizes and may be ordered customized through the manufacturer.

Angle adjustable footrests (E & J) are available to accommodate limitations of plantar flexion and dorsi-

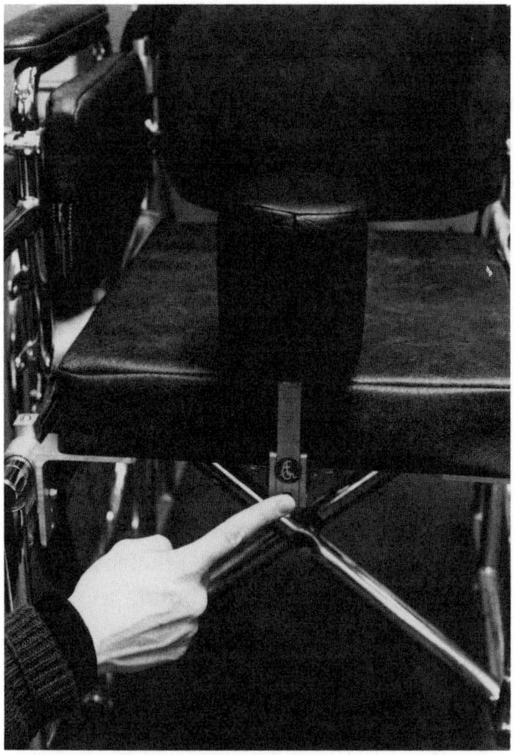

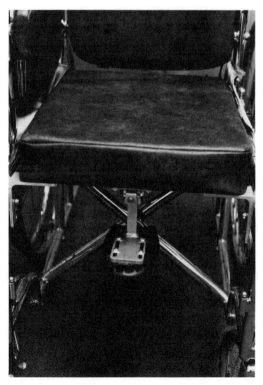

Figure 8–4 The pommel in the locked position can be released by pressing the button.

Figure 8–5 The pommel in the flipped down position for transfers or urinary care

flexion. These provide full surface contact to the sole of the foot and allow for modifications as ROM is gained. Ethafoam blocks can also be used for foot support. Heel loops may be necessary to keep the foot from sliding back on the footrest.

Ankle straps may assist in holding the foot in place (Figure 8–6). The strap should be placed at a 45° angle across the ankle and provide a downward, backward pull (Bergen & Colangelo, 1985). Excessive extensor tone may cause pressure against the strap, creating a potential for skin breakdown. In these cases, strapping may be contraindicated. If the patient's feet pull into crossed extension, a piece of Ethafoam placed on a foot board between the feet may prevent the feet from crossing each other.

TRUNK/BACK

The trunk should be supported as symmetrically as possible to provide stabilization, allowing for increased upper extremity function and head control. Flexible spinal deformities may be corrected, while accommodations must be made for those that are fixed.

Firm Back

Just as the sling seat affects the pelvis and the lower extremities, hammocking of the sling back promotes a kyphotic spine and provides little trunk stabilization (Bergen & Colangelo, 1985). A firm back may provide support to the spine to encourage back extension. Commercial backs can be attached with Velcro or strapped to the chair. A firm board covered with foam and then upholstered can be mounted on the frame with adjustable drop hooks. This is the alternative most commonly used at RIC, as modifications can be made in the desired angle of recline.

For some individuals, a firm upright back may be too rigid, causing pressure at the mid-thoracic level of the vertebrae. This may be modified by:

- changing the contour of the back
- decreasing the firmness of the back
- modifying the lordodic support
- tilting the individual back in space

In some cases, semirigid material or closed cell foam can be inserted between the patient's back and the upholstery to provide a firm surface without a hard board.

Back Height

Back height is determined by the individual's head, trunk, and upper extremity control. Individuals with poor trunk control may require back support to the top of the shoulders. This allows for attachment of a headrest or shoulder straps. For patients with poor trunk control but with functional use of their upper extremities, back support to just below the inferior angle of the scapula is recommended.

Lumbar Supports

The lumbar area is gaining increased attention as professionals are becoming attuned to wheelchair user's complaints of low back pain or the development of a slumped posture. Zacharkow (1984) and Hage (1985) promote using lumbar supports for individuals with passively mobile lumbar spines. These help stabilize the pelvis at the desired tilt while supporting the lower back. Measurements can be taken of the lordodic space created when the individual is positioned appropriately in the seating system. The thickness and height of the lumbar roll should be according to the natural curve of the patient's spine. A lumbar roll that is too thick or that extends too far into the thoracic area tends to push the individual out of the chair or to promote hyperextension of the spine. Lumbar supports are commercially available, or can be custom made, and should be stabilized to prevent slippage.

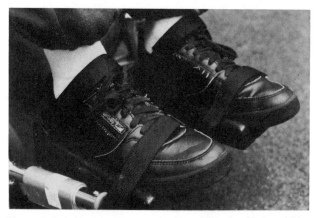

Figure 8–6 Ankle straps are attached at a 45° angle with the addition of toe straps.

Lateral Trunk Supports

Trunk supports provide stability to prevent lateral flexion and free the patient's arms for function. Placement of the trunk supports should not be determined until the individual is positioned in the seat and back with proper lower extremity support. In some cases, the stability the individual receives from the seat and back make lateral supports unnecessary.

Trunk supports should be placed a minimum of four fingerwidths below the axilla to avoid brachial plexus injury. The higher and closer the supports are in relation to the trunk, the greater the external stability provided. Bilateral trunk supports are suggested as they provide three points of control, one at either side and one posteriorly (Trefler, 1984). By providing support on both sides of the trunk, the individual is less likely to lean into or away from a trunk support. The trunk supports may be positioned slightly away from the trunk to encourage dynamic trunk movement and should allow for trunk expansion and warm clothing.

Trunk supports can be placed obliquely or symmetrically, depending on how the individual responds to the tactile input. Oblique trunk supports are often used for individuals who lean excessively to one side or who are beginning to establish a spinal curve. The higher trunk support is placed on the flexed side of the trunk, and the lower support acts as a counterbalance.

Considerations for determining the type of trunk support to use are:

- durability and strength needed to support the body
- availability of mounting space on the firm back
- ease of removal for transfers
- thickness of the trunk pad
- cosmesis

A trunk support system therapists have found effective was designed by Kozole and Hedman of the Rehabilitation Engineering Department at RIC. It consists of a piece of Kydex, which is padded, upholstered, and attached to a double-hinged hardware system that is screwed into the backrest. The trunk support system is durable, easy to use, and flips away to allow for lateral transfers (Figure 8–7).

Commercially available hardware can be used with the Kydex trunk supports. The hardware attaches to the firm back, and the support is removable. It is often used when the solid back is not wide enough for mounting of

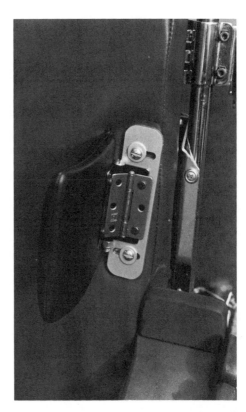

Figure 8–7 The RIC lateral trunk support attachment hardware allows for quick release for ease in transfers.

the RIC trunk supports (Figure 8–8). Otto Bock trunk supports attach to the uprights of the chair and swing away. They can be used when hardware cannot be attached to the firm seat or when greater height adjustability is desired (Figure 8–9).

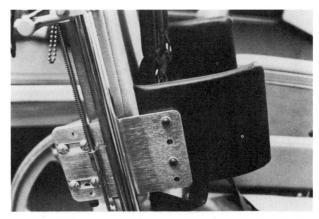

Figure 8–8 The removable lateral trunk hardware by Creative Rehabilitation Equipment attaches Adaptive Engineering Laboratory lateral trunk support pads to a firm back.

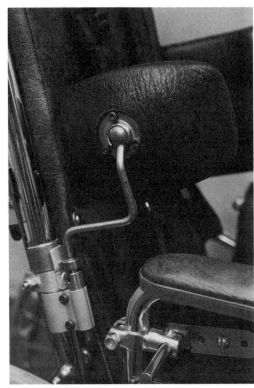

Figure 8–9 Otto Bock swing away lateral trunk supports attach to the wheelchair uprights.

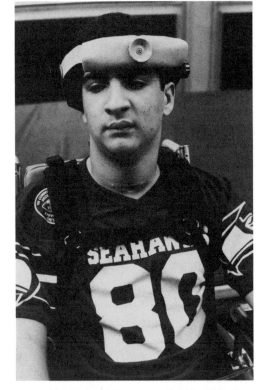

Figure 8–10 An H-strap has foam padding at the shoulders for comfort. The top and bottom straps are attached to the firm back of the wheelchair.

Anterior Chest Supports

The H-strap and butterfly vest provide a backward pull at the shoulders and are used to prevent forward flexion of the trunk. The H-strap depicts an "H" as two vertical straps are attached to the backrest at the top and at the bottom. The horizontal portion crosses the chest, connecting the vertical straps (Figure 8–10). Bergen and Colangelo (1985) suggest one-inch straps for children and two-inch straps for adults. A butterfly vest provides greater surface support at the chest. It is used when a firm anterior counterforce is needed (Figure 8–11). The straps used for the H-strap or butterfly vest can provide joint approximation through the shoulders. If the backrest ends slightly below the shoulders, approximation will occur when the straps are attached to the backrest. If the backrest is higher than the shoulders, the straps should be attached to the anterior of the backrest, behind the scapula.

HEAD POSITION

The optimal position for the head is in slight ventroflexion in midline, while neutrally aligned with the

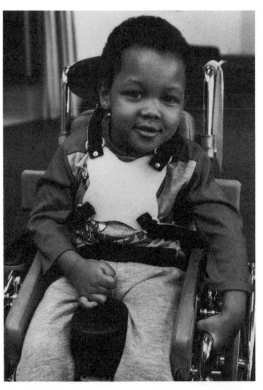

Figure 8–11 The butterfly vest is used primarily with children.

shoulders. Many patients in early stages of recovery have poor head control, generally influenced by abnormal tone or muscle weakness. The body should, therefore, be positioned optimally before deciding on intervention for the head.

Posterior Support

Posterior support is the most common intervention for weak neck extensors. While addition of a standard head extension may be all that is needed, it often does not provide enough support to maintain the head in the vertical position against the effects of gravity or abnormal tone. Commercially available or customized headrests may prevent this. Equipment commercially available includes:

- Otto Bock head and neck supports that can be attached to a firm back or uprights of the wheelchair (Figure 8–12)
- Miller Special Products headrest that attaches to the firm back and drops down to allow intermittent use (Figure 8–13)
- MEDCO hardware that attaches to a firm back

All offer adjustability for height, angle of support, and anterior/posterior movement. If a patient responds adversely to the tactile stimulation in the occipital region by hyperextending the head, a neck ring is suggested.

Anterior Head Support

A forehead strap is available on the Miller headrest and can be attached to the Otto Bock when greater anterior support is needed. However, when abnormal tone in the neck flexors is severe, an anterior forehead band may irritate the skin. Slightly reclining the patient's position in space decreases the effects of gravity and may assist in positioning the head. A neck collar providing additional anterior support may also be effective. A soft collar combined with posterior support may be effective in patients with minimal tone but is usually not enough to counteract severe flexor tone. A Plastizote collar reinforced with low-temperature plastic or commercially available anterior neck supports (Danmar) can be effective. A modified cervical orthosis may also be considered and is cosmetically more acceptable than a plastic collar.

Lateral Head Support

Lateral flexion of the head and neck can be prevented by the use of lateral blocks attached to an extended firm-back chair. Lateral supports should not obstruct the visual field or push against the ear. Commercially available models provide adjustable hinges on the supports (STC, MEDCO), allowing variable angle placement, dependent on the individual's needs. Intarsia manufactures a headrest that provides posterior support to the occiput combined with lateral head support. It is made of Kydex and can be cut to the desired length and heated to adjust the angle of lateral support.

UPPER EXTREMITY POSITIONING

The scapula must be able to move freely to allow full humeral motion. If the arms require support, the lap

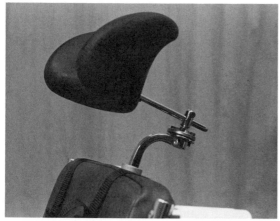

Figure 8–12 The Otto Bock headrest.

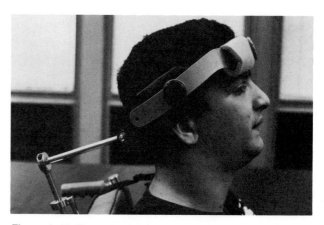

Figure 8–13 The Miller Special Products headrest with forehead strap attached

board or armrests should be placed at a height that will maintain the integrity of the glenohumeral joint without pushing the shoulder girdle into elevation or allowing subluxation.

Scapular and Shoulder Intervention

Abnormal muscle tone in the upper trunk can produce scapular retraction, protraction, or humeral extension. When the scapula is retracted, protraction blocks can be incorporated into the seating system by building up the surface of the hard back or attaching wedges before upholstering (Bergen & Colangelo, 1985). Protraction blocks work best when they extend from the medial border to the superior lateral border of the scapula. This cups the scapula, promoting the protraction necessary for forward reach.

If the upper extremities are pulled into excessive protraction and internal rotation, retractor pads will assist in bringing the scapula back into a neutral position (Bergen & Colangelo, 1985). Retractors should provide a gentle pull at the clavicle and head of the humerus. Commercially available devices (Theradyne, Mullhulland) can be attached to a customized seating system.

Shoulder extension at the humeral joint can be counteracted by mounting humeral blocks on the lap board. The length of the block is determined by the amount of surface area needed to control the upper extremities (Figure 8–14). Blocks are fabricated from Ethafoam, covered with pressure-reducing foam, and then upholstered.

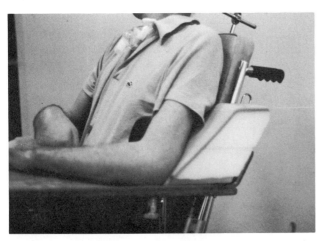

Figure 8–14 Humeral blocks attached to the patient's lap tray can be removable or permanently attached.

Arm Boards and Lap Trays

Support provided for the upper extremities through the use of arm boards and lap trays may improve posture by decreasing the pull of gravity on the arms, causing forward flexion of the trunk (Bergen, 1986b). Arm boards or arm troughs attach to the armrests. Both are commercially available or can be custom fabricated. They are the choice for individuals whose arms can be placed in neutral without severe increased elbow flexor tone pulling the arm medially into internal rotation. This allows the arms to be supported without "cutting the body in half," as a lap board does. Webbing straps may be used for stabilization.

A lap board provides greater surface area for placement of objects when arm function is limited. Lap boards made of Plexiglas allow the patient to view the lower extremities and see where they are going. Communication systems, environmental control units, or electric wheelchair controls may be incorporated onto the surface of the lap board. When upper extremity function is limited, disciplines must cooperate and set priorities with the patient as to placement of switches for optimal function.

Overhead Slings

Overhead suspension slings are made of cuffs at the elbow and wrist that attach to a rod fastened to the wheelchair. They are used to facilitate upper extremity movement by placing the arm in a gravity-eliminated position. The available arc of motion is determined by the distance between the point of suspension and the cuffs. The longer the distance, the greater the arc. Shoulder abduction, horizontal abduction and adduction, and elbow flexion and extension can be assisted by the use of overhead slings (Taylor, 1986). They are frequently effective in controlling edema. With a flaccid extremity, periodic checks to ensure glenohumeral alignment should be made.

NONLINEAR CONTOURED CUSTOMIZED SYSTEMS

For individuals with contractures, boney prominences, spinal curvatures, or other boney deformities of the trunk, linear systems may not provide enough surface contact with the body. This results in undue pressure and skin problems on the parts of the body coming in contact with the seating system. By contouring the system, greater surface area for support can be provided, producing comfort, decreased pressure, and greater stability. Some of the following systems require specialized training and equipment to use. It is suggested that the therapist contact the manufacturers directly to obtain further information.

Methods of providing a contoured system include:

- hand-carved foam
- high-temperature plastic formed from plaster body casts (Payette et al., 1985)
- foam in place, which is a two-piece seating system fitted in the wheelchair. Custom cushions are created using a chemical mixture poured into bags which produces a foam that rises to form around the patient.
- matrix, developed by the Bioengineering Center of University College, London, which is a sheet of plates held together by metal washers and screws. The highly adjustable sheets allow for repeated modifications.
- bead seat, developed by the University of Tennessee, uses vacuum consolidation to mold the cushion. Beads that are enclosed in bags are mixed with epoxy. Then, the desired patient position is determined. The vacuum maintains the position until the epoxy sets (Hobson, Heinrich, & Hands, 1983; Hobson, Taylor, & Shaw, 1986).
- contour-U, which is a simulator frame with separate rubber bags for the seat and back filled with beads. Air is evacuated to allow shaping to the patient. Plaster molds are taken of the formed bags and used to fabricate the foam cushions. This system uses a centralized process.

ALTERNATIVE POSITIONS

Bed Positioning

Proper bed positioning is a critical factor involving nursing, therapists, families, and caretakers. A program consisting of pillow propping and frequent turning is started upon the individual's admission to the hospital. In most cases, sleep promotes relaxation, and pillows suffice as props. However, with some individuals, a predominance of tone still exists while at rest, which may lead to abnormal patterning of the trunk, head, and extremities. Discomfort, contractures, decubiti, or deformity may result from uncorrected posturing.

When pillows are not firm enough to prevent tonal influences of position, definitive positioning pieces of Ethafoam and T-foam can be fabricated to provide the necessary support. The therapist should determine the position that promotes the most relaxation. Supine positioning generally requires little intervention with the exception of pillow placement or firm guides along the side of the bed to prevent rolling. For positioning in sidelying, a single bed with side rails is recommended. Ethafoam is cut into the shapes conforming to the desired positions, padded with pressure-reducing foam, and upholstered. Pieces are attached with straps to the side rail for stabilization. Other pieces to promote extremity flexion or extension are attached either to the positioning bolster at the trunk or to the opposite side rail (Figures 8–15 and 8–16).

Sidelyers

Static positioning, even in a well-designed seating system, can be detrimental if it is the only position provided (Bergen & Colangelo, 1985; Trefler, 1984; Ward, 1983). An individual will begin to "look like the chair" and may develop contractures and muscle tightness if not offered position changes during the day. Position changes are suggested to alter the gravitational pull on the body, allow the individual to move muscles not used in the seated position, and provide diversified environmental stimulation. Definitive equipment may be suggested to assist in maintaining the individual in various positions. Sidelyers are frequently used with children and can be incorporated into home, school, and therapy programs allowing for play. Sidelyers are occasionally used successfully with adults but are often cumbersome. Many families of adults opt for intervention that incorporates sidelying in bed.

Sidelying is an excellent position for the severely motorically involved individual as it places the head, arms, and body in a gravity-eliminated position. This may break up abnormal tone and encourage increased function (Bergen & Colangelo, 1985; Trefler, 1984). The sidelyer generally consists of two main pieces, one horizontal and one vertical. The individual lays on his side on the horizontal portion with the vertical piece angled against the body. The therapist must decide if the angle desired should be acute, perpendicular, or obtuse, depending on the therapeutic goals and the indi-

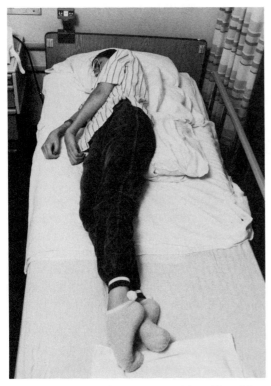

Figure 8–15 The patient's position in sidelying without intervention

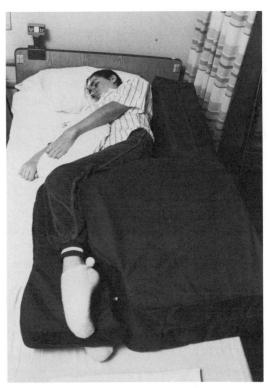

Figure 8–16 Positioning bolsters attached to side rails of the hospital bed reduce some of the patient's extensor tone.

vidual's comfort. A pelvic strap across the iliac crest assists in maintaining the sidelying position. Additional pieces can be added to position the head, legs, and arms. Once the individual is placed in sidelying, the therapist should evaluate the lower extremities to determine if reciprocal or symmetric placement is desired. Pieces can be attached with Velcro where desired to enable the individual to be positioned on both sides.

THE POSITIONING PROGRAM

Positioning intervention must be integrated into the therapy program and daily regimen of the individual. Education of staff and primary caregivers is essential to ensure carryover for positioning goals.

Once positioning intervention takes place, a written schedule should be provided for the staff. It will vary as the individual adjusts to and builds tolerance for the equipment. In the beginning stages, the positioning system may be used only during therapy to allow the therapist to monitor effectiveness closely and make modifications before allowing the individual to use the equipment on the nursing floor or at home.

Family and staff teaching should include:

- instruction in the purpose and benefits of using the provided equipment
- proper handling for placement of the patient in the system
- schedule for use of equipment and position changes
- precautions
- care of equipment

The teaching is usually done verbally with visual demonstration of the equipment or with the patient. A pictorial and/or written program may assist with follow through and use of equipment.

RIC has developed a generic pictorial home program detailing the purpose, placement, and care for each piece of positioning equipment issued for wheelchair seating systems. Each piece is described on separate sheets of paper, allowing the therapist to provide the caregiver with information illustrating only the equipment issued. Polaroid pictures of the patient in the system are also provided. A follow-up plan should be formulated with the family and therapists to monitor the positioning system for modifications that may become necessary.

A positioning system does not take the place of therapy but is an adjunct to it. The ideal positioning system provides optimal support, body alignment, and function with the minimum amount of equipment. It reflects the needs of the patient without being an equipment burden to the patient's caregivers. A positioning system can be very effective, yet the patient will benefit from time out of the system during therapy and rest periods. This enables him to experience the sensory input and mobility often unavailable to one confined to a wheelchair or a positioning system.

REFERENCES

Anderson, B.S., Murphy, R., Ortengran, R., & Nachemson, A.L. (1979). The influence of backrest inclination and lumbar support on lumbar lordosis. *Spine, 4*(1), 52–58.

Bergen, A.F. (1986a). The prescriptive wheelchair: An orthetic device: 1–4. *Home Care, 2–4* May-August.

Bergen, A.F. (1986b). Seating assessment and options. Instructional Course. Minneapolis: Rehabilitation Engineering Society of North America, Association for the Advancement of Rehabilitation Technology.

Bergen, A.F., & Colangelo, C. (1985). *Positioning the client with central nervous system deficits: The wheelchair and other adapted equipment* (2nd ed.). Valhalla, NY: Valhalla Rehabilitation Publications.

Bergman, J. (1986). *Position in life is everything or is it?* Birmingham, AL: Tutorial Sparks Center.

Brunswic, M. (1984). Ergonomics of seat design. *Physiotherapy, 70*(2), xx–xx.

Butcher, B. (1985). Foot support with 90° knee flexion on adult wheelchairs. *Proceedings of the Eighth Annual Conference on Rehabilitation Technology.* Memphis, TN: Rehabilitation Engineering Society of North America, Association for the Advancement of Rehabilitation Technology.

Hage, M. (1985). *Ischial and femoral weight bearing during anterior and posterior sitting postures.* Unpublished master's thesis, PT School, Northwestern University, Evanston, IL.

Hill, J., & Presperin, J. (1986). Orthotic management and positioning. In J. Hill (Ed.), *Spinal cord injury: A guide to functional outcomes in occupational therapy.* Rockville, MD: Aspen Publishers.

Hobson, D.A., Heinrich, M.J., & Hands, S.F. (1983). Bead seat insert and seating system. *Proceedings of the Sixth Annual Conference on Rehabilitation Technology.* Washington, D.C.: Rehabilitation Engineering Society of North America, Association for the Advancement of Rehabilitation Technology.

Hobson, D., Taylor, S.J., & Shaw, G. (1986). Bead matrix insert system: A follow-up clinical report. *Proceedings of the Ninth Annual Conference on Rehabilitation Technology.* Minneapolis, MN: Rehabilitation Engineering Society of North America, Association for the Advancement of Rehabilitation Technology.

Midwest Regional RESNA/AART Special Interest Group on Seating and Wheelchairs. 1986. Proceedings of Fall Meeting, Iowa City, Iowa. Washington, D.C.: Rehabilitation Engineering Society of North America, Association for the Advancement of Rehabilitation Technology.

Nwaobi, O., & Smith, P. (1986). Effect of adaptive seating on pulmonary function in children with CP. *Proceedings of the Eighth Annual Conference on Rehabilitation Technology.* Washington, D.C.: Rehabilitation Engineering Society of North America, Association for the Advancement of Rehabilitation Technology.

Payette, M., Albanese, M.K., & Carlson, J.M. (1985). "Custom seating at Gillette Children's Hospital. *Proceedings of the Eighth Annual Conference on Rehabilitation Technology.* Washington, D.C.: Rehabilitation Engineering Society of North America, Association for the Advancement of Rehabilitation Technology.

Saftler, F., Vaugn, K., & Hart, J. (1986). Therapeutic seating for the developmentally disabled. *Proceedings of Therapeutic Equipment Specialist Regional Workshops,* Orlando, Florida.

Siekman, A.R., & Flanigan, K. (1983). The anti-thrust seat: A wheelchair insert for individuals with abnormal reflex patterns or other specialized problems. *Proceedings of the Sixth Annual Conference on Rehabilitation Technology.* Washington, D.C.: Rehabilitation Engineering Society of North America, Association for the Advancement of Rehabilitation Technology.

Taylor, S.J. (1986). *Adapted seating for adult and pediatric clients.* Lecture, Brick, NJ.

Trefler, E. (1984). *Seating for children with cerebral palsy: A resource manual.* Unpublished manuscript, University of Tennessee, Rehabilitation Engineer Program, Memphis.

Trombley, C., & Scott, A. (1977). *Occupational therapy for physical dysfunction.* Baltimore: Williams & Wilkins.

Ward, D. (1983). *Positioning the handicapped child for function: A guide to evaluate and prescribe equipment for the child with CNS dysfunction.* St. Louis: Phoenix Press.

Zacharkow, D. (1984). *Wheelchair posture and pressure sores.* Springfield, IL: Charles C Thomas.

Part IV

Daily Living Skills

Self-Care and Homemaking

Anita Van Dam-Burke, OTR/L
Karen Kovich, OTR/L

The goal of occupational therapy (OT) for each patient is to promote the maximum level of independence in daily living skills. In everyday life, through repetition, a routine is established, enabling individuals to complete self-care with little thought or effort. While these tasks remain familiar to the head-injured patient, a combination of cognitive, sensory-perceptual, and motor deficits may make it difficult for him to complete tasks as he did before the injury. Cognitive and sensory-perceptual deficits may cause a loss of the ability to draw on previously learned patterns of behavior that allow for performance of tasks at an automatic level. Persistent motor deficits may make it necessary for the patient to use adaptive equipment or alternative techniques. Daily living skills training is a comprehensive program that integrates evaluation results and short-term goals from all related areas. Training programs are designed for each patient, taking into consideration individual roles, interests, and responsibilities.

Several principles may be applied when working with head-injured patients toward a goal of maximum independence.

- The most effective method of assistance must be determined for each patient.

Various types and amounts of assistance may be used. These include cueing, physical assistance, and adaptive equipment. Cueing may be verbal, tactile, or visual. It is important to identify deficits in the sensory system to determine which type of cueing will be most effective. Tactile cues, hand-over-hand assistance, and verbal sequencing may be more beneficial than visual imitation in helping patients with severe motor planning deficits relearn motor patterns. Patients with speech and language deficits may benefit more from a combination of visual and tactile cues than verbal cues. An agitated patient may respond to verbal and visual cues yet be unable to tolerate frequent tactile cues. Cognitive and sensory-perceptual deficits may limit the use of adaptive equipment. A dressing stick, which is helpful for a patient with limited hip range of motion (ROM), may complicate task performance if motor planning deficits are present or if the patient has difficulty learning new tasks. A button hook, frequently indicated for patients with decreased fine motor control, may be difficult to use with visual perceptual deficits.

- The patient's potential for new learning must be determined before deciding on specific techniques for intervention or adaptive equipment.

It is important to gain information on the potential for new learning. This can be determined through observation of the patient's performance of unfamiliar tasks. Formal testing by the clinical psychologist may also provide helpful information on learning style, such as the patient's potential to learn a new technique and use adaptive equipment or the amount of repetition necessary for new learning.

- Quality and efficiency of performance of daily living skills must be considered in determining realistic expectations for each patient.

Although patients are encouraged to be as independent as possible, lack of quality and efficiency may limit functional capabilities. A patient may have the motor control required to get a toothbrush to his mouth yet be unable to brush enough to insure adequate oral hygiene. A patient who can feed himself may require 2 hours to complete a meal. The therapist must determine whether the skills of the patient are at a level that ensures safe, healthy, and timely performance of daily living tasks.

- Repetition and consistency of approach are vital to the learning and carryover of daily living skills.

Tasks are practiced on a daily basis, using the same techniques, equipment, position, and amount of cueing. This information is conveyed to nursing staff, family members, and others working with the patient to aid in incorporating newly learned techniques into the daily routine.

At the Rehabilitation Institute of Chicago (RIC), OT programming in self-care activities focuses on the following areas of function.

- feeding
- grooming
- dressing
- bathing
- meal preparation
- light homemaking

The results of the initial evaluation and periodic reevaluations in these areas form the framework for the self-care program.

Self-care training is an ongoing program during rehabilitation. It begins with patients at the awakening level. At this level, prefunctional tasks are emphasized to establish participation and the component skills necessary to begin more formal self-care training. As the patient progresses and component skills improve, self-

care training continues, following a graded progression, toward the goal of maximum independence. Increasing the patient's independence in activities of daily living (ADL) may reduce reliance on caregivers, improve self-esteem, and facilitate return to premorbid roles, interests, and responsibilities.

RATING PERFORMANCE IN DAILY LIVING SKILLS

At RIC, performance of daily living skills is rated on initial and discharge evaluations according to the Rehabilitation Institute of Chicago Functional Assessment Scale (RIC-FAS). This seven-point scale was developed by the Institute and is shown in Table 9–1. It is used to rate performance of functional activities specific to each discipline.

Exhibit 9–1 is the rating form used on the OT initial/discharge evaluation. Major daily living tasks addressed in OT are listed in bold face as core items. Below each core item, subskills necessary for completion of the item are listed. Upon initial evaluation, each subskill is rated by placing an "A," indicating admission status, under the appropriate level of performance. A total rating for the item is then determined based on performance of the subskills. After the initial rating, the therapist sets a long-term goal by placing a "G" in the rating of expected performance. On initial evaluation, all core items must be rated with the exception of meal preparation, homemaking, and community inte-

TABLE 9–1   Functional assessment scale

Rating	Level of performance
7	Independent
6	Independent with equipment or adapted environment
5	Independent with set-up
4	Minimal assistance: patient performs 75% of the task or greater, or requires intermittent supervision or cueing
3	Moderate assistance: patient performs 50% to 75% of task, or requires continuous supervision or cueing
2	Maximal assistance: patient performs 25% to 50% of task or performs less than 25% but can direct care
1	Dependent: patient requires total physical assistance

Exhibit 9–1 Initial rating form

REHABILITATION INSTITUTE OF CHICAGO
OCCUPATIONAL THERAPY DEPARTMENT (PAGE 3)

Patient _John Smith_

RIC No. _____

Date _____

[X] Initial ☐ Re-evaluation ☐ Discharge

V. SELF-CARE ACTIVITIES

KEY
7 = Independent
6 = Independent with equipment
5 = Independent with set-up
4 = Minimal assistance (patient performs 75% or >)
3 = Moderate assistance (patient performs 50 to 75%)
2 = Maximal assistance (includes dependent but can direct care) (patient performs 25 to 50%)
1 = Dependent (25% or <)
0 = Not applicable or patient not responsible for these tasks. Only selectable for certain items.

ALL CORE ITEMS NOTED WITH BOLD LETTERING MUST BE RATED. If skills vary within component groups, the more dependent rating is used for the core item functional level. If there is *NO goal*, or the patient is already at his/her expected level, rate the goal the same as the functional level. *Meal Preparation, Homemaking and Community Re-integration,* may be deferred until they may be appropriately addressed. On discharge, the date the goal was set shall be noted in the Date Column.

A = ADMISSION STATUS   G = DISCHARGE GOAL   CIRCLE = DISCHARGE STATUS

	0	1	2	3	4	5	6	7	Comments/Equipment
FEEDING	■				A		G		
Hand to Mouth								A	
Utensil Use						A			
Cup Use						A			
Cut Food		A							
UE DRESSING	■				A			G	
UE On					A				
UE Off								A	
Fastners					A				
LE DRESSING	■			A		G			
LE On				A					
LE Off					A				
Socks/Shoes				A					
TOILETING	■			A		G			
Manage Clothes					A				
Manage Leg Bag		A							
Hygiene				A					
GROOMING	■					A	G		
Wash Face/Hands							A		
Brush Teeth						A			
Comb/Brush Hair						A			
Shave/Make-up						A			
BATHING	■			A	G				
Sponge						A			
Shower		A							
Tub				A					
COMMUNICATION	■			A			G		
Writing				A					
Telephone					A				
Typing				A					
MEAL PREPARATION Date	A								
Basic									
Complex									
HOMEMAKING		A							
Light Homemaking									
Heavy Homemaking									
COMMUNITY INTEGRATION		A							
Planning									
Resource Utilization									
Money Management									
Safety Considerations									

Page 3   Therapist _____   Date _____

Exhibit 9–2 Discharge rating form

REHABILITATION INSTITUTE OF CHICAGO
OCCUPATIONAL THERAPY DEPARTMENT (PAGE 3)

Patient _John Smith_
RIC No. _____
Date _____

☐ Initial   ☐ Re-evaluation   ☒ Discharge

V. SELF-CARE ACTIVITIES

KEY 7 = Independent
6 = Independent with equipment
5 = Independent with set-up
4 = Minimal assistance (patient performs 75% or >)

3 = Moderate assistance (patient performs 50 to 75%)
2 = Maximal assistance (includes dependent but can direct care) (patient performs 25 to 50%)
1 = Dependent (25% or <)
0 = Not applicable or patient not responsible for these tasks. Only selectable for certain items.

ALL CORE ITEMS NOTED WITH BOLD LETTERING MUST BE RATED. If skills vary within component groups, the more dependent rating is used for the core item functional level. If there is **NO goal**, or the patient is already at his/her expected level, rate the goal the same as the functional level. **Meal Preparation, Homemaking and Community Re-integration,** may be deferred until they may be appropriately addressed. On discharge, the date the goal was set shall be noted in the Date Column.

A = ADMISSION STATUS   G = DISCHARGE GOAL   CIRCLE = DISCHARGE STATUS

	0	1	2	3	4	5	6	7	Comments/Equipment
FEEDING	■				A		(G)		
Hand to Mouth								0	
Utensil Use								0	
Cup Use								0	
Cut Food						0			
UE DRESSING	■				A		(G)		
UE On								0	
UE Off								0	
Fastners								0	
LE DRESSING	■			A		G	0		
LE On								0	
LE Off								0	
Socks/Shoes						0			
TOILETING	■			A	(G)/0				
Manage Clothes									
Manage Leg Bag		0							
Hygiene							0		
GROOMING	■				A		(G)		
Wash Face/Hands								0	
Brush Teeth								0	
Comb/Brush Hair								0	
Shave/Make-up								0	
BATHING	■			A	G	0			
Sponge								0	
Shower					0				
Tub									
COMMUNICATION	■			A			(G)		
Writing								0	
Telephone								0	
Typing									

	Date	0	1	2	3	4	5	6	7	Comments/Equipment
MEAL PREPARATION	Date				A	(G)				
Basic	8/1					A				
Complex				A						
HOMEMAKING	8/1				A	(G)				
Light Homemaking						A				
Heavy Homemaking				A						
COMMUNITY INTEGRATION					A	(G)				
Planning					A					
Resource Utilization					A					
Money Management					A					
Safety Considerations					A					

Page 3   Therapist _____   Date _____

gration. Initial rating on these may be deferred to a time when they are more appropriately addressed. Should the ratings of these items be deferred, the date the initial status and goal was determined must be noted in the date column on the discharge evaluation.

At the discharge evaluation, admission ratings and goals of core items are transferred from the initial evaluation form. Status at discharge is indicated by placing a circle in the appropriate level of performance (Exhibit 9–2). Through this method, the discharge evaluation clearly shows the patient's initial status, the goal that was set, and the progress the patient made.

FEEDING

Feeding includes all aspects of eating and drinking, such as sucking, chewing, swallowing, using appropriate utensils, opening containers, and pouring liquid. Feeding training may relate to the facilitation and development of normal oral motor movement in patients who exhibit abnormal patterns as a result of injury. Another focus may be self-feeding. The goal in both cases is to maximize independent function. For some patients, a comprehensive feeding program may include short-term goals in both areas. In other cases, self-feeding may need to be delayed until oral motor function is optimized. The therapist uses evaluation results in all areas related to feeding to design and implement a successful program.

Cognitive Considerations

General level of arousal and attention span are important to consider when designing a feeding program. To begin feeding training, the patient must be alert, able to respond to the presence of food in the mouth, and actively attempt to control it. Alert patients must be able to attend to a task for 5 minutes. With attention deficits or behavior problems, such as agitation, feeding begins in a low-stimulus environment, such as the patient's room. Verbal cueing may be necessary to redirect attention back to the task. If the patient becomes agitated or upset during a meal, eating is briefly discontinued until he is calm and able to be redirected. As attention increases and behavior problems subside, eating is attempted in a more stimulating and social environment, such as the patient dining area or cafeteria. The patient may require increased verbal cueing to maintain attention.

Impulsivity, demonstrated by an inability to monitor the rate and amount of food intake, is often seen in self-feeding. Verbal and tactile cues, serving one item of food at a time, or using small portions provide the patient with an external monitoring system. Instructing the patient to put the utensil down after every one or two bites until the mouth is cleared may also help slow the rate of eating.

Memory deficits may interfere with independent feeding. A patient may be unable to remember compensation techniques from one meal to the next. He may also forget when the last meal was eaten or how long it is until the next. If the patient uses a memory book, it is helpful to record the time of each meal and the specific foods that were eaten. The therapist or caregiver can then refer the patient to the memory book rather than answer repeated questions regarding the time of the next meal.

Sensory-Perceptual Considerations

Apraxia or motor planning deficits may be marked by an inability to bring the hand to the mouth, use utensils correctly, or properly sequence the task. If these deficits are severe, verbal sequencing of the task before beginning may assist the patient in conceptualizing it. Hand-over-hand assistance may be required to help the patient develop a more automatic hand-to-mouth pattern. With mild apraxia or improved motor planning, tactile or verbal cues may be sufficient.

Decreased visual scanning or field deficits may interfere with a patient's ability to locate food in front of him. Patients with both deficits may attend to food on only one section of the plate. Before starting, it may be beneficial to have the patient identify all items of food in the meal. Verbal cues may be used to direct the patient to scan all areas of the table rather than moving all food into the limited field of vision. Tactile cues, such as gently turning the patient's head, may also improve visual scanning.

Decreased sensory awareness may lead to pocketing of food in the cheek. Tactile cues, such as touching or rubbing the outside of the cheek, may increase the patient's awareness of food in the mouth. Verbal reminders or visual cues, such as demonstrating how to use a finger to clear the mouth, may also be helpful.

Motor Considerations

The optimal position for feeding is sitting with 90° of hip flexion, feet supported, and trunk and neck in midline. The neck should be slightly flexed (10°) to allow for ease of swallowing (Figure 9–1) (Farber, 1982). Feeding is contraindicated if the head is in extreme flexion or extension. It is difficult and dangerous to swallow in this position. If correct positioning cannot be maintained independently, external supports such as those pictured in Unit 8 may be necessary. In the absence of external supports the therapist can support the patient's head with one hand while feeding him with the other. In case of severe tone, which may make head positioning difficult, feeding may require two people with one person holding the patient's head in the optimal position while the therapist attempts feeding. As head and trunk control improve, external supports may be eliminated and assistance decreased.

Effective oral motor control is essential to feeding. A thorough evaluation must be completed to identify specific deficits that interfere with feeding (Unit 2). Once evaluation establishes that the individual can take food by mouth, training begins. The program may be two-tiered. Specific facilitation and inhibition techniques are used to normalize oral motor patterns. At the same time, foods are graded to require the patient to use increasingly more complex motor patterns. The combination of approaches allows the patient to move toward self-feeding.

Feeding training often begins with small amounts of food (1/2 teaspoon) of pureed consistency, such as pudding or baby food. Thick liquids, such as nectars or juices, thickened with baby food are preferred over thin liquids, which are often the most difficult to swallow (Figure 9-2). The consistency of food usually progresses from pureed to soft ground to soft chopped to regular as oral motor control improves.

Coughing before, during, or after swallowing may indicate food in the trachea. Initially, a therapist should supervise feeding until it is determined that the process is safe for the patient and the performance is consistent.

Patients with tracheostomies present special problems. To assist in determining whether the patient is aspirating, the food is dyed with small amounts of food coloring. The patient's phlegm is then observed for traces of color, which may indicate food in the lungs.

The therapist records the amount of food eaten by the patient during feeding training. This assists in determining caloric intake and provides information used to adjust supplemental feedings.

Successful self-feeding requires adequate muscle tone, voluntary movement, and functional arm placement in at least one upper extremity to bring the hand to the mouth. This hand-to-mouth pattern requires 40° to 130° of active motion at the elbow. Long-handled utensils may be used to compensate for lack of elbow flexion. When upper extremity control is limited by abnormal muscle tone, hand-over-hand assistance may be indicated. Limitations in forearm rotation may be compensated for with swivel utensils. If deficits in muscle strength exist, a balanced forearm orthosis (BFO) or Swedish sling may assist by eliminating the effects of gravity. These are used primarily when arm placement is limited due to muscle weakness and are generally not recommended for use with abnormal muscle tone.

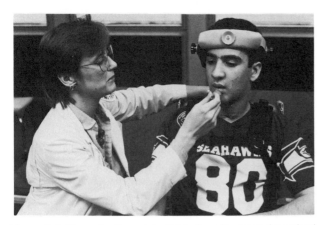

Figure 9–1 The patient's neck is slightly flexed to create the optimal position for swallowing.

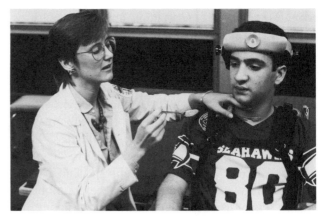

Figure 9–2 Swallowing can be facilitated by gently stroking the patient's neck in a downward direction.

Movement disorders such as ataxia limit motor control. As a result, feeding may be difficult, messy, or unsafe. Increased control may be achieved by placing a two- to three-pound weight on the wrist. This increases proprioceptive input to the extremity and may improve control. When the ataxic effects are noted proximally, stabilizing the arm on a surface such as a table top or wheelchair armrest may increase control. This is not a normal position for feeding, however, and the patient may require cueing to keep the elbow placed while completing the hand-to-mouth pattern. Cueing is decreased as the patient begins to use the technique more consistently. When ataxia affects the distal portion of the extremity, a cockup splint to stabilize the wrist may increase control. For ataxia in the trunk and head, a headrest may be indicated. This provides a point of contact that may improve upper extremity control even in the patient with independent vertical head control. When ataxia is severe and presents problems in safety, the patient should be carefully evaluated for the ability to use utensils near the face. If ataxia cannot be adequately overcome to allow for safe or neat utensil feeding, the patient may have to be fed or resort to finger foods in social situations.

The hand function components of grasp, release, and manipulation are important in self-feeding. Abnormal muscle tone may result in decreased fine motor coordination or interfere with hand function, making feeding difficult. Splints, adapted utensils, or other equipment may be indicated. When the amount of grasp is difficult to control, rigid plastic or Tupperware glasses are used. Styrofoam and breakable glasses are avoided for safety reasons. Cups with lids prevent spills, and a long straw eliminates the need to pick up a cup. Scoop dishes or plate guards may assist the patient with getting food onto a utensil. Utensil cuffs and built-up handles help compensate for decreased grasp. For some patients, hand function may be enhanced when the wrist is supported. These patients may benefit from a custom-made or commercial wrist cockup splint.

ORAL-FACIAL HYGIENE AND GROOMING

Oral-facial hygiene and grooming refer to personal care tasks such as washing hands and face, brushing and combing hair, shaving and applying makeup, brushing teeth, and nail care. They are frequently the first to be addressed in self-care training.

Cognitive Considerations

A patient must be able to attend to a task for 5 minutes, with redirection as necessary, to perform oral-facial hygiene functionally. Awakening or agitated patients not at this level may benefit from prefunctional tasks. These include:

- using a toothette or lemon glycerine swab to provide sensory stimulation to the mouth or lips
- identifying or matching familiar self-care items such as a brush, comb, toothbrush, soap, etc.
- communicating the purpose of self-care items
- attempting to see if the patient will automatically use self-care items correctly, such as bringing a washcloth to the face or a brush to the hair
- performing simple tasks such as washing the face or brushing the hair with hand-over-hand assistance (Figure 9–3)

If attention or arousal is insufficient to complete oral-facial hygiene, the patient may be required to perform

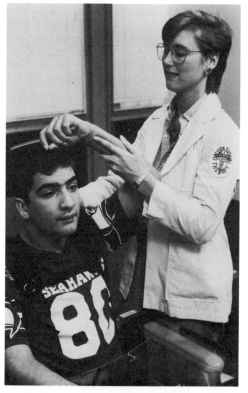

Figure 9–3 Hand-over-hand assistance may be necessary during self-care training.

only one task. In general, washing the face and brushing the hair require less cognitive and motor abilities than shaving or brushing the teeth and, therefore, may be more successful. Oral-facial hygiene is usually practiced in the patient's room rather than the clinic area. The room provides a low-stimulus, familiar atmosphere. A mirror may assist in keeping the patient's attention.

Impulsivity may be demonstrated by a patient rapidly performing any task with little attention to quality or safety. He may require verbal or tactile cues to slow down. Handing the patient one item of equipment at a time may also slow the rate. The therapist may need to point out areas that require additional attention. A mirror gives the patient visual feedback on the quality of the performance once the task is completed.

Memory deficits may interfere with oral-facial hygiene. The patient may be unable to define the tasks to be completed or the steps of a task already performed. A checklist assists with recall (Figure 9–4). The list is handed to the patient with self-care items or is posted by the sink.

Lack of initiation may also be seen. This is evidenced by the patient who completes only one step of a

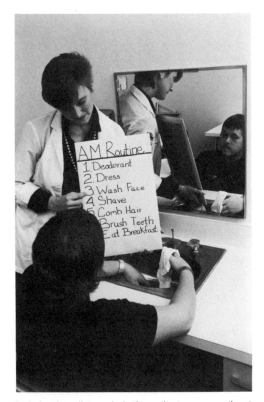

Figure 9–4 A written list can help the patient sequence the steps of a task.

task, such as putting toothpaste on the brush, and then stops. Verbal cueing between each step may be required to keep him engaged in the activity. Tactile cues may be useful in helping him initiate a motor sequence by putting cueing on a less cortical level. Safety and judgment issues arise primarily in shaving with an electric or safety razor. While electric razors may be indicated for patients who are impulsive, judgment in using the razor around water must first be determined.

Sensory-Perceptual Considerations

The inability to plan motor movements may interfere with oral-facial hygiene and grooming. Apraxia may be demonstrated by the inability to position a toothpaste tube correctly to get paste onto the brush. Hand-over-hand assistance may be necessary to help the patient establish patterns of movement such as bringing a toothbrush to the mouth or manipulating a shaver to reach all areas of the chin and cheeks. If the patient is unable to conceptualize or sequence the steps of the task, verbal sequencing may be useful.

Visual field deficits, unilateral neglect, or lack of bilateral integration may cause a patient to groom or apply makeup to only one side of the face. When deficits are severe, tactile cues such as rubbing the cheek area that is not shaved or touching the head where the hair is not combed may be beneficial. For some patients, verbal cues are helpful in orienting them to areas that need further attention.

Motor Considerations

The optimal position for oral-facial hygiene and grooming from a wheelchair is sitting upright with 90° of hip flexion, feet supported, and trunk and neck in midline. If this position cannot be maintained independently, external supports may be used. Prefunctional oral-facial tasks may be practiced with the patient in supine or propped in sitting in bed or on a mat.

Adequate arm placement and endurance in at least one upper extremity are required for oral-facial hygiene. Initially, due to abnormal muscle tone, the patient may require hand-over-hand assistance to guide the hand to the face or to maintain the required position. The therapist gradually decreases manual contacts as control increases. Placing the elbow on a stable surface, such as the sink or wheelchair armrest, assists in decreasing the proximal demands of arm placement. If arm placement is hindered by limited ROM, long-handled equipment may be indicated. When muscle weakness prevents adequate arm placement, a BFO may assist by eliminating the effects of gravity. If decreased control secondary to movement disorders, such as ataxia, is evident, stabilizing the elbow may assist in increasing control (Figure 9–5). A two- to three-pound weight placed at the wrist increases proprioceptive input to the extremity and may improve control. This technique may be used alone or in conjunction with proximal stabilization. If ataxic effects are noted distally, a wrist cockup splint may be indicated. Suction brushes and soap stabilizers also decrease the amount of distal control needed.

Fine motor control is necessary to manipulate grooming equipment. Rapid alternating movement is required for certain tasks, such as effective toothbrushing and some makeup application. If fine motor control or rapid alternating movements are impaired, discretion should be used in encouraging participation in activities that may be dangerous, such as shaving with a safety razor or applying eye makeup. To compensate for decreased grasp, a terrycloth wash mitt with a D-ring closure can be fabricated or purchased. Commercially available foam may be used to build up the handle of a toothbrush, comb, or makeup applicator. Thermoplastic materials can be used to fabricate handle adaptations for electric razors or brushes. Straps of Velcro and webbing attached to equipment also aid weak grasp.

DRESSING

Dressing refers to upper and lower body dressing. It includes clothing, manipulating fasteners, and the donning and doffing of orthoses.

Cognitive Considerations

To begin functional dressing training, a patient must be alert and able to attend to a task for 5 to 10 minutes, with redirection as necessary. For the awakening or agitated patient who is not at this level, prefunctional dressing tasks may be used. These include:

- naming items of clothing and the corresponding body part with which each is identified
- reaching for objects in directions that encourage functional arm placement necessary for dressing, such as over the head, behind the back, and to the feet
- encouraging participation in component skills such as assisting in pulling up pants during routine toilet activities
- practicing with large fasteners on a shirt placed in the patient's lap
- placing or removing large rings from extremities

Dressing training should occur in a low-stimulus environment. Through our experience, it is most beneficial when practiced as part of the morning self-care routine. Dressing at a familiar time often increases the patient's willingness to participate and assists in basic orientation. Patients may require frequent verbal redirection to the task, even in a low-stimulus environment.

Difficulty in identifying the steps of a task and sequencing them are common problems. Initially, undressing may be more successful than dressing. This sequence is less demanding and often does not require the use of adaptive techniques.

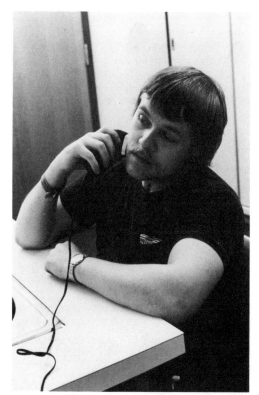

Figure 9–5 Stabilizing the elbow can reduce upper extremity tremors for the patient, allowing him to perform tasks such as shaving.

When dressing, a patient may require verbal cues to choose the correct article of clothing. The therapist may hand pieces of clothing individually to the patient or place them on the bed in the proper order to assist with sequencing. A written checklist may also be used and is best used when handed to the patient with the clothing. The list may include:

- remove pajamas
- put on underwear
- put on shirt and fasten
- put on pants and fasten
- put on socks and shoes

As sequencing skills improve, the use of lists and cues decreases and is eventually discontinued.

Deficits in problem solving may be observed in dressing. The patient may be unaware that the hand will not fit through a sleeve because the cuff is buttoned. Verbal cueing may be required to assist in identifying the problem. Once the problem is identified, the patient may require assistance in determining a feasible solution. Initially, the focus is on the patient determining one solution and carrying it out with assistance, if necessary. As problem-solving ability improves, the patient is required to identify two alternative solutions.

One of the most important cognitive factors in developing dressing skills is the ability to learn new or alternate methods of performing tasks. Problems with new learning often limit the use of adaptive equipment. Significant memory impairments may make it difficult for patients to recall the sequence or techniques used in dressing. Daily practice sessions with the therapist using consistent techniques and equipment facilitates carryover of new skills. Information is provided to nursing staff and family members to ensure that the routine remains consistent, including the sequence of dressing, the amount and type of cueing, and the specific techniques used.

Impulsive patients must be closely monitored during dressing to insure safety. Deficits are often apparent in patients who assume positions that are unsafe, such as standing to pull up the pants when balance is poor. Encouraging the patient to define the consequences of his actions verbally may help improve safety awareness during a task. Impulsivity is also demonstrated in inattention to the details of dressing, such as not remembering to check fasteners or forgetting to tuck in a shirt. Verbal cues and supervision are used to monitor the quality and slow the rate of performance. Handing one article of clothing to the patient at a time assists with proper pacing. Mirrors may be helpful for patients who require visual feedback to judge their final appearance.

Sensory-Perceptual Considerations

Patients with impaired visual processing or visual field deficits may have difficulty distinguishing between the parts of an article of clothing, such as the sleeve or the front or back. They may also have difficulty with tasks such as lining up fasteners or finding individual items of clothing in a drawer or closet. To compensate for visual impairments, the patient may be encouraged to locate buttons or a label to serve as a landmark in determining the position of clothing (Figure 9–6). Using tactile and verbal cues and removing other articles of clothing from the visual field may be helpful.

Motor planning deficits are often evident in dressing tasks. They may be demonstrated by an inability to place the arm into a sleeve or difficulty in orienting a shirt correctly to put it on. Initially, the patient may benefit from direct hand-over-hand assistance. This is gradually decreased as the patient can respond to verbal cues or plan the task independently.

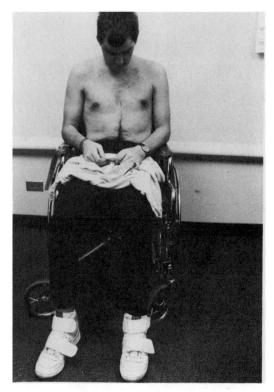

Figure 9–6 Cues such as shirt labels can help a patient when planning how to perform an activity such as dressing.

Unilateral neglect and limited bilateral integration become more evident in tasks that demand bilateral movements, such as dressing. The therapist should provide assistance from the more severely affected side. Right and left body awareness is encouraged through tactile and verbal cues. Patients may require hand-over-hand assistance to cross the midline or to position and work with the more involved extremity.

Motor Considerations

The amount of independent head and trunk control, balance, and equilibrium a patient demonstrates often determines the most effective position for dressing training. Dressing may be performed in supported or unsupported sitting or in standing. In evaluating the positions used for dressing, static and dynamic balance are observed. A patient who can sit unsupported at the edge of a bed may be unable to maintain that position during an activity such as lifting his arms overhead to put on a shirt.

While the patient may initially practice dressing in supine or supported sitting in bed, he is encouraged to perform the task in sitting as soon as possible. Sitting promotes normal postural tone, weight shift, and balance and equilibrium reactions at an automatic level. Sitting in a wheelchair to dress is an option for patients who do not exhibit the dynamic balance required for unsupported sitting. Incorporating lower extremity support and symmetric weight bearing in sitting aids in increasing stability. As trunk control increases, the patient begins to dress in unsupported sitting at the edge of the bed. In this position, gravitational demands are increased, but the task is made easier when the bed is placed at a height that allows the lower extremities to contact the floor.

During all phases of dressing training, the therapist should insure that the patient is in a proper position to facilitate normal postural tone and minimize the chance of increasing abnormal muscle tone secondary to excessive effort. Figures 9–7 through 9–16 show a patient completing upper and lower extremity dressing as the therapist incorporates facilitation techniques (Gee & Passarella, 1985).

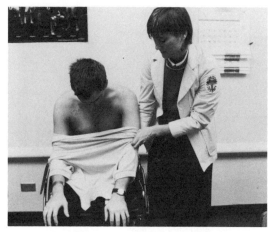

Figure 9–8 The affected upper extremity can be placed in a supported position during functional tasks.

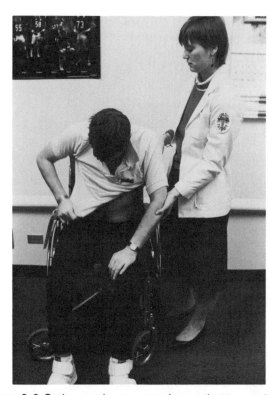

Figure 9–9 Cueing may be necessary for a patient to complete a task.

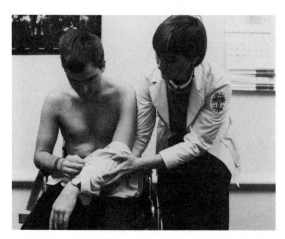

Figure 9–7 The patient sits in a supported position as the therapist provides assistance from the more affected side.

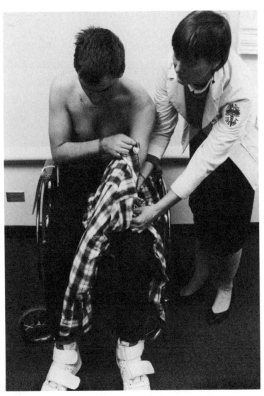

Figure 9–10 Protraction and extension of the upper extremity are facilitated during dressing.

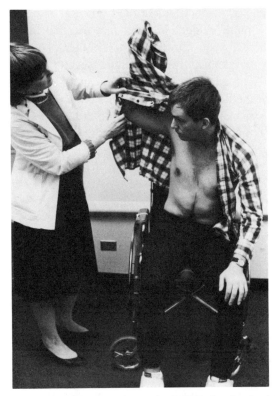

Figure 9–11 Assistance may be required with the less involved side if perceptual or cognitive deficits are present.

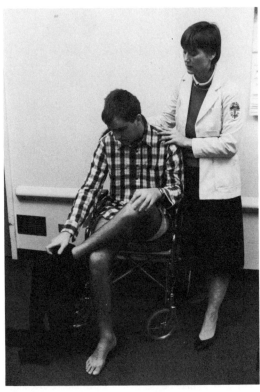

Figure 9–12 Pants are started over the more involved extremity.

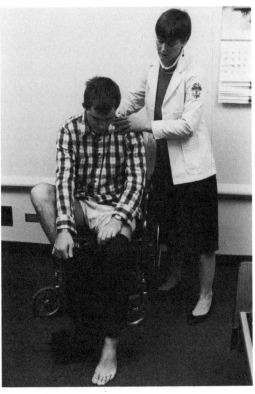

Figure 9–13 The trunk is stabilized as the patient performs more difficult steps of the task.

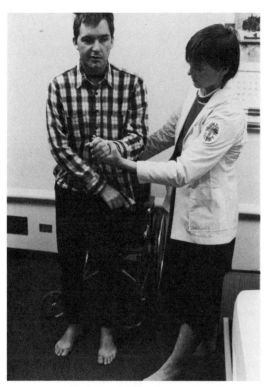

Figure 9–14 The upper extremity is supported and bilateral weight bearing is encouraged when the patient stands to complete his dressing.

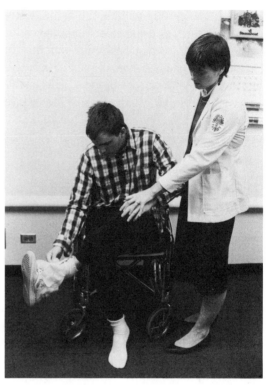

Figure 9–15 Often it is easier to cross the affected lower extremity as the patient's weight is supported on his nonaffected side.

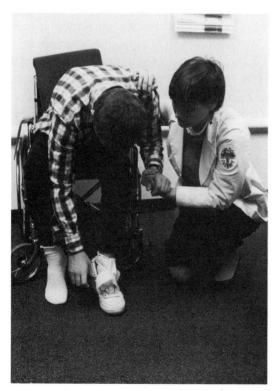

Figure 9–16 Facilitation is used to encourage symmetric weight bearing.

BATHING

Bathing includes washing the entire body and shampooing the hair. The activity may take place in a tub, shower, or a bed bath, as appropriate.

Cognitive Considerations

Bathing is normally performed in a low-stimulus environment. This limits the amount of distraction for patients with deficits in attention. Patients with sequencing deficits may have difficulty planning the steps required for bathing. To assist with sequencing, the therapist may ask the patient to identify the steps of the task verbally before beginning. She may also hand the patient bathing items such as soap, washcloth, and towel in the proper order. As sequencing skills improve, verbal cues are decreased.

Bathing requires significant safety awareness and judgment. These skills are often limited after head injury. The patient may require constant supervision, cueing, and hands-on assistance to ensure safety. Impulsive patients are often unable to anticipate the consequences of their actions, such as trying to walk on a slippery floor, getting into the tub before testing the water temperature, or using electric appliances around a shower or bath. When beginning bathing training with patients who demonstrate impulsive behavior, it is often beneficial to perform a dry run. This enables the therapist to determine which steps of the task require assistance for safety. Verbal and tactile cues and close supervision assist in slowing the rate of performance. Before bathing, the patient may be asked to state the consequences of unsafe actions presented verbally by the therapist. As safety awareness improves, close supervision and minimal cueing are decreased. Due to the inherent safety issues in bathing, the patient must have insight into his behavior and demonstrate no problems with safety or judgment before allowed to bathe independently.

Problem-solving deficits may be demonstrated by the inability to figure out how to get into or out of the tub or to adjust the water temperature. Such patients may be asked to identify one or two strategies to solve problems that arise. For example, if the water is too hot, the patient may identify adding more cold water or waiting until the water cools. The patient is then encouraged to choose the alternative he feels is most viable and carry it through. The effectiveness of alternative solutions is then discussed. As problem-solving ability increases, patients may require cueing only for less routine problems.

Sensory-Perceptual Considerations

Apraxia may interfere with the ability to bathe as demonstrated by an inability to motor plan how to apply soap to a washcloth or how to position body parts to wash. Hands-on assistance to provide tactile input may be helpful. Verbal rather than visual cueing may also be beneficial and may be used in conjunction with hands-on assistance or in place of it as praxis improves.

Unilateral disregard and lack of bilateral integration may inhibit the patient's ability to wash all body parts independently. If deficits are severe, the patient may require hands-on assistance to locate a body part with the washcloth or to cross the midline. This is decreased as body awareness and integration improve.

Motor Considerations

Active trunk control is essential to tub bathing. The tub provides only minimal support. For bathing the patient with severe motor involvement, shower chairs may be adapted with seat belts or trunk supports to enable the caretaker to have both hands free to wash the patient. Commercially available plastic trunk supports with webbing straps can be riveted to the upright posts of the shower chair. Foam liners commonly found in these supports should be removed and replaced with terrycloth material. This protects the skin and cuts down drying time. Seatbelts of 2-inch webbing can be attached to the chair or tied around the trunk to help stabilize the patient. With limited trunk control, tub benches with backrests are recommended. Even with a bench, lack of trunk balance may limit the individual's ability to wash the lower extremities.

Patients with adequate trunk balance to maintain unsupported sitting may use bath benches with or without a backrest. A hand-held shower nozzle is useful to wet and rinse the body for such patients.

Patients with good balance and equilibrium reactions may shower while standing. Nonslip adhesive strips are recommended for the tub in all cases. Grab bars should also be installed to assist in maintaining the standing position or to aid with transferring into and out of the tub.

To ensure adequate hygiene, the patient must be able to reach all body parts, requiring full arm placement. Long-handled sponges or brushes may be useful in reaching the lower extremities and back in the absence of full arm placement. Equipment may also be useful for reaching the lower extremities for the patient whose ROM is limited secondary to contracture or ectopic bone.

Decreased fine motor control may interfere with using a washcloth or with manipulating soap. In these cases, a wash mitt or soap-on-a-rope is recommended.

LIGHT HOMEMAKING TASKS

Maintaining one's living environment requires the performance of activities such as laundry, bed making, vacuuming, sweeping, dusting, and washing dishes. Generally, these tasks are less demanding than meal preparation because they are more repetitive and have fewer steps and variables. A patient may be able to assume responsibility for certain aspects of homemaking even if he cannot assume the total responsibility for a household. Participation in these tasks is often suggested so that the patient can play a more productive role in household activities.

Cognitive Considerations

When memory or sequencing deficits are mild, a daily or weekly checklist of homemaking activities may serve as a reminder. The therapist should suggest appliances that may be used safely by a patient with mild memory deficits, such as an iron with an automatic shut off. With more severe deficits, the patient may participate in homemaking tasks as a treatment modality rather than to meet a functional goal. Tasks are included that require one-step completion and are repetitive, such as folding clothes or drying dishes. Limiting steps may decrease the amount of verbal cueing required.

Impulsivity may affect the quality and safety of performance. Cues to slow down or to review the quality of work after a task is completed may be helpful. Providing the patient with a sample, such as a correctly folded piece of clothing, may also provide direction.

Sensory-Perceptual Considerations

Patients with significant sensory-perceptual deficits may participate in homemaking tasks as a treatment modality. Deficits in bilateral integration and motor planning may interfere with the ability to use both upper extremities spontaneously. Tasks such as washing and drying dishes and folding and hanging clothes that require bilateral integration may be used as training activities.

Motor Considerations

Most homemaking tasks can be performed from a wheelchair. The therapist should recommend equipment to make the job easier. Canister vacuum cleaners are easier to use from a wheelchair than upright models. Front-loading washers and dryers are more easily accessible. Instruction in energy conservation techniques may be helpful to both patients in wheelchairs and those who ambulate with assistive devices. Furniture can be arranged to provide for easier mobility in a wheelchair.

MEAL PREPARATION

Meal preparation includes planning and safely using the tools and appliances necessary to prepare a meal.

Cognitive Considerations

The ability to independently plan and prepare meals is most often limited by cognitive and sensory-perceptual deficits rather than physical limitations. Depending on the severity of these deficits, meal preparation may be used as a treatment modality or as a primary goal. With moderate to severe cognitive impairment, meal preparation is used in treatment to address a variety of component skills, such as sequencing, problem solving, or the ability to follow directions. For patients at this level, the role as a helper in meal preparation may be developed in treatment and suggested to the family to encourage carryover. The patient assists with mixing, peeling, and measuring, while the planning and organization of the meal is the primary responsibility of a family member. At the alert oriented level, various degrees of participation are possible. Patients may be able to prepare cold meals independently but be unable to use the stove or oven due to deficits in safety awareness.

When meal preparation is a primary goal, the patient's level of participation will depend on previous roles, preference, and necessity. A patient responsible solely for preparing lunch while family members are at work may focus on cold rather than hot meals. An individual whose role includes preparing meals for a family needs to develop a full range of planning and organizational skills in this area.

The ability to sequence and follow directions is a component skill of meal preparation. When working on simple sequencing, one-, two-, or three-step items, such as pouring a glass of juice or making a cold sandwich, may be used. These skills are graded by the gradual addition of multistep tasks. A meal planning checklist developed at RIC by Sullivan (1982) ranks meal preparation activities from simple to complex. Activities become more complex due to increased cognitive demands.

1. Prepare one cold item (glass of juice or sandwich).
2. Prepare two cold items (glass of juice and sandwich).
3. Prepare one stove-top item (eggs, canned soup, tea).
4. Prepare one simple oven item (frozen dinner, stir-and-frost cake).
5. Prepare one complex oven dish (cookies from scratch, meatloaf, casserole).

6. Prepare one hot and one cold item (macaroni and cheese and a salad).
7. Prepare two hot items (soup and grilled cheese sandwich).
8. Prepare three item dinner (main dish, vegetable, and potato).

It may be beneficial to have the patient verbally identify the steps of the task before beginning. A written list may be helpful for patients with memory deficits. If written directions are provided, such as a recipe or box cake mix, it may benefit the patient to read through all directions before beginning (Figure 9–17). Lists are discontinued as the patient refers to them less frequently. As patients are able to sequence a task consecutively, they should be required to sequence a task simultaneously, such as preparing two or three hot items at the same time.

As activities become more complex, written recipes or more involved lists may be required. If the patient's ability to follow complex recipes or lists is limited, and meal preparation is a goal, it may be helpful to develop a cookbook that lists simple main dishes, vegetables, and desserts. A variety of simple cookbooks are also available commercially.

Planning and organizational skills are necessary to create menus and identify ingredients. Initially, patients may be required to plan simple meals, such as soup and a sandwich, list the ingredients, and obtain them from the hospital cafeteria or a nearby store. As patients demonstrate the ability to plan simple meals, more complex meals are planned and prepared. Long-range planning and organization can be practiced by planning a weekly grocery list for a family of a specific size.

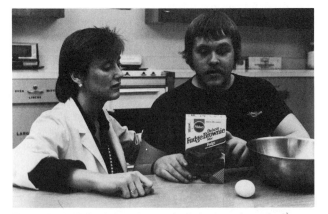

Figure 9–17 Following a written recipe helps organize and sequence cooking tasks and encourages short-term recall.

Safety issues are significant with meal preparation and include:

- ability to demonstrate good judgment while working with sharp objects, including awareness of finger placement when working with a knife and cutting with the knife positioned away from the body
- ability to monitor food as it is cooked, including using the proper intensity of heat, recognizing by sight, sound, taste, or smell when food is boiling, burning, or needs to be removed from the heat
- using safe body mechanics when removing food from the oven
- demonstrated awareness of temperature precautions such as use of hot pads, not setting objects on or near a stove top in use, and awareness of sensory deficits and proper compensation techniques
- demonstrated ability to recall that food is in the oven or that the oven needs to be turned off when meal preparation is completed
- ability to react to an emergency situation in a timely manner (i.e., grease fire, broken glass, pot holder or towel catching fire)

Impulsivity and the inability to determine the consequences of actions severely limit safety awareness in the kitchen. Such patients require close supervision. Verbal cues to slow or stop performance or discussion of the consequences of actions when poor judgment is shown may assist in improving safety awareness. Patients who do not develop these skills should be restricted in kitchen activities.

Meal preparation can be used as a modality to remediate deficits in simple problem solving, such as what to do when egg shells get into the batter or the proper sized pan to use. Higher level problem-solving skills are necessary as the complexity of the meal increases. When working on complex skills, the patient may be able to identify the problem but may require verbal assistance to define solutions. The therapist should require the patient to determine one, two, or three solutions to a given problem and decide which option to choose after weighing each. A therapist may observe and provide verbal cues to encourage a patient's use of anticipatory problem solving in meal preparation. This may entail placing foil in the oven beneath a dish that is very full or removing food from the dish.

Memory deficits may be addressed through meal preparation, such as recall of verbal directions to a task or monitoring the time of food baking in the oven. While written lists, timers, and verbal reminders may assist the patient with mild memory deficits, patients with moderate to severe deficits will require constant supervision to function in the kitchen (Figure 9–18).

Sensory-Perceptual Considerations

Sensory-perceptual deficits interfering with meal planning and preparation include slowed or impaired sensory processing time, which may impact on safety. The inability to process visual, olfactory, auditory, or tactile input may delay the patient in recognizing that the intensity of heat needs to be adjusted or that food is burning. Cueing to attend and respond to environmental stimuli may increase patient awareness. If a patient has a deficit in one primary sensory modality, such as olfaction, compensation techniques can be taught using other senses, such as increasing visual monitoring of food as it is cooking.

Bilateral integration and motor planning are necessary to use upper extremities simultaneously, such as lifting a pan from the oven, stabilizing a bowl with one hand while mixing with the other, or identifying and using various kitchen utensils. Meal planning should not be a goal when patients have moderate to severe deficits in either area but can be used as a modality to encourage bilateral use of the upper extremities.

Motor Considerations

For the patient preparing meals from a wheelchair who lacks trunk control sufficient to enable both upper

extremities to be used in a functional task, external supports may be added to the wheelchair. When working from a wheelchair, instruction is provided on placement of the chair for proper body mechanics and safety. When working at a stove or counter, the wheelchair should be positioned beside the work surface with the more functional arm toward the surface. When obtaining food from the oven, the wheelchair should be placed to the right or left of the oven to avoid reaching over the door.

As patients develop standing balance, kitchen tasks performed in standing are incorporated into treatment (Figure 9–19). Initially, the patient may use the wheelchair for mobility in and around the kitchen and stand only when supported by the table or countertop. Gradually, the patient should practice all skills in standing as appropriate.

Table-top arm placement is required to perform activities such as cutting, mixing, stirring, etc. Forward and overhead arm placement is required for obtaining items from cupboards or the oven. Reachers can be useful when arm placement is limited. When

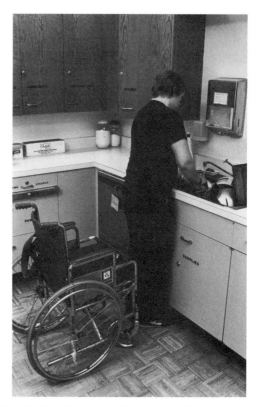

Figure 9–19 Standing can be incorporated into many daily living tasks. The therapist checks for symmetry in weight bearing and appropriate weight shift when the patient reaches off center.

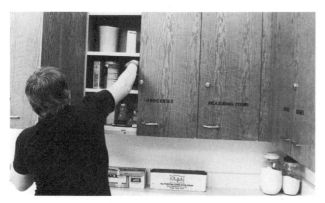

Figure 9–18 Labels on cupboards and drawers can help a patient with cognitive or perceptual deficits locate necessary items.

ataxia limits control, safe meal preparation is often not possible unless the deficits are minimal. Stabilization of the elbow on the table or wheelchair armrest may increase control.

Patients may prefer a microwave rather than a conventional oven. Its countertop height makes it easier to reach into. The microwave offers increased safety in that there is no exposed heat source and it does not need to be shut off when cooking is completed.

Hand function and fine motor coordination are necessary to manipulate food and utensils and to open containers. Dycem is commercially available and is useful for stabilizing bowls, plates, or pans on table-top surfaces. Utensils adapted with built-up foam or webbing handles help compensate for decreased grasp. Handles fabricated from orthotic material must be made of high-temperature plastics, such as Kydex, to enable them to be washed in hot water or used in cooking.

CONCLUSION

Functional improvement in motor, sensory-perceptual, and cognitive skills is reflected in improved performance of ADLs. This is often used to measure the success of OT intervention. The ability to care for personal hygiene needs independently and participate in home and leisure activities adds to the patient's feelings of self-esteem. Family members can assist the occupational therapist in targeting specific skills that will be needed by the patient post-discharge. The therapist can help the family by sharing with them those tasks the patient can perform independently and allowing them to observe the types of cueing or assistance needed by the patient. Independence will not be achieved by many severely injured patients; however, the occupational therapist can help them become as functional as possible.

PROBLEM AREA: ACTIVITIES OF DAILY LIVING

Subcategory: Self-Care

Self-care refers to feeding, oral-facial hygiene, grooming, dressing, bathing, and toileting. Each task should be rated separately.

Long-term goals and indicators	Short-term goals	Treatment ideas
1. Patient is dependent in self-care tasks (no goal). • does not participate cognitively or physically in any part of task • little response to environment.	1. Patient will participate in prefunctional self-care task.	1. Provide instruction to nursing/caregiver.
2. Patient will perform self-care with maximal assistance. • requires physical and cognitive assistance for more than half of task • participates in prefunctional self-care tasks.	For short-term goals, address subskills of each core item listed on initial evaluation by grading: • amount of physical assistance given • amount and type of cueing given • equipment used • position in which the task is performed • amount of time given to perform task • environment in which the task is performed.	2. • See above. • Refer to component deficits most significantly interfering with function and provide remediation as indicated. • Provide equipment, physical or verbal assistance, and supervision as necessary. • Provide repetition for safe performance.
3. Patient will perform self-care with moderate assistance. • requires physical assistance for approximately half of the task • continuous verbal cueing and close supervision is necessary.		3. • See above. • Update position in which activity is performed as motoric ability allows.

Subcategory: Self-Care continued

Long-term goals and indicators	Short-term goals	Treatment ideas
4. Patient will perform self-care with minimal assistance. • physically performs more than half the task • requires supervision to ensure safety and intermittent cueing for performance.		4. See above.
5. Patient will perform self-care independently with set-up. • may require intervention during unpredictable occurrence • no physical assistance needed.		5. See above, with no physical assistance.
6. Patient will perform self-care independently with equipment or adapted environment: • may require equipment due to physical limitations • no verbal or physical assistance required.		6. See above, with no physical assistance or supervision.
7. Patient performs self-care independently. • no equipment or verbal or physical assistance required • consistent quality of performance in all settings.		7. No treatment necessary.

Subcategory: Home Management

Home management refers to meal preparation, laundry, and cleaning.

Long-term goals and indicators	Short-term goals	Treatment ideas
1. Patient is dependent in home management skills (no goal). • shows little response to environment • does not participate cognitively or physically in any aspect of task.		1. Patient is not involved in home management at this level.
2. Patient will perform home management skills with maximal assistance. • requires physical or cognitive assistance for more than half the task • participates in task as a modality to address skills rather than in a functional manner.	For short-term goals, address specific tasks or portion of by grading: • amount of physical assistance given • amount and type of cueing given • equipment used • position in which the task is performed • amount of time given to perform the task • environment in which the task is performed • amount of supervision required.	2. • Refer to component deficits most significantly interfering with function and provide remediation as indicated. • Provide instruction to caregiver on ways patient can be involved in portions of task as a modality to address cognitive or physical skills. • Provide equipment, verbal and/or physical assistance, and supervision as necessary.

Subcategory: Home Management continued

Long-term goals and indicators	Short-term goals	Treatment ideas
3. Patient will perform home management skills with moderate assistance. • requires physical assistance for approximately half of the task • cognitive and physical deficits limit potential for independence in activities • participates in task as a modality to address deficits rather than in a functional manner • continuous verbal cueing and close supervision necessary.		3. • See above. • Provide repetition of activity using consistent method of performance. • Instruct in energy conservation techniques. • Suggest modifications to home environment.
4. Patient will perform home management skills with minimal assistance. • physically performs more than half the task • requires supervision in the home to ensure safety and intermittent cueing for performance.		4. See above.
5. Patient will perform home management independently with set-up. • no physical assistance needed • may require intervention during unpredictable occurrence.		5. See above, with no physical assistance.
6. Patient will perform home management skills independently with equipment or adapted environment. • may require equipment, adapted environment, and use of energy conservation techniques due to physical limitations • no verbal or physical assistance required.		6. See above, with no physical assistance or supervision.
7. Patient to perform home management skills independently. • consistent, time efficient quality of performance of all tasks • no equipment or physical or verbal assistance required.		7. No treatment necessary.

REFERENCES

Farber, S. (1982). *Neurorehabilitation: A multisensory approach.* Philadelphia: W.B. Saunders.

Gee, Z., & Passarella, P. (1985). *Nursing care of the stroke patient: A therapeutic approach.* Pittsburgh, PA: A.R.E.N. Publications.

Sullivan, B. (1982). *Meal preparation checklist.* Rehabilitation Institute of Chicago.

Community Reintegration

Lorie Cripe, OTR/L
Marlene Morgan, MOT, OTR/L

The degree to which the head-injured patient can manage in the community will ultimately determine his level of functional independence. For patients who progress to an alert oriented level, or whose expected outcome falls into the moderate disability to good recovery range, rehabilitation does not take place exclusively in the clinic, nor does the process end when they are discharged. This is the population for which a community reintegration program is particularly suited. These individuals may be able to expand their life styles by participating actively in the community either independently or with minimal supervision.

When planning to address community reintegration, the therapist incorporates information from varied sources. Information regarding the patient's present and projected psychosocial, cognitive, sensory-perceptual, motor, and activities of daily living (ADL) status is critical to the development and timing of the reintegration program. Information from other disciplines regarding communication status, ambulation status, vocational plans, and adjustment to disability are incorporated into the plan. In this way, deficits that may limit the patient's independence in the community can be identified early and targeted for remediation or compensation. The goal of community reintegration is to enable the patient to resume a meaningful life style.

At the Rehabilitation Institute of Chicago (RIC), community reintegration is addressed in three phases. During the first phase, the patient works in the clinic on building and mastering basic skills. The second phase incorporates trips into the community. During the third phase, the patient assumes primary responsibility for planning and organizing outings. As the patient progresses through each phase, the focus is on developing or improving skills in areas identified as critical to independent community functioning. For the head-injured patients treated at RIC, areas addressed by occupational therapy (OT) are:

- orientation
- communication
- money management
- community mobility
- prevocational/vocational/educational areas
- self-management

Planning for and offering a community reintegration program involves the entire team. The occupational therapist may rely on staff from physical therapy, speech and language pathology, nursing, or therapeutic recreation to participate in trips and to provide information as to the patient's status, assess performance, and set goals. Before trips are scheduled, several logistical factors must be considered and approved by the administration. Orders from the physician may need to be obtained before patients can leave the hospital. Staffing issues for both individual and group trips need to be assessed to ensure that the staff-to-patient ratio facilitates goal attainment and assures patient safety. This ratio depends on the level of function of the patients involved. Generally, if more than two patients are to participate in an outing, two staff members are required. Groups are usually limited to five patients in order to evaluate performance and ensure safety. All patients should be properly identified, and the staff should be aware of the proper procedures established by the facility in the event that a patient becomes injured or lost.

ORIENTATION

The ability to maintain orientation is critical for independent functioning. Initially, community reintegration interfaces with cognitive remediation. Consistent orientation to person, place, and time is a prerequisite for the higher-level orientation required for independence in the community. Once patients show these skills, the focus shifts to topographic orientation and time awareness and management.

Topographic orientation is the ability to place oneself in the environment and navigate within it. A progression of topographic orientation may include:

- orientation on the unit. This may involve the patient finding his room, the nurses' station, the physician's office, and the elevator.
- orientation off the unit. This may involve the patient finding his way to treatment rooms, the cafeteria, and the gift shop.
- limited orientation outside the hospital. This may involve the patient traveling within two blocks of the hospital and back.
- extended orientation outside the hospital. This will be different for each patient depending on his level of function and is designed to meet the patient's needs after discharge.

During the first phase of reintegration, patients practice topographic orientation in the clinic. Activities are graded to require increased independence. Activities in the clinic include directional games, map-reading games or exercises, and using the hospital directory to practice locating places by identifying environmental cues. These types of activities build skills and provide structured practice. They also assist the therapist in determining strategies the patient may use to compensate for deficits.

Initially, the therapist may need to structure activities highly by pointing out landmarks, such as the nurses' station or the elevators, and cueing the patient to use them. Orientation strategies include encouraging the patient to make and use maps or written directions, training along consistent routes, using repetition, and encouraging the identification and use of environmental cues. Strategies must also incorporate practice in asking for help. The therapist assists in problem solving a contingency plan for times the patient may become lost or disoriented.

Using the designed strategies, the patient practices topographic orientation in the hospital. The therapist continually grades and evaluates the orientation strategies for effectiveness and modifies them if necessary. Supervision is gradually reduced until the patient can function independently or requires only minimal supervision.

During the second phase, the patient practices orientation during a series of community outings. The patient and therapist prepare for the trips by mapping out routes and determining transportation needs and the amount of time required. Initially, these trips are scheduled one-on-one with the primary therapist. This allows the therapist to determine how the patient performs and helps determine his appropriateness for a group.

Once skills and deficiencies are identified, patients may progress to a group, and the group leaders are informed of their status. The therapist is sensitive to the fact that trips outside the hospital may be stressful and grades them accordingly. As the level of stimulation increases in a complex or unfamiliar environment, the patient's processing may become slowed. A patient who used a map as an orientation aid in the hospital and could follow a fairly complex set of directions would be required on initial outings to follow only a simple map. As the patient shows increased comfort in the community, the complexity of the trips is increased. The patient may travel farther from the hospital or be required to use public transportation.

On these trips, the therapist evaluates the patient for indicators that will be critical in determining whether he will be independent in the community or will require supervision on a long-term basis. Problem-solving abilities, memory, the use of environmental cues, such as street signs and buildings, reactions to unexpected events, and the patient's emotional reactions to being in the community are important to note.

During the third phase, patients prepare and assume increased responsibility for trips. By using a city map or directory, the patient chooses a destination, locates it on a map, determines a route, and makes a map or lists directions that include landmarks or bus routes. The patient may also be required to plan an alternate return route. On the trip, the patient follows through with the plan, using good judgment and problem-solving skills. The therapist provides supervision as necessary to ensure his safety. The therapist continues to evaluate the patient and to note which situations require supervision and/or assistance. At the conclusion of the trip, the patient and therapist discuss what happened and develop additional strategies for dealing with problems that were encountered.

Few individuals who rely on aids or compensation techniques for topographic orientation will be completely independent in the community. Most will be independent for only selected outings or will be able to travel over familiar routes or for short distances, such as going to school, to therapy, or to work and back. For safety reasons, they will continue to require supervision for extended trips or trips to unfamiliar destinations. Making the family aware of the patient's level of function and educating them in his use of orientation aids or techniques are important parts of the reintegration program. This helps ensure patient safety after discharge. The area around a hospital is usually unfamiliar to many patients. The family may report that orientation is improved once the patient returns home and is engaged in a simple daily routine.

Awareness of time and the ability to manage it are critical to orientation. Difficulty structuring time is frequently seen. The ability to structure time depends on the prerequisite skills of basic orientation, an awareness of time, insight into what is meaningful or fulfilling, and memory sufficient to remember having completed a sequence of activities.

To prepare the patient for community reintegration, the therapist initially works with him to improve the skills of memory and orientation as related to time. Patients are provided with a daily schedule prepared by the team. It designates hours for therapy, rest, meals, and leisure activities. The patient is oriented to the use of the schedule by all team members and is encouraged to use cues such as clocks, calendars, and watches. As the patient becomes proficient at following the schedule, he is required to take more responsibility in developing it. The therapist continues to provide the framework while the patient makes decisions concerning free time and leisure activities. It may be helpful to have the patient keep a daily log to compare with the

schedule. This can provide the basis for discussion between the therapist and the patient regarding time management and problem areas.

As the patient progresses into the community, he is encouraged to use time-structuring skills in planning trips. Initially, the therapist helps determine a realistic schedule, including travel time and time required at the destination. During the trip, the therapist assists the patient with monitoring and following the agenda and keeping to the schedule. Throughout the trip, the therapist evaluates the effectiveness of the time-management strategies devised by the patient and notes the level of time awareness demonstrated.

At the highest level, the patient is responsible for scheduling and executing a trip. Guidelines as to the time that can be spent away from the hospital are established by the therapist. In addition to evaluating the patient's use of time-management strategies, the therapist looks for evidence of his ability to grasp the abstract concept of general time awareness and the passing of time. Treatment goals may include reducing the number of aids or compensation techniques required for independent functioning. Developing a sense of time is important, particularly if discharge plans include school, employment, or a diversified life style of daily activity necessitating a flexible schedule.

COMMUNICATION

The ability to communicate and interact with others is important for reintegration into the community. Communication skills include verbal and interpersonal skills and the ability to use the telephone and to write. Each area allows the patient access to the community at large. Patients may lack basic skills necessary for effective communication and social interaction. Factors contributing to this deficit may include:

- use of a communication device
- difficulty with initiation
- articulation difficulties
- inability to self-monitor behavior

To incorporate communication into a community reintegration program, the therapist must be aware of the patient's communication deficits and techniques or equipment he requires. For example, if the patient uses an electronic alternate communication system, the program must include ways to incorporate it into social encounters. If the patient exhibits word-finding problems or is difficult to understand, role playing may be used to focus on how to handle problems socially.

The patient may demonstrate inappropriate social interactions. For patients with insight into their disability, a tape recorder may be helpful. This allows them to evaluate their actions objectively and comment.

Role playing provides the opportunity to practice social interactions in preparation for community encounters. Through role playing, areas may be identified that require further remediation, such as organization and clarity of thought or appropriateness of topics. Role playing situations should be concrete, practical, and related to encounters the person will have after discharge.

When the patient is comfortable with role playing, and the therapist feels his basic skills are adequate, he may be given assignments in the hospital. These may include going to the cafeteria or gift shop to purchase an item, asking for help or directions, or giving information. Telephone skills are also practiced. The patient may be required to call a store or business to determine its location and hours of operation or the transit authority to confirm the bus route to a destination. If the patient is hesitant about such face-to-face or telephone encounters, the situation may be practiced or specific questions or comments written down for self-cueing.

After the interaction, the therapist and the patient critique the performance together. The areas to be examined include etiquette, clarity of questions or answers, and the accuracy of the patient's report.

After practice sessions in the hospital, the patient uses his skills to plan and participate in trips designed to include graded levels of interaction. During the trips, the therapist determines whether his communication status will be a limiting factor in the patient's ability to function independently.

MONEY MANAGEMENT

Managing money is an important part of adult living. Having and managing money increases an individual's feelings of independence and control. Money management involves a variety of activities ranging from using money to make a simple purchase to budgeting and complex financial management. The patient's ability to manage money independently may fall at any point along the continuum. To be independent in handling money at the basic level, the patient must have adequate mathematical skills. To assist the patient with developing money management skills, the therapist may first assess his ability to identify coins and compute the value of money.

These skills may be addressed by using games that involve money, such as "Pay Day" and "Monopoly," solving mathematical puzzles, or performing addition and subtraction problems. As the patient begins to grasp the monetary and mathematical value of money, simulated situations are introduced. The patient may practice shopping and gain confidence in counting money and making change. Next, the focus shifts to the value of money. The patient develops simple shopping lists, such as for a week's groceries, and estimates the cost using newspaper advertisements to assist with pricing.

Trips into the community may initially involve making selected purchases from local stores, attending events that charge admission, and ordering at restaurants. Community outings are graded in complexity, with the patient required to develop more complex lists and budgets. Sound judgment in spending is stressed. In the budgeting process, patients are encouraged to think about their needs versus their wants and to set priorities for purchases.

COMMUNITY MOBILITY

The ability to move freely is an important aspect of community reintegration. The issue of mobility is addressed broadly and includes not only physical skills and use of ambulation aids and wheelchairs but also safety issues involving judgment, the ability to problem solve, the ability to maintain orientation and use environmental cues, and the ability to drive a car or use or arrange public transportation.

In the clinic, the therapist works with the patient to practice mobility skills, such as transfer training and physical endurance activities, that are prerequisites for meeting the demands of reintegration activities. In the hospital, the patient is encouraged to walk or wheel independently between therapies, following the daily schedule. In addition to serving as a conditioning activity and building endurance, this helps make the patient aware of the limits of his physical capacity, how far he can travel without stopping, and the time required to go from place to place. Initially, a patient may need cues to incorporate energy conservation techniques or to stop and rest as he learns to pace activity more efficiently. These factors will be important for the patient to consider when he plans outings. The patient is encouraged to use environmental cues and to determine the most efficient route between two points. The therapist monitors for evidence of safety awareness, impulsivity, and problem-solving skills. Patients who remain impulsive or who show decreased awareness of safety and judgment or poor problem-solving skills may require continual supervision in the community to ensure safety.

During this in-hospital training period, the therapist encourages the patient to incorporate all of the subskills he has learned into the mobility activities. He practices compensation techniques for perceptual, cognitive, and communication deficits. For example, if left-sided neglect is a problem, the patient is cued to look to the left and scan the environment until it becomes a habit. Before the first trip, the therapist reviews and reorients the patient to safety cues that may be found in the environment, such as stop signs, traffic lights, and crosswalks.

The patient prepares strategies to deal with safety problems that may occur on the outing. A list of tasks is compiled, and the trip is planned to ensure that the patient makes good use of his physical resources. During the trips, the therapist evaluates the effectiveness of his mobility in new situations. These may include moving through a crowded store, managing curbs, observing traffic signals and safety regulations, pushing a shopping cart, trying on clothing, or transferring into or out of public transportation. When problems arise, the therapist acts as a resource in helping the patient solve them and notes areas that require future planning or remediation.

It is at this level that the therapist and team may explore the issue of driving. Many patients are incapable of operating a motor vehicle. A variety of deficits may restrict driving: physical problems, medications or integration problems that slow reaction or cause drowsiness, poor judgment, visual-perceptual disturbances, and altered mental states. These may be temporary or permanent. Formal driving evaluations and training programs are available. At RIC, the therapist provides information regarding the patient's motor, sensory-perceptual, and cognitive status that may impact on driving ability. The results of the driving evaluation and training program will, to a large degree, determine whether the patient will rely on an automobile, other

drivers, or public transportation for his primary means of extended mobility.

The patient plans excursions and participates in complex activities, such as locating and using public transportation, hailing a taxi, scheduling transport on the shuttle system for the disabled, or taking the bus or train. This includes telling the driver or conductor the destination and handling the money for a fare. The patient is required to demonstrate effective use of mobility aids, good judgment, safety awareness, and the ability to verbalize or demonstrate contingency plans. The therapist carefully evaluates patients who require supervision. Many patients will continue to require supervision in at least selected areas of community mobility to ensure safety. It is important that these supervision issues be made clear to both the patient and the family or caregivers.

AVOCATIONAL, PREVOCATIONAL, EDUCATIONAL AREAS

Early in the patient's hospitalization, the therapist works with him concerning the issues of avocational interests and prevocational and educational plans. Leisure interest inventories and activity configurations are used to determine the patient's time utilization and interest patterns before injury. Whenever possible, the patient is encouraged to continue activities he found fulfilling. In some cases, this will require an adaptive device or that the activity itself be adapted. The patient may work with the therapist on a one-to-one basis or may be part of an avocational group. Changes in activity patterns, such as the possibility that time previously spent working will now be leisure time, are incorporated into the plan. Leisure activities may also serve a therapeutic purpose. Many avocational activities may be used to work on the remediation of cognitive and perceptual skills. The therapist needs to be aware of the role an activity played in the person's life and respect that position so as not to change an activity that once brought pleasure to the patient into one he no longer looks forward to or appreciates.

During the hospital stay, the patient may have the opportunity to participate in and experience a variety of new activities in a supervised setting. Therapeutic recreation may sponsor wheelchair sports, adapted games, or field trips. Patients are encouraged to participate in these activities whenever possible. Before discharge, the therapist and patient may make a list of resources for leisure activities near home. This includes social service agencies, civic groups, clinic-based activity programs, special park district classes, or the names of individuals who may serve as resources. This resource network is important, as a person's interest in leisure activities changes as he develops and matures. Activities that are appropriate at the time of hospitalization may not meet recreational needs later.

For many patients, continuing to pursue vocational and educational goals is important. Deficits in cognition, motor function, communication, or behavioral or emotional disorders may reduce or prohibit their access to competitive employment or education. Individuals work with vocational rehabilitation to formalize educational and vocational plans. Many factors must be considered. These include their work experience, the competition inherent in a job, the level of skill required, and the predicted structure required, such as a sheltered workshop.

Prerequisites to successful return to work are dependent on the type of vocational placement. These may include good interpersonal communication skills, memory, cognition, awareness of deficit areas, the ability to learn new information, reliable transportation, and adequate self-care skills. Through clinical interaction, the therapist evaluates the patient in skill areas that will be important indicators of his ability to return to work. The therapist works with him on work-related behaviors, such as filling out job applications, role-playing job interviews, and exploring vocational strengths and weaknesses. Specific jobs may be simulated to assess patient performance. Formal discussion sessions may allow patients to discuss their fears about returning to work or school and to plan strategies for coping with anticipated problems. Group activities may be structured as in an assembly line with each patient responsible for completing a part of the task that will benefit the group.

For many patients, their plans for return to work or school may need to be modified or adapted to fit their new life style. For example, the individual may be able to work only part time or may be required to take only one or two courses per semester. Volunteer work may be a satisfying substitute for competitive employment. In evaluating or adapting the workplace or school, the therapist may make a site visit with the vocational counselor. A plan for adapting the job environment or the job site is explored with the employer and patient. Plans made to return the patient to a job or to school must be carefully monitored for their long-term feasibility after discharge. The employer must be informed of factors that may affect the patient's performance. Community resources for the patient and the employer must be identified to ensure the ongoing success of reintegration.

SUPERVISION AFTER DISCHARGE

Many patients will require supervision to interact in the community at the time of discharge. The level of supervision and the circumstances in which it is required vary for each patient. Family members and caregivers need to be told the level of supervision the patient requires for safety. The patient and the family need to be oriented to the global nature of community reintegration and educated concerning the skills required for the patient to be safe.

It is often helpful for the family to accompany the patient on supervised outings into the community. They can then interact with the patient and the therapist and gain a practical understanding of the barriers to independence that the patient may face and learn appropriate compensation techniques. The family is encouraged to take the patient on community outings when on home passes and to discuss with the therapist problems that were encountered. The treatment team must be in close contact with the family to determine how comfortable they feel with their responsibility for the patient's safety and the patient's level of independence. As discharge approaches, and plans for outpatient therapy are formalized, the family provides critical information as to the patient's post-discharge schedule and the level of supervision they will be able to provide in community situations.

SELF-MANAGEMENT

The self-management aspect of community reintegration is an extension of the ADL skills developed in the rehabilitation setting. It is a combination of the patient's ability to complete self-care, demonstrate insight into his disability, and demonstrate an awareness of cultural norms.

As an extension of the dressing program, the patient practices wardrobe planning with an emphasis on dressing appropriately for the season and occasion and choosing flattering styles and complementary colors. The importance of grooming and hygiene is stressed, with an emphasis placed on its importance in interacting with others, in creating a positive impression, and in preventing illness and disease.

Independent feeding is expanded to include elements of proper nutrition and diet and the skills required for ordering and dining in restaurants and other public places. Good health and prevention of illness are incorporated into a program designed to educate the patient as to his disability and to encourage responsible behav-ior in taking medications and in balancing work, play, and leisure to promote a well-rounded life style.

Social norms, as represented by the rules of conduct and etiquette, are examined and incorporated into the areas in which the patient is evaluated and receives feedback throughout the reintegration process.

Issues of self-management are not approached in the same systematic method as the other aspects of reintegration. They are incorporated at the opportune time into both clinic-based treatment sessions and community trips.

PROBLEM AREA: ACTIVITIES OF DAILY LIVING

Subcategory: Community Reintegration

Community reintegration refers to obtaining goods and services, topographic orientation, money management, transportation, time and self-management, and interaction in the community.

Long-term goals and indicators	Short-term goals	Treatment ideas
1. Patient is dependent in all community reintegration tasks (no goal). • does not participate cognitively or physically in any part of the task • family/caregiver totally responsible for trips outside the home.		1. Patient not involved in community reintegration tasks at this level.
2. Patient will perform community reintegration tasks with maximal assistance. • requires physical and cognitive assistance for more than half the task • in community setting for enjoyment rather than for functional outcome.	For short-term goals, address specific tasks or positions by grading: • amount of physical assistance given • amount and type of cueing given • equipment used • position in which the task is performed • amount of time given to perform the task • environment in which the task is performed • amount of supervision required.	2. • Refer to component deficits most significantly interfering with function and provide remediation as indicated. • Provide instruction to caregiver on methods of facilitating safe performance. • Involve patient in planning and practicing community tasks in a structured setting. • Provide graded physical assistance, cueing, equipment, or supervision as necessary.
3. Patient will perform community reintegration tasks with moderate assistance. • requires physical assistance for approximately half the task. • continuous verbal cueing and close supervision required at all times.		3. See above, progressing to practice of tasks in an open environment.
4. Patient to perform community reintegration tasks with minimal assistance. • physically able to perform more than half the task • requires supervision to ensure safety and intermittent cues to maintain orientation.		4. See above.

Subcategory: Community Reintegration continued

Long-term goals and indicators	Short-term goals	Treatment ideas
5. Patient will perform community reintegration tasks with set-up. • requires supervision for orientation to new or difficult situations • set-up may include preplanning task or transportation • may require intervention in unpredictable occurrences.		5. See above, with no physical assistance.
6. Patient will perform community reintegration tasks with equipment. • may require equipment due to physical limitations (communication, transportation) • no verbal or physical assistance required.		6. See above, with no physical assistance or supervision.
7. Patient will perform community reintegration task independently. • no equipment or verbal or physical assistance required • consistent and safe quality of performance in all settings.		7. No treatment necessary.

Subcategory: Prevocational/Vocational

Long-term goals and indicators	Short-term goals	Treatment ideas
1. Patient will perform some work tasks not necessarily related to previous or potential employment with cues in a highly structured setting. • requires concrete, repetitive task • tasks are more basic than those performed in work environment • needs direction to move from one step or task to the next.	1. • Patient will perform the following simulated job task(s): _____ in a structured setting (*with, without*) (*assistance, supervision*) for _____ (*minutes/hours*).	1. • Address performance of prevocational skills such as time management, appearance, social skills, attention, response to supervision, awareness of quality of performance, and physical requirements • Divide vocational tasks into component skills to use as a modality to improve vocational potential.
2. Patient will perform some work tasks relevant to previous or potential job in a structured setting with close supervision. • may function in workshop or supervised job environment • can perform simple component tasks related to previous job • other indicators as above except that tasks are related to former or potential job duties.	2. • See goal 1. • Patient will initiate transition from one job task to the next (*with cues, with written instruction, independently*). • Patient will identify component skills relevant to previous job.	2. • See above, more directly related to previous or potential job. • Use vocational rehabilitation services to assist in defining realistic expectations of job potential.
3. Patient will perform all work skills relevant to previous or potential job in a minimally structured setting and/or with work site modifications. • environment may need to be less distracting • supervision required to monitor quality of performance.	3. • Patient to identify (*one, two, three*) job tasks that may require modification.	3. • See above. • Conduct job site visit. • Provide instruction to patient/employer on modifications necessary for performance. • Provide suggestions on gradual return to work.

Subcategory: Prevocational/Vocational continued

Long-term goals and indicators	Short-term goals	Treatment ideas
4. Patient will perform all work skills relevant to previous or potential job in appropriate work environment. • may require limited work hours initially • may require supervision for new tasks.	4. • See goal 3.	4. • See above.

Subcategory: Leisure Skills

Long-term goals and indicators	Short-term goals	Treatment ideas
1. Patient will participate in leisure activities with assistance. • may require modification of task or environment • supervision required.	1. • Patient will participate in _____ task with (*cueing, assistance*).	1. • Determine previous interests and new interests within capabilities. • Modify to enable participation. • Repeat to facilitate independence. • Instruct the family on methods of assistance.
2. Patient will participate in leisure activities independently with assistance to structure free time. • can participate in activity when directed • supervision may be required.	2. • Patient will participate in _____ task (*following instruction when initiated by others*).	2. • See above. • Assist patient in planning free time with balance of work and leisure.
3. Patient will participate in leisure activities and structure free time independently. • does not require direct supervision in performance of tasks • can perform task with adequate problem solving and good safety skills.	3. • Patient will use daily schedule to plan activities for leisure time. • Patient will plan and initiate daily schedule of leisure and ADL activities.	3. • See above.

Technical Aids

Janet Bischof, OTR/L

A technical aid is a tool used by a patient to compensate for a decreased ability to accomplish a task. When used properly, technical aids can play a critical role in the treatment of the head-injured patient. They can maximize independence and function in many areas, including cognition, communication, motor function, and daily living skills. They may also improve problem-solving and sequencing skills or facilitate the communication of feelings and needs. This unit describes the referral and assessment process for a technical aid for the head-injured patient. Commercial devices that can be used and options for mounting them are addressed.

The referral and assessment process includes the following steps.

- referral
- evaluation
- determination of the control and device for trial
- training
- determination of the mounting system
- equipment ordering and fabrication
- family and attendant education
- follow up

REFERRAL

Inpatients at the Rehabilitation Institute of Chicago (RIC) are typically referred for a technical aids evalua-

tion by the physician or team member, but a physician's order must be obtained before evaluation. Outside referral sources may include family members, teachers, vocational counselors, health professionals, personal care attendants, physicians, community agencies, and independent living centers. A referral form should be used to gather information from the referral source. This information should include a summary of the following areas.

- motor status, including head and neck control and upper and lower extremity active movement and control
- status of wheelchair positioning
- medical status, complications, and precautions
- cognitive and perceptual status, including orientation, memory, and visual skills
- communicative status, including yes/no reliability and whether the patient is verbal or is using an augmentative communication system
- the needs and expectations of the patient and family
- discharge date and environment

EVALUATION

Involving the patient's occupational therapist, physical therapist, and speech and language pathologist in the technical aids evaluation is strongly recommended.

This helps facilitate optimal results. Variables such as unusual patterns of behavior and the effects of medications can be quickly identified, and the patient's motor, sensory-perceptual, and cognitive status can be determined. The evaluation process addresses the following six areas.

1. *Psychosocial:* The patient's awareness of his deficits and his subsequent adjustment to disability will affect the evaluation and its impact on the justification for ordering equipment. Alertness and motivation are required for functional incorporation of a device in activities of daily living (ADL). These factors are critical in using an environmental control unit (ECU) or alternate communication system.

2. *Cognitive/sensory-perceptual status:* Results of formal and informal evaluations in these areas from the referral source should be obtained when possible. Informal observations rather than specific evaluations are used during the evaluation when possible. Cognitive skills to be evaluated include the understanding of cause-and-effect relations, sequencing, the ability to accomplish new learning, initiation, judgment, attention, and impulsivity. Sensory-perceptual skills include somatosensory and visual processing and perceptual and motor-planning abilities. During the evaluation, modifications can be attempted to compensate for deficits. For example, large switches or a color contrast between the device and the table surface may compensate for figure-ground deficits. A light touch switch may be easier to motor plan than a pneumatic switch. Labeling buttons on the device with pictures or large words may help compensate for memory deficits.

3. *Motor:* Information on the patient's motor status, including wheelchair positioning, should be available from the referral source. The motor component of the evaluation for an augmentative communication device and other aids should be performed after the patient is positioned appropriately. A functional motor assessment includes:

- head and neck active range of motion (AROM) and control
- upper extremity arm placement, coordination, tone, reflexes, hand function, endurance
- lower extremity AROM, coordination, tone, reflexes, endurance
- ambulation status
- need for formal wheelchair seating and positioning evaluation

- use of orthotics, such as a wrist and hand orthosis
- facial and tongue movement in the case of pneumatic switch evaluation

When determining the motion the patient will use to operate a switch, it is essential to note the effect of the movement on the entire body. Changes in tone, abnormal reflex patterns, efficiency of movement, fatigue, and the ability to maintain eye contact and attention to the device and switch should be observed. These observations will play an important role in the choice of the access mode. For example, a patient may have the motor control to activate a switch with the hand but doing so may cause his head to fall into flexion. For this patient, a head switch may be chosen as it would allow him to maintain eye contact with the device. In another case, a patient may be able to use a head pointer to access a communication device. If, however, the patient must rely on a caregiver to don the head pointer, he may be more functional using a slower method, such as pointing with his hand.

4. *Educational/leisure/vocation:* The patient's educational, vocational, and recreational interests and goals will affect the type of device or ECU recommended. The environment in which the activities will take place is critical in determining how the device will be set up. For example, for a child who uses a communication device in a classroom, two equipment set-ups are possible. If the child changes classrooms during the day, the device must be mounted onto the wheelchair. However, if the child spends the entire day in one classroom, mounting the equipment onto the wheelchair may be unnecessary and an added complication for the caregivers.

5. *Funding:* A letter of justification from the therapist and the physician that accompanies the equipment order may be critical in obtaining approval for funding. The letter should be as detailed as possible and should include a description of the device, a brochure, if available, and the change in the patient's functional status that can be expected. It should also stress the cost-effectiveness of the device if decreased attendant care is expected. Some inexpensive technical aids, such as battery-operated devices and switches, may be paid for by the family. Other funding sources include church organizations, clubs, community organizations, and funding drives. The patient's social worker may help identify funding sources.

6. *Family involvement:* The family or caregivers need to be involved in the evaluation process to ascer-

tain their attitude toward the patient's use of equipment. Family involvement is critical because carryover, in most cases, will depend on them. The entire process, including evaluation, training, and procurement of funds, can be positively or negatively affected by the attitudes of the family.

DETERMINATION OF THE CONTROL AND DEVICE FOR TRIAL

By compiling the results of the evaluation, the therapist can determine the devices and methods of control that should be tried with the patient. A trial period is conducted with all appropriate devices when possible. Frequently, equipment can be obtained on loan from vendors for periods of up to 1 month at no cost. Information should also be provided to the patient and family regarding equipment that is not available for trial.

Methods of Operation

A control and a method of operation are required to operate electronic equipment. The switch is the control, and the method can be either direct selection or scanning. In direct selection, one-switch activation indicates one item. For example, hitting a computer key produces one letter on the monitor. Scanning requires multiple switch activations to indicate one item. For example, in a simple computer scanning system, one-switch activation is required to start scanning, and another is required to stop scanning and select the item. The method of operation should be analyzed to ensure the best method is chosen for the patient. Direct selection requires less cognitive skills than scanning. For the patient with intact motor skills, it also provides a faster rate of input. However, for the patient with severe motor involvement, it may result in a large number of errors or fatigue.

Direct Selection

A head or chin pointer provides a method for direct selection for patients who cannot use their upper extremities due to abnormal tone, reflexes, ataxia, or paralysis. Use of a head or chin pointer requires fair to good head and neck flexion, extension, and rotation. Custom-made head pointers provide the best fit and can be more cosmetically pleasing. Ease of application may be a significant factor in the incorporation of a head

pointer into a patient's daily life. Head pointers are an efficient means of accessing a keyboard or a variety of pushbutton devices, such as a telephone or an ECU.

One custom design (Figure 11–1) fabricated by the rehabilitation engineering department at RIC is made from two strips of Kydex with a Velcro band behind the head and under the chin. After the components are attached, the Kydex is heated and molded to fit the patient. The head pointer is then lined with pressure-sensitive foam.

The viewpoint optical indicator also provides direct selection. It is a device mounted on a headband that emits a light beam. The patient moves his head to shine the light on a desired spot, i.e., a word on a communication board. Figure 11–2 shows a nonverbal patient using another device, an optical indicator, to operate a communication device.

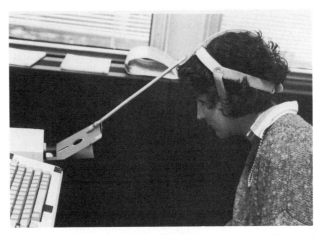

Figure 11–1 The ability to adjust the length of this custom-designed head pointer allows the client to access the entire keyboard and load floppy disks.

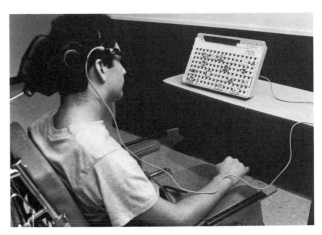

Figure 11–2 The optical indicator, a light sensor, is mounted on a headband and provides a method of direct selection to activate the Light Talker communication system.

Scanning

Scanning methods fall into two categories: traditional, or automatic, scanning and step scanning. In the first method, activation of a switch causes a cursor or light to scan an array of items. When the desired item is reached, the switch is activated again. In step scanning, the switch must be activated repeatedly to advance the cursor or light. When the desired item is reached, selection is indicated by either pressing a second switch or allowing a specified amount of time to elapse without closing the switch. Dual-switch input systems require significantly higher cognitive skills than one-switch systems. They are required for devices such as ECUs. A patient who has only one efficient control site for switch activation and needs a dual switch unit will need to explore computer options or contact a rehabilitation engineering department to adapt the device. It is often possible to adapt a commercial device from two- to one-switch activation.

Some commonly used commercial switches for ECUs or single-device controls are listed in Table 11–1, which compares features to assist with switch selection. While most devices provide either visual or auditory feedback, some patients benefit from the additional auditory feedback a switch provides.

Some switches, such as the infrared, eyebrow wrinkle, and electromagnetic (EMG), require a significant amount of a caregiver's time for placement, adjustment, and care. For example, a patient using an EMG switch to operate a computer requires someone else to place the electrode on his forehead when he wants to operate the computer. An eyebrow switch may require periodic readjustment of the headband to which

it is mounted. An infrared switch can be activated by an eye blink but is extremely sensitive to changing light. The patient may need a visor to minimize this problem. These switches are extremely sensitive. Maintenance may be a problem for a patient who has multiple caregivers because all must be well trained in placing the switch in the correct position.

Battery-Operated Devices

Battery-operated devices, such as toys, appliances, and buzzers, controlled by a switch can be easily incorporated into treatment to improve a wide range of cognitive, communication, and motor activities. They can be used with the awakening patient as a yes/no communication system. Battery-operated toys offer the head-injured child the chance to play. A buzzer can offer a head-injured adult a way to signal basic needs, such as hunger or toileting. Self-esteem and independence may be enhanced, as the patient no longer needs to ask for assistance to perform activities such as turning on the radio. Learning to control a battery-operated device using a single switch may be the first step in learning to operate a more sophisticated system, such as a communication device, an ECU, or an electric wheelchair.

Commercial battery-operated toys and appliances can be adapted for use with a switch through two methods. The first and simplest is to make or purchase a battery adapter. This requires no adaptation of the toy, and it may be removed easily and used with several toys. With a battery adapter, the toy operates only when the switch is activated and stops when the switch is released (Figures 11–3 and 11–4).

TABLE 11–1   Switch options

Switch	Single/dual	Body parts used for operation	Feedback
Pneumatic	Single	Mouth	None
Sip-n-Puff	Dual	Mouth	None
Light touch lever	Dual	Arm, hand	None
Leaf	Single	Head, arm, hand, knee	None
Tread	Single	Head, arm, elbow, hand, knee, foot, toe	Auditory
Finger light touch	Single	Finger	Auditory
Large round	Single	Elbow, hand, finger	None
Single rocker	Single	Head, arm, elbow, hand, knee, foot, toe	Auditory
Dual rocker	Dual	Hand, finger	Auditory
Mercury	Either	Head	None
P-Switch	Single	Eyebrow, jaw, upper or lower extremities	Auditory (optional)
Infrared	Single	Eye blink	None
Eyebrow wrinkle	Single	Eyebrow	Auditory

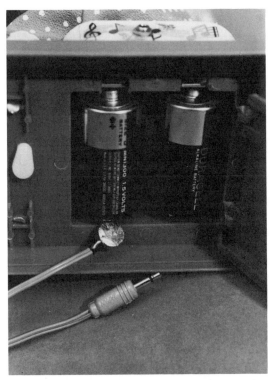

Figure 11–3 The metal disk on one end of the battery adapter is slipped between the battery and the battery contact. The miniature plug on the opposite end is inserted into a switch.

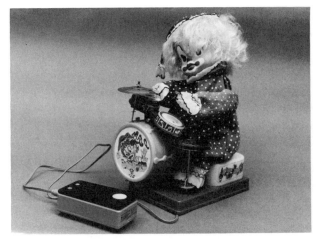

Figure 11–4 The toy's switch remains in the "on" position when connected to a battery adapter although the toy runs only upon activation of the switch.

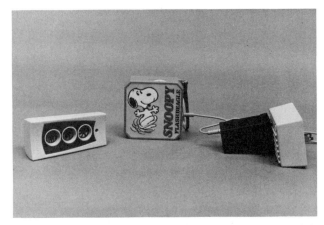

Figure 11–5 This adapted radio can be controlled via a single switch or through an ECU. The latter requires a cable connecting the toy to a MED switch module plugged into the TASH ECU receiver (right). The transmitter (left) can control three appliances or toys through ultrasonic signals to the receivers.

The second method is to install a miniature phone jack. A switch is connected to the jack using a miniature telephone plug. Once adapted, the device can be controlled only by a switch. The on/off switch is left on, and the device operates only as long as the switch is activated (Figure 11–5). Toys can be adapted by parents or the therapist by following a simple set of instructions. Adapted toys can be purchased from several sources (see Exhibit 11–1) or obtained on loan from a lending library. Rehabilitation engineers or individuals with experience in electronics may be willing to adapt toys and appliances. Liability should be explored before pursuing this option.

To have the toy or appliance remain on when the switch is not held, a switch latch mechanism can be used (Figure 11–6). This device has two miniature phone jacks at either end, enabling it to be connected to one or two switches. The toy or appliance is connected to one end and the switch to the other. A single-switch activation turns on the device, and it remains on until the switch is activated again. The switch latch is recommended for persons with limited endurance and as a component for training in the use of a communication or ECU system.

Application. By structuring the treatment session with a specific goal in mind, adapted toys and appliances can be incorporated to promote cognitive, sensory-perceptual, motor, and communication skills. Visual tracking can be addressed by using a moving toy. Object permanence and attention span can be emphasized by having a toy disappear behind a cover and then reappear. Memory and sequencing skills can be promoted by having the patient control two toys with two switches. Motor goals may be addressed through the use of adapted toys and switches. Head control may be promoted in a variety of positions by using a mercury switch (Figures 11–7 and 11–8). Arm placement is facilitated by critical placement of a switch in any

Exhibit 11–1 Equipment sources

ADAPTED TOYS

Ablenet, 360 Hoover Street, N.E., Minneapolis, MN 55413

Crestwood Company, P.O. Box 04606, Milwaukee, WI 53204–0606

Toys for Special Children Catalog, Steven Kanor, Ph.D., Medical Engineer, 8 Main Street, Hastings-on-Hudson, NY 10706

COMPUTER KEY GUARDS AND KEY LATCHES

Don Johnston Developmental Equipment, 981 Winnetka Terrace, Lake Zurich, IL 60047

Extensions for Independence, 635-5 N. Twin Oaks Valley Road, San Marcos, CA 92069

Prentke Romich Company, 1022 Heyl Road, Wooster, OH 44691

TASH, Inc., 70 Gibson Drive, Unit I, Markham, Ontario, Canada L3R 2Z3

COMPUTER PERIPHERALS

Adaptive Peripherals, 4529 Bagley Avenue North, Seattle, WA 98103

Koala Technologies, 3100 Patrick Henry Drive, Santa Clara, CA 95050

ECUs AND BUZZERS

Don Johnston Developmental Equipment, 981 Winnetka Terrace, Lake Zurich, IL 60047

DU-It Control Systems Group, Inc., 8765 Township Road 513, Shreve, OH 44676-9421

Fordham Radio, 260 Motor Parkway, Hauppauge, NY 11788 (electronics catalog)

Medical Equipment Distributor, Inc. (MED), 3223 S. Loop 289, Lubbock, TX 79423

Prentke Romich Company, 1022 Heyl Road, Wooster, OH 44691

Radio Shack

Rehab Technology, Inc., 498 S. Plymouth, P.O. Box 185, Aviston, IL 62216

Sears

TASH, Inc., 70 Gibson Drive, Unit I, Markham, Ontario, Canada L3R 2Z3

X-10 Inc., 185A LaGrande Avenue, North Vale, NJ 07647

ELECTRIC PAGE TURNERS

Medical Equipment Distributors, Inc. (MED), 3223 S. Loop 289, Lubbock, TX 79423

Maddock, Inc., 6 Industrial Road, Pequannock, NJ 07440

J.A. Preston Corp., 60 Page Road, Clifton, NJ 07012

Touch Turner, 443 View Ridge Drive, Everett, WA 98203

Zygo Industries, Inc., P.O. Box 1008, Portland, OR 97207

EMERGENCY CALL SYSTEMS

AT&T National Special Needs Center 3, 2001 Route 46, Parsippany, NJ 07054

Independent Living, Inc., 770 Frontage Road, Suite 118, Northfield, IL 60093-9990

Lifeline Systems, Inc., One Arsenal Marketplace, Watertown, MA 02172

SPEAKER PHONES AND INTERCOMS

McDade and Company

Prentke Romich Company

Radio Shack

Service Merchandise

Telephone companies

SWITCHES (Refer to ECU sources)

Luminand, Inc., 8688 Tyler Boulevard, P.O. Box 268, Mentor, OH 44060-0268

Zygo Industries, Inc., P.O. Box 1008, Portland, OR 97207

VOICE RECOGNITION SYSTEMS

Key Tronic, P.O. Box 14687, Spokane, WA 99214

Prentke Romich Company, 1022 Heyl Road, Wooster, OH 44691

The Voice Connection, 17835 Skypark Circle, Suite C, Irvine, CA 92714

Voice Machine Communications, Inc., 10522 Covington Circle, Villa Park, CA 92667

---

developmental position. Incorporating a variety of switches into the treatment plan, such as different-sized push, squeeze, or pull switches, may facilitate hand function. Switches can be incorporated into a strengthening program by being graded to be activated with varying amounts of pressure. Weight bearing in the developmental positions can be facilitated by having the patient stand, kneel, or push down on a flat switch.

Adapted toys are used to promote communication skills. The speech and language pathologist may use toys to encourage interaction or to assist in the development of expressive and receptive language skills. For the nonverbal patient, adapted toys can be used for switch training as a precursor to using a communication aid. Learning to operate a communication device with a switch that requires new and controlled motor move-

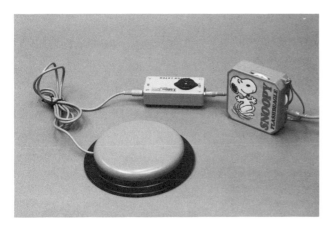

Figure 11–6 The switch latch is connected to the battery-operated device and the switch.

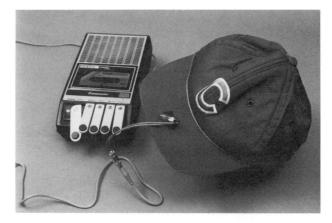

Figure 11–7 A mercury switch mounted on a baseball cap controls the on/off switches of the tape recorder. The music will turn off when the head is tilted to an undesirable angle.

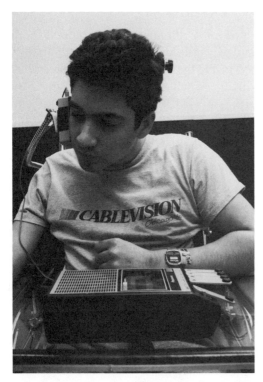

Figure 11–8 Switch training with a tape recorder is a precursor to a communication device and a means of facilitating head control.

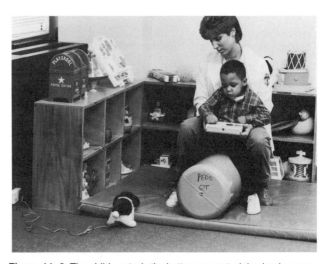

Figure 11–9 The child controls the battery-operated dog by depressing one of the four large colored circles on the TASH Ultra 4 ECU transmitter.

ments may be overwhelming. Switch training before operating the device may make the transition easier (Figure 11–9).

Call Systems

For the nonverbal patient, a call system may be one of the first technical aids required. Four categories of call systems are described. They are most appropriate for the oriented patient who has severe motor deficits.

Call buzzers and intercom systems may also be useful for the nonoriented patient.

Nurse Call System

For the patient with severe motor impairment, an adaptation of the conventional call system may be required. Some systems allow the interchange of commercial switches, including light touch, head activated, and pneumatic switches (Figure 11–10). If the switch cannot be easily interchanged, a switch-operated buzzer system mounted in the hallway outside the patient's room may be considered. A cable attaches the bedside switch to the buzzer. Some switches can be mounted on the bed with a gooseneck or retractable arm. It can be positioned for head, shoulder, or hand

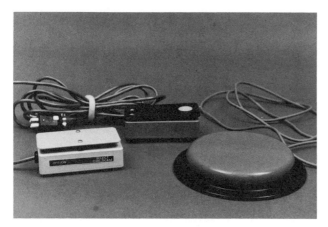

Figure 11–10 Switches (left to right): dual rocker switch, light touch plate switch, round plate switch.

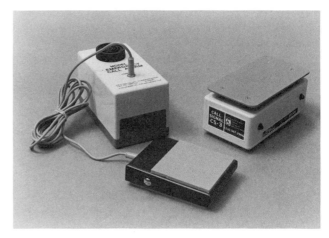

Figure 11–11 Zygo call alarm interfaced with a tread switch (left). PRC CS-3 Call Signal, which can be activated with or without a switch (right).

activation. The call system can also be activated by an eyebrow switch. However, this switch may require frequent repositioning to ensure reliability.

Buzzer

A buzzer can serve a variety of purposes. It is portable and can be used in many settings. It can be used as a call alert system or as a simple communication device to signal yes or no. A battery-operated buzzer can be operated independently or interfaced with a variety of switches. A buzzer can be fabricated from low-cost materials from a hardware or electronics store. Simple instructions are available in manuals on homemade switches or battery-operated toys (see Reading and Resource List).

Commercial buzzers vary in cost, ability to be adapted for switch control, ease of mounting onto a wheelchair, and compatibility with ECUs. The Zygo call alarm and the Prentke Romich Company (PRC) call system (Figure 11–11) can interface with any switch having a miniature phone plug. The PRC model can also be activated independently of a switch by depressing a touch plate.

The mounting location of a buzzer system may be influenced by a patient's cognitive status. For an oriented patient, the buzzer may be attached with Scotchmate or Velcro to the wheelchair armrest or lap board. If there is a question about the patient's ability to use a buzzer appropriately due to perseveration or deficits in initiation, a trial period is recommended during which the patient is carefully monitored by the team as to his purposeful use of the device. To decrease nonpurposeful activations, the buzzer may be mounted out of full sight. Some buzzers can be placed in a holder

fabricated of Orthoplast. The holder can then be attached with Velcro to the wheelchair uprights, attached inside the armrest, or placed in a wheelchair bag with the switch attached to the patient or the chair frame (Figure 11–12). Alternatives to battery-operated buzzers are a desk call bell or a dinner bell, which may need to be adapted to allow for easier activation (Figure 11–13).

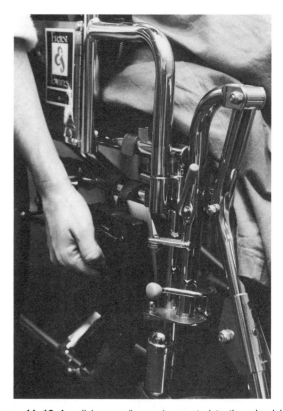

Figure 11–12 A call buzzer (beeper) mounted to the wheelchair frame

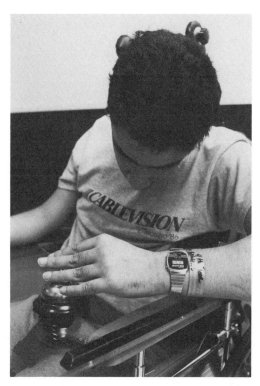

Figure 11–13 Desk call bell mounted to a lap board for a nonverbal client

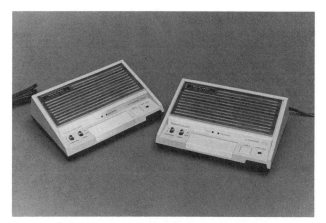

Figure 11–14 A wireless intercom system enables monitoring of a person's need for assistance from another room.

Intercoms

Wireless intercoms may benefit patients at home who are dependent on wheelchair mobility or who require monitoring from bed. For the verbal patient, they can be used to communicate with a family member in another room. For the nonverbal patient, they permit family members to monitor him and pick up distress signals from another room. Because monitors can be placed in several rooms, these systems allow caregivers to attend to household tasks. Commercial systems operate by having the patient activate a touch plate to talk and release it to listen. The amount of pressure required varies with each system. Some systems can be locked in the listening position. With the system locked, the caregiver can monitor sounds from the patient's room on an ongoing basis (Figure 11–14). Nursery monitors, which are available from toy stores, may be an alternative for some patients.

Emergency Call Systems

A variety of emergency call systems have been designed to aid the patient with severe motor involve-

ment who may be left alone for short periods. An emergency call system is any device that notifies someone outside the home of the patient's need for immediate assistance. Each system varies as to the method of input, cost, and installation and the process through which help is obtained. Evaluation of the system and careful matching of the most appropriate system to the patient is critical. Some systems require that the patient function at a high cognitive level. Others may be used by a patient who is oriented but lacks certain skills in problem solving or sequencing.

Most emergency call systems, including Lifeline and the Ezzie system, work through a transmitter worn or carried by the patient. The transmitter activates an automatic telephone dialing mechanism, sending a recorded message to a central monitoring station. Upon receiving the message, the center contacts an emergency medical team, a family member, or a neighbor listed in the patient's file. The pushbutton on the system can be adapted for the patient with limited hand function by building up the button or attaching a lever. The transmitter can be mounted with Velcro on the wheelchair armrest or headrest. A pneumatic switch is available with the Lifeline system for the patient with severe upper extremity limitations. This system is activated by a pushbutton and can be rented for a reasonable monthly fee. The Ezzie system is activated when the monitor worn by the patient tilts. It detects falls and, therefore, may be appropriate for patients who are inpulsive with transfers or those with decreased balance reactions. AT&T and Radio Shack offer pushbutton remote transmitter systems that activate preprogrammed telephone numbers and send a taped distress message (Figure 11–15).

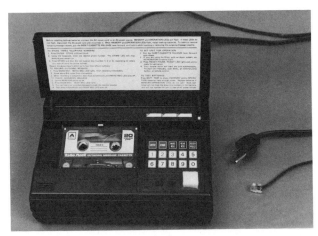

Figure 11–15 The Automatic Message Dialer automatically dials up to three preprogrammed telephone numbers upon pushbutton activation and plays a custom-recorded tape.

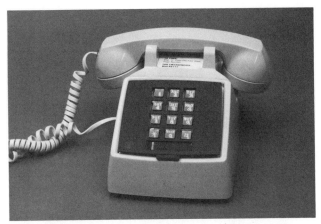

Figure 11–16 AT&T key guard on a standard desk telephone

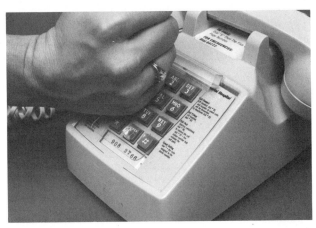

Figure 11–17 The operator is dialed when this clear plate (AT&T) covering all keys is depressed.

Telephone Systems

Patients may be able to operate standard telephone systems independently with only minor adaptations. For patients with fine motor control or visual deficits, key guards or enlarged key pads are available. AT&T offers a free key guard that fits over a standard desk or wall telephone (Figure 11–16). Custom key guards can be fabricated by a rehabilitation engineer or occupational therapist. Large number stickers can be placed over a standard key pad or rotary dial. Telephones with enlarged key pads are available commercially. For patients who have difficulty in completing a call, AT&T offers a faceplate that depresses the operator button when touched (Figure 11–17). The caller can then request assistance to dial the number. This service is provided free with an application signed by a physician.

Memory deficits may limit a patient's ability to use the telephone. Several strategies have proven helpful. Frequently dialed numbers can be listed next to the telephone. Speed calling requires only one or two numbers to be depressed to complete a call and is available as a monthly service from most telephone companies or may come as a built-in feature in some telephones. Speed calling may be made easier if photographs of persons or locations that correspond to the programmed numbers are placed next to the numbers on the telephone pad.

For patients with limited upper extremity function, a speaker phone or amplifier eliminates the need to hold the receiver. For the nonverbal patient, they may be used in conjunction with an augmentative communication device that has speech output. While a speaker phone allows for hands-free conversation, it does require the patient to depress one button to answer and disconnect a call. It also compromises privacy. Speaker phones may be equipped with features, including automatic redial of the last number dialed, speed calling, and a privacy button, which allows the caller to converse with someone in the room without the other party being able to listen in. Many companies manufacture speaker phones with quality and price directly related. The patient should try the telephone before purchasing. A standard pushbutton telephone can be inexpensively converted to a speaker phone by replacing the receiver with an amplifier.

A hands-free telephone called the Directel is offered by AT&T. It features a microphone and operator-assisted calling. To reach the operator, the patient sips or puffs into a tube. The same sip or puff allows him to hang up. Goosenecks, shoulderrests, and headphones eliminate the need to hold a receiver. Goosenecks, available from medical supply companies, have a table clamp on one end and hardware on the other that allows the telephone receiver to be easily slipped in and out. To answer or hang up the telephone, the patient depresses a toggle switch that operates the switch hook (Figure 11–18).

Electric Page Turners

An electric page turner may be recommended for patients unable to turn pages due to upper extremity limitation. Page turners operate by activation of either a single switch or a series of four switches. In the single-switch operation, one page is turned forward with each switch activation (Figure 11–19). The four-switch method allows for forward and backward page turning.

The features available vary, and all systems should be examined before a decision to purchase is made. Features to examine include direction of turning (forward and reverse), number of switches required, cognitive skills required, types of compatible switches, ability to interface with an ECU, adjustable viewing angle, types of reading material accommodated (textbooks, paperbacks, magazines), maintenance, com-

plexity of set-up for each reading session, and cost. See Exhibit 11–1 for specific equipment information.

Environmental Control Systems

ECUs offer the patient with severe motor deficits and mild cognitive deficits the ability to control selected aspects of his immediate environment. There are a number of commercial ECUs as well as custom units designed by rehabilitation engineering centers. Nine of the commercial systems are described in Table 11–2. The more comprehensive systems are not included, as the high-level cognitive skills required to operate them often preclude their use with head-injured patients. (Refer to Exhibit 11–1 for further references on these systems.) Note that the Rehab Technology ECU and the TASH Ultra 2T are the only systems that pair a switch with a direct selection method (Figure 11–20). The switch options list includes those most commonly interfaced with each device and is not inclusive.

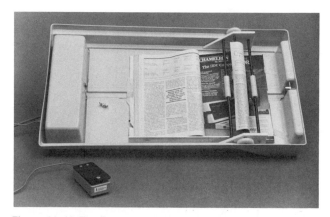

Figure 11–19 The Brussee electric page turner turns one page forward upon one-switch activation.

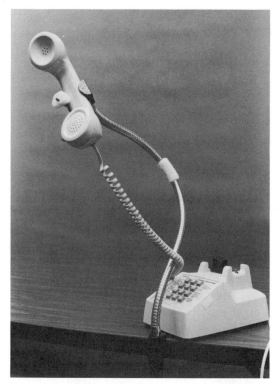

Figure 11–18 A gooseneck telephone holder and toggle switch facilitate independent use of a standard desk telephone.

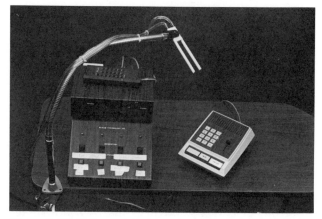

Figure 11–20 Puffing and sipping on the two straws control the on/off switches of four appliances through the Rehab Technology ECU.

TABLE 11–2   Environmental control units

System	Selection method	Switch options	ECU/user interface		ECU/appliance interface	Feedback	Appliance number			Options	Cognitive skills required	Source
			Portable transmitter	Stationary console			Latch	Momentary	Either			
Switch-it	Direct selection	None	Ultrasonic		Ultrasonic signal to receiver in same room (A)	Visual	3	0	0	None	Initiation, orientation to place and person, fair to good long term memory	VSC Corp.
TASH Ultra 2T	Direct selection	Pneumatic, light touch, dual rocker, joystick	Ultrasonic		Ultrasonic signal to receiver in same room (A)	None	2	0	0	Wheelchair Fortress Scientific Controller	Same as above	TASH
TASH Ultra 4	Direct selection for switch-activated joystick, hand-held and large button transmitters	Pneumatic, light touch	Ultrasonic		Ultrasonic signal to receiver in same room (A)	None	4	0	0	Same as TASH Ultra 2T	Same as above	TASH
X-10 Command Console	Direct selection	None		Key pad	House wiring, remote control (A,B)	Visual	16	0	0	None	Above, plus fair sequencing skills	Radio Shack, X-10, MED, Sears
X-10 Mini-Controller	Direct selection	None		Key pad	House wiring, remote control (A,B)	Visual	8	0	0	None	Same as Switch-it	X-10, MED
Home Control Center	Direct selection	None	Key pad		Radio transmission, house wiring (A,B)	Auditory	4	0	0	None	Same as Switch-it	Radio Shack
X-10 ECS-8	Two-switch step scanning	Pneumatic, light touch, rocker, leaf, tread		Connected to switches	House wiring, remote control (A,B)	None	8	0	0	None	All above, plus good sequencing skills	X-10, MED
Rehab Technology	Direct selection	Pneumatic: adaptations for other switches possible through manufacturer		Connected to switches	Appliances plugged into ECU	Visual, auditory	0	0	4	Television, telephone	All above, fair to good judgment, fair to good problem solving	Rehab Technology Inc.
Rehab Technology	Two switch	Pneumatic: adaptations for other switches possible through manufacturer		Connected to switches	Appliances plugged into ECU	Visual, auditory	0	0	8	Television, telephone	All above, fair to good judgment, fair to good problem solving	Rehab Technology Inc.

Another differentiating feature of ECUs is the user-ECU interface, which describes the location of the patient. Systems are classified as having either a portable transmitter or a stationary console. The stationary console is connected to an outlet, and the patient must be at the console to operate the ECU (Figure 11–21). A portable transmitter is wireless and can be used away from the ECU; some, such as the Switch-it or the Ultra 4, can be hand held (Figures 11–22 to 11–24).

The ECU-appliance interface refers to the transmission of signals from the ECU to the device being controlled. Appliances may be plugged directly into the ECU or into a remote receiver, which is then plugged into an outlet. Many ECUs use X-10 modules as their receivers. The three most commonly used types of X-10 modules are for appliances, incandescent lamps, and wall switches (Figure 11–25). For example, a radio to be controlled by an ECU would be plugged into a module. The module would be plugged into the electrical outlet (Figure 11–26). X-10 modules operate up to at least 50 feet on the same transformer and allow the appliance to be controlled from any room. Each

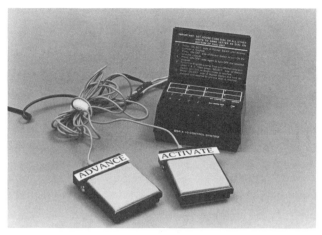

Figure 11–21 The X-10 ECS-8 ECU is a stationary console controlled by two switches. One tread switch advances to the desired numbered appliance and the second turns the appliance on and off.

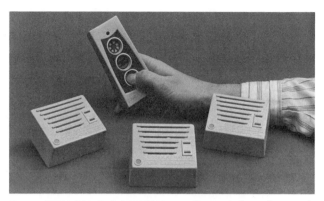

Figure 11–22 The Switch-it ECU transmitter controls appliances via ultrasonic signals to its three color-coded receivers. Each appliance is plugged into one of the three receivers.

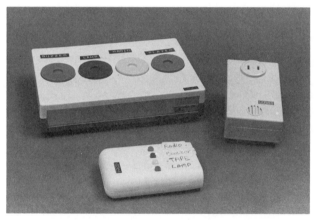

Figure 11–23 The TASH Ultra 4 ECU has a hand-held (front) and a large pushbutton transmitter (back), which send ultrasonic signals to color-coded receivers (right).

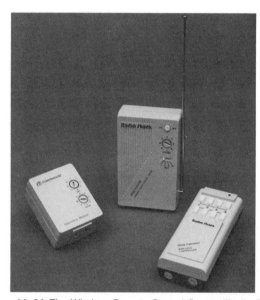

Figure 11–24 The Wireless Remote Control Center (Radio Shack) features a hand-held four-button transmitter (right), which sends a radio signal to the plugged-in receiver (middle). The receiver sends a signal over existing house wiring to a corresponding module into which each appliance is plugged.

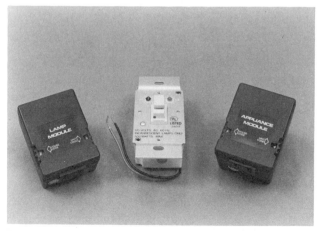

Figure 11–25 X-10 modules: (left to right) lamp, wall switch, appliance

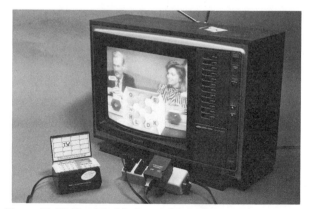

Figure 11–26 The television's on/off function is controlled through the X-10 Command Console ECU (left) by plugging it into an appliance module.

module is manually set to a house code and a number that corresponds to the settings on the transmitter (Figure 11–27). These set-ups can be easily reset at any time.

Appliances can be controlled via two modes: latching or momentary. Latching refers to switch activation where a device remains on when the switch is activated and released and goes off only when the switch is activated again. Momentary refers to switch activation where a device remains on only when the switch is held and turns off when the switch is released.

Computer Adaptations and Alternate Access

Using a computer as a therapeutic modality is becoming increasingly common. The computer may serve as a tool for cognitive remediation or to facilitate motor skills. It may be used as an augmentative or alternative communication system or to fill avocational or vocational needs. A patient with minimal to moderate motor deficits may require only simple adaptations to operate a computer system through a standard keyboard. For the patient with severe motor deficits, an alternative may be needed. Keyboard emulators provide access to the computer so that it responds as though the input were coming from the keyboard. They allow the patient to have access to all software for a particular system.

Computer Adaptations

On/Off Switch Adaptation. Most on/off switches are located on the back of the computer. This makes it difficult for patients with limited arm placement or head pointers to activate the equipment. This can be

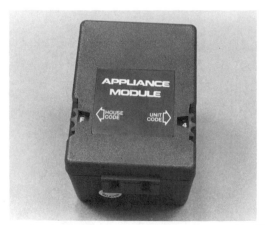

Figure 11–27 The X-10 appliance module set on house code "F" and unit code "4."

addressed by plugging all the computer hardware into a multiplying outlet and then mounting the outlet in a position that makes the on/off rocker switch on the power strip easily accessible. Another solution may be to mount a power controller beneath the monitor. The hardware is plugged into the back of the power controller, and the patient turns each peripheral on and off through corresponding pushbutton switches on the front panel.

Keyboard Adaptations. Key guards can enhance the speed and accuracy of operation, especially when the patient has ataxia and requires a head or hand-held pointer. Key guards prevent the fingers or pointers from slipping or hitting a wrong key. They also serve as a resting place for a head or hand-held pointer and help prevent accidental key activation while the patient is reviewing or resting. Proficient head and hand-held pointer users may be slowed down by a key guard. Key guards are available for many computers, including the Apple II series, Atari 800, Franklin ACE 1000, Epson Hx 20, Commodore 64, and IBM PC. Custom key guards can be fabricated for other computer systems.

Latching mechanisms for keys such as the control and shift keys are built-in on some key guards. The mechanism allows the key to remain depressed without the user holding the key down manually. It is designed as a lever and is activated or released as the patient presses on alternate sides of the latch. This design permits the patient to use a head or single pointer to activate more than one key at a time, which is necessary with many software programs. Key latches that easily attach with adhesive strips or Scotchmate are also available. They are particularly useful for keys, such as the control keys, that are usually located outside the periphery of a standard keyboard. Other key latches attach with screws. Therapists and owners are cautioned to examine the warranty of the machine before drilling into its body to attach screws. Disturbing the body of the device may invalidate the warranty.

Inserting Software. Many adaptations are available to help the person with adequate arm placement but limited control insert a floppy disk into a disk drive. They consist of an extended shelf on the drive. The patient drops the disk onto the shelf and pushes it into the slot with one finger or a head or hand-held pointer. The door may be opened or shut with limited upper extremity control or by using a pointer. See Exhibit 11–1 for information on commercial disk guides (Figure 11–28).

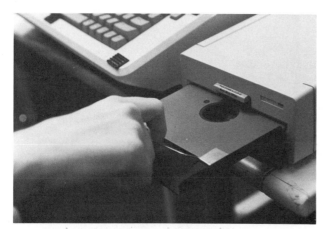

Figure 11–28 The disk guide and wire loop attached to the floppy disk (Extensions for Independence) facilitate independent operation.

Positioning of Devices. Positioning of the computer and peripheral devices is critical. It can be the determining factor between the patient using a standard keyboard or needing an adaptation. Proper positioning can also increase the efficiency of operation and duration. Selecting a table for computer hardware for a patient in a wheelchair needs to take into account the height and length of the wheelchair arms, the angle of recline, and the angle of the user's legs. An additional factor to be considered for patients who use head pointers is the method of accessing the keyboard. Adjustable-height tables and U-shaped work stations generally provide good working areas. Some patients may require an elevating table to position the computer between their wheelchair armrests. Detachable keyboards can be angled to the optimum position by using a bookrest. Monitor arm supports are available that support the monitor, allow it to be adjusted to any angle, and allow it to be swung away from the computer. Monitor arms should be carefully checked for use with the patient's specific system before purchase. Some arms may be unable to support the weight of the selected monitor (Figures 11–29 and 11–30).

Alternate Access

Adaptive Firmware Card. This hardware provides transparent access to the Apple II and IIe and serves as a transparent keyboard emulator for individuals unable to use the keyboard. This allows information to enter the computer from sources other than the standard keyboard, thus permitting use of all standard software for the computer. The interface consists of a printed circuit card that is inserted in the computer and a small plastic box that is screwed onto its side (Figures 11–31 and 11–32). This box contains two minijacks for switch interfacing and a thumbwheel, which is manually turned to the selected mode of input. Sixteen input modes are available to accommodate the variety of needs of the disabled. All may be applicable to a wide range of motor skills. The keyboard remains active and can be used at any time.

The process cannot be controlled only through one-switch activation. The software must first be inserted in the disk drive. The second step is to turn on the computer. The program does not load immediately but requires keyboard input for the timing or scanning rate.

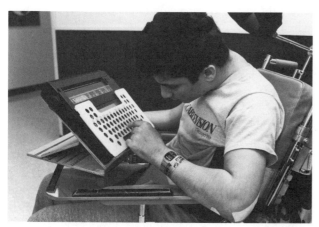

Figure 11–29 Mounting of a portable lap-sized computer or communication device is on a slantboard secured to a lap board with Scotchmate.

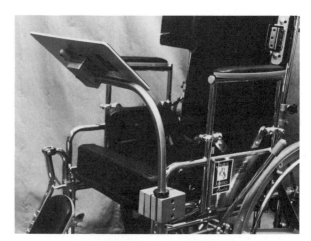

Figure 11–30 The Wheelchair Mounting Kit (Prentke Romich Company) offers a mounting option for lap-sized computers and communication aids. It allows a variety of positions, including the angle of the device, and is easily swung away for transfers.

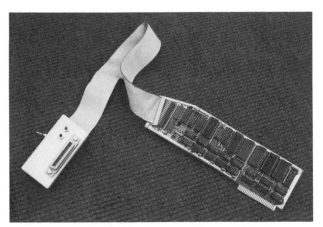

Figure 11–31 The Adaptive Firmware Card consists of a switch interface box on the left and a printed circuit card on the right.

The individual can then use the selected input method through his control switch. The input modes include three types of one-switch scanning; morse code, with one or two switches; two-switch scanning; and modes to accept peripherals, such as a miniature or expanded keyboard. The speed of the cursor and the required reaction time of the user can be accelerated or decelerated at any time. The Firmware Card provides access to games, word processing, or educational programs for individuals with limited arm placement and head control.

One- or two-switch inputs are possible through a variety of switches, including pneumatic, eyebrow, eye blink, or EMG. The expanded keyboard can be activated by hand, foot, or orthosis. The miniature keyboard is activated by a probe that can be attached to a head pointer or a hand orthosis.

Computer Entry Terminal (CET-1). The CET-1 provides transparent access to a variety of computer systems, including the IBM PC, IBM XT, and the Apple II series. This lightweight portable device, which is divided into 128 squares, provides a method of direct selection with an optical head pointer. This is mounted on a headset and requires fair to good head control. Each activation of the head pointer selects a single character, a computer control function, or a phrase previously stored by the user. The single character or phrase is immediately displayed on the monitor and on the CET-1 display. Single-switch row-column scanning and joystick control are options.

Eyetyper Model 200. The Eyetyper provides a method of direct selection through eye gaze. The user is positioned in front of a lightweight display consisting

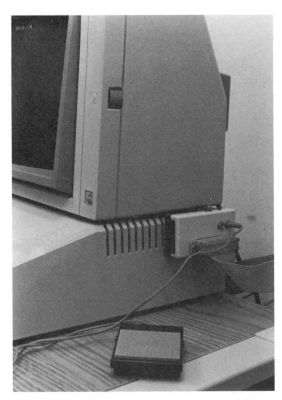

Figure 11–32 A tread switch connected to the Adaptive Firmware Card allows for a single-switch scanning method.

of a lens, set-up light, eight eye-gaze sensor positions, and a box that displays the selected characters. Movement of the user's eyes to the desired item on one of the sensor positions will display the item; it can also be spoken into the built-in speech synthesizer. Ability to maintain the head in one position is critical to using this device, as movement of the eye away from the lens necessitates constant readjustments. However, the person may be able to operate a computer at a significantly faster rate and with greater endurance than with a single switch.

Voice Recognition Systems. Voice recognition systems are one of the newer developments in data entry. They were designed to increase its speed and to make the learning of complex software easier. Many new systems compatible with a variety of computers are entering the market. Therapists are advised to look into these systems carefully before purchasing. Some are designed to run only particular software, while others are machine specific and provide access to all software packages designed for a particular computer. In evaluating these systems, one should consider the accuracy of its voice recognition, the amount of vocabulary, the length of training required, and the price.

The systems operate by the user speaking a word or phrase into a microphone (also available in a headset and as a wireless microphone). The computer recognizes the input and responds to it as though it were given through a keyboard. Before running a program, the user builds the necessary vocabulary for it and trains the computer to recognize his voice speaking the selected words. In the training process, the user speaks each word or phrase at least three times. Additional training of up to ten repetitions may ensure greater accuracy in recognition. When pronunciations that differ from the voice patterns to which the machine has been trained are used, repetition of commands may be necessary. For example, a problem may occur if the user's voice is unusually hoarse. For a patient with speech and language deficits that result in inconsistent voice patterns, the system may not be feasible.

These systems were designed to be used concurrently with keyboard access. This dual access decreases the necessity of hitting several keys for one action. For the disabled, however, input solely through voice recognition is possible. The input time for a voice recognition system must be compared with that of other systems. It is not indicated for every patient, as reliability, needs, and the user's ability to build and train vocabulary are significant factors in determining its effectiveness for the user. Four systems compatible with the Apple and IBM are listed in Exhibit 11–1.

Koala Pad. The Koala Pad is an electronic video sketch pad that allows for the creation of a variety of multicolor graphics. It can be used with any Apple II series computer through a game port. To operate the system, a stick or a finger is moved across the pad. Two-touch switches also need to be activated. They can be adapted with a latching mechanism to keep them depressed until they are released. This may be necessary for programs that require the user to move the stick while simultaneously holding the switch down. The stick can be attached to an orthosis or head pointer if necessary. Maintained pressure is required to activate the Koala Pad. It can be used as a miniature keyboard through custom-developed software. Software that can be used includes games, drawing, educational and graphic design packages, and programming options.

Light Pen. A light pen allows the user to access the computer by holding the pen next to the monitor and pushing a small button at the end of the pen to activate it. This is currently not a functional alternative for patients with limited hand function or abnormal muscle tone. The pen may be operated using unilateral or bilateral hand function. When two hands are used one hand is used to place the pen while the other hand pushes the button. Upper extremity endurance is also a factor to consider. Fatigue may become a factor in keeping the pen accurately placed on the monitor.

TRAINING

Because of memory and learning deficits, training in the use of switches and devices may be time-consuming and necessitate numerous repetitions. A longer training program for the use of simple low-cost devices, such as buzzers or battery-operated toys, may be justified. It is helpful to have some of these devices available for evaluation purposes and to loan to the patient during training. Effective incorporation of devices into the patient's daily routine may be required to justify purchase. Extensive training with expensive devices, such as an ECU, may not be justified if the funding source has not been established. Extensive training may frustrate the user if funding is denied and the claim is deemed unacceptable for third party reimbursement.

DETERMINATION OF THE MOUNTING SYSTEM

The results of the motor evaluation are integrated with educational and vocational needs to determine the type of mounting system most appropriate for the patient. Mounting sites include the wheelchair, walker, bed, table, desk, or floor. Rehabilitation engineering services may be required to design and fabricate a custom mounting system or to adapt a commercial device. One device may need to be interchanged throughout the day among a variety of mounting systems, as in the case of a patient who may spend time on the floor, in a wheelchair, and in bed.

EQUIPMENT ORDER AND FABRICATION

When the evaluation and trial periods have been completed, and all options have been discussed with the patient and family, definitive equipment is ordered or fabricated. To ensure use of the equipment, the patient and family should be involved in all aspects of selection. This may include the color or mounting of the device. Before ordering, an appraisal of all costs, including the cost of adaptations, should be completed.

FAMILY AND ATTENDANT EDUCATION

Upon delivery of the equipment, the patient, family, and/or attendant are educated as to the use, care, and set-up of the device. Other involved persons, such as the patient's teachers, coworkers, or therapists, may also require training. In some cases, equipment set-ups can be demonstrated adequately enough to allow a family member to set up the system in the discharge environment. When possible, a rehabilitation engineer and the patient's therapist should be available to set up more complex systems. This will help ensure that training is complete and that appropriate modifications can be made by a person familiar with the patient. The patient and family should be notified of appropriate resources for equipment repair and replacement. While some vendors offer to set up equipment for a fee, a primary therapist who is more familiar with the patient's functional status should accompany the vendor and incorporate necessary adaptations when practical.

FOLLOW UP

After set-up of the equipment, periodic rechecks are recommended. This helps ensure that the client is using the device optimally and allows the therapist to monitor ongoing changes. Cognitive, sensory-perceptual, motor, and language skills may change significantly enough to warrant the ordering of more complex devices and control methods. Equipment needs for a patient may change if he returns to work or school. If a device is found to be faulty, it should be repaired or replaced as soon as possible. Many vendors provide loaner units to patients whose devices are being repaired.

Therapists recommending technical aids for their clients must remain up-to-date in their knowledge of available equipment. It may be most efficient for one or two therapists in a facility or a geographical area to develop specialty skills in technical aid evaluation and recommendation. At RIC, the team is composed of the occupational therapist and the speech language pathologist, with consultative services as needed from rehabilitation engineering, physical therapy, and vocational rehabilitation. Resources in this area are growing and include national and regional conferences, disabled consumer groups, equipment companies, national computer data system networks, rehabilitation and research facilities, and specialized publications.

Computer Use for the Remediation of Cognitive, Perceptual, and Fine Motor Deficits

Russ Hollander, OTR/L

INTRODUCTION

Given the statistics regarding the young age of many head-injured patients, computers and video games are often familiar aspects of their premorbid life style. Given the technology that allows for nontraditional access to the computer and the relative ease with which therapists can be trained to use hardware, new options are available in the treatment of cognitive, perceptual, and fine motor impairments. A variety of software is available to help therapists guide patients through portions of the rehabilitative process. See Exhibit 11A–1 for a partial list of resources listing journals and newsletters that address computer use. Factors to consider when choosing a software package include variable skill levels, specific skill or goal area addressed, and cost. The key is to select appropriate software to meet specific treatment goals. Reviews of specific programs are beginning to appear to help therapists select appropriate software (Kreutzer, Hill, & Morrison, 1987). Some of the journals listed include programs which can be typed in free of cost. Other options to reduce the cost of acquiring software include programs that are considered public domain and can be legally copied. Many user groups have a number of these programs available to members.

While the clinical observations and involvement of trained professionals allow a more complete picture of the patient, this same human element may skew and interfere with evaluation and treatment efforts. With the possible exception of some evaluations with standardized testing protocols, methods of presentation, cueing, and interpretation vary. Even standardized tests do not always consider variations as subtle as voice, tone, and volume, or background colors. Consistent, nonspontaneous formats of presenting information such as those found in some software programs can be beneficial in comparing clients against either their own performance over time or those of others. Depending on the program selected, computer assisted therapy (CAT) can provide this consistency or random variation of stimuli where indicated. The computer's methods of presenting information and recording responses may bring more objective data to the rehabilitation format.

Computer use may also be viewed as a cost- and time-efficient modality from a staffing standpoint. According to a survey of centers using CAT ("Cognitive Rehabilitation," 1984), 21 percent employ the format on a client self-directed basis, 41 percent as part of group treatment, and 11 percent as a component of home programs. Though the vast majority (95 percent) of the centers engage clients in a one-to-one treatment situation, the additional CAT skill reinforcement sessions frequently result in lower patient cost. CAT can continue as part of a home program for patients who have access to equipment. Follow up can be provided by periodic outpatient rechecks to evaluate progress and the continued appropriateness of suggested programs.

Exhibit 11A–1 Computer resources

Microcomputers: Clinical Applications, E. Nelson Clark, MS, OTR, Editor
    Slack Incorporated
    6900 Grove Road
    Thorofare, NJ 08086

The OT's Computer, published bimonthly
    Denis Anson, MS, OTR
    3685 N.E. Olympic Street
    Hillsboro, OR 97124

Computer Disability News, free, one copy per agency
    National Easter Seal Society
    2023 W. Ogden Avenue
    Chicago, IL 60612

AOTA Information Packet on Computers
    AOTA Products
    11383 Piccard Drive
    Rockville, MD 20850

Cognitive Rehabilitation, A Publication for the Therapist, Family and Patient, published bimonthly
    NeuroScience Publishers
    655 Carrollton Avenue
    Indianapolis, IN 46220

Rehabilitation Technology Review, newsletter of the Association for the Advancement of Rehabilitation Technology (RESNA), free with RESNA membership or $25 per year for nonmembers
    RESNA
    1101 Connecticut Avenue, N.W. Suite 700
    Washington, DC 20036

Compute! The Journal for Progressive Computing
    Compute! Publications, Inc.
    825 7th Avenue
    New York, NY 10019

Assistive Devices Information Network
    University of Iowa
    Division of Developmental Disabilities
    University Hospital School
    Iowa City, IA 52242

CURRENT APPROACHES TO COGNITIVE-PERCEPTUAL RECOVERY

In reviewing the theories of cognitive-perceptual recovery, two approaches are representative of current practice at RIC. One theory recognizes that the brain has some plasticity and proposes that damaged areas regain their functional ability over time (Glassman, 1970). In following this theory, therapists often provide graded stimulation and use facilitation techniques to impact deficit areas positively. Techniques are incorporated into a treatment plan based on the patient's deficits and the principles of normal development in which the patient is encouraged to progress through the developmental stages. Treatment efforts, at times, may encourage the patient to function at a lower developmental level rather than disrupt the normal progression by using compensatory methods.

A functional substitution theory accepts the brain's ability to compensate for deficits and proposes that nondamaged areas take over the function usually performed by damaged areas (Luria, 1948; Rosner, 1970). Following this theory, a treatment program focuses on compensatory techniques and recognizes the patient's ability to use his functional and undisturbed strengths to manage deficit areas. Frequently, therapists mix facilitation and compensation techniques based on their clinical experience and the patient's response.

Regardless of the theoretical framework employed, the therapist's ability to control the environment is crucial. To appreciate and understand the relation of the stimulus or treatment to a patient's performance, the therapist must be able to:

- control the intended stimulus
- reduce extraneous stimuli
- grade a new stimulus based on the patient's performance
- provide feedback

This ability to manipulate and control the variables of an environment and provide immediate feedback is a positive feature of CAT.

Current trends in health care emphasize the need for time-efficiency and cost-effectiveness. When dealing with the remediation of cognitive and perceptual deficits, it is often difficult to track and monitor patient improvement. This is due in part to the fact that cognition and perception are components of more comprehensive functional levels.

CAT programs may enable the therapist to:

- isolate specific cognitive-perceptual skills in evaluation and treatment to ensure the directness of treatment efforts

- recognize subtle changes in performance using an objective system for monitoring treatment response and for justifying treatment effort
- provide additional treatment time in a supervised setting
- monitor the impact on functional skills

Table 11A–1 outlines some of the advantages and disadvantages of the CAT format.

TABLE 11A–1   Advantages and disadvantages of CAT

Advantages	Disadvantages
Objectivity	
Consistent stimulus pattern	Not empathetic to patient/ environment (i.e., frustration, noise, glare)
Consistent method of grading responses	Lacks creativity, spontaneity, flexibility
Technical format and structure	Fails to appreciate quality factors or clinical observations
Cost/time-effectiveness	
After purchase of system	Initial set-up costly
Cost-effective reinforcement sessions	Repair of hardware costly
Few expendable items	
Specificity of results/ data illustrates progress to third party payers	
Printouts of test results may minimize documentation time	
Psychological	
Mature: may appear consistent with other technology in the health care setting	Intimidating to some staff and clients
	May not fall within sociocultural realm
May relate to premorbid exposure to video games	May not reinforce patient's efforts, only results
Adaptability	
Various modes of input available	Does not respond to all modes of input
	Positioning of set-up may not accommodate some clients

Manipulation of Variables/Test Parameters

The control of the treatment environment is essential to the clinician. Similar to traditional treatment environments, CAT may allow the therapist to alter and manipulate specific aspects of the stimulus or background environment to stimulate or train for desired performance. While many cognitive-perceptual programs offer controlling factors as menu items, some make automatic adjustments to the task depending on the user's performance. In these situations, the individual "teaches" the computer his abilities. This may be frustrating to the client who cannot perform at the baseline level or who excels beyond that point and must "work up to" a challenge.

Adjusting the variables as pretest or menu items makes it possible for the session to begin at a predetermined skill level. Selections may be based on clinical observations or previous attempts. Aspects that may be altered or options selected include:

Stimulus	Background/feedback	Other Options
Size	Auditory feedback	Review of results
Speed/timing	Visual feedback	Data analysis
Color	Overall test time	Printout of results
Shape		Storage/filing
Patterns		Mode input
Random		
Systematic		
Level of difficulty (from a developmental progressive sequence)		
Extinct/nonextinct		

Methodology for Setting Parameters

1. Start at basic level (preprogrammed *or* predetermined level) based on clinical observation or previous performance.
2. Review results.
3. Manipulate variables so as to upgrade or downgrade difficulty:

   - background unchanged, stimulus adjusted
   - background adjusted, stimulus unchanged
   - background and stimulus changed
   - background and stimulus unchanged, overall quality or efficiency monitored

COMPUTER USAGE AT RIC

It is the philosophy at RIC that CAT is a modality or adjunct to the rehabilitation process rather than a treatment in and of itself. Just as motor-based exercises are not functional tasks, cognitive-perceptual activities on a computer may facilitate skill development to the point of evaluating a client's functional status only when those skills are mastered in the context of a functional task. Additionally, the objective data received can be fully appreciated only when combined with the clinical observations of a trained professional.

Some deficits appear more conducive to remediation using computer software than others. For example, patients with strictly visual-perceptual deficits may benefit more than patients with more global sensory-perceptual dysfunction. Programs related to specific cognitive tasks, such as problem solving or arithmetic reasoning, may be effective in providing the patient with a variety of problems and immediate feedback.

Other skills addressed, such as arousal or attention, motor planning, and memory, need to be closely monitored in terms of functional carryover. A common problem noted in head-injured patients is poor generalization, which may be evidenced by improved computer scores but limited or no functional improvements. More research and reviews are needed to assist therapists in selecting appropriate software, determining which patients could benefit the most, and confirming functional applications and carryover. Local OT or other user groups can be a good source of information when beginning to use computers with patients. Table 11A–2 illustrates some of the skill areas for which we use CAT at RIC.

We have found it helpful to develop a support and steering committee with the following objectives:

- determine and monitor department hardware and software needs
- focus on the areas of perceptual and cognitive functioning most responsive to retraining through technology
- act as a central resource network for orientation, problem solving, adaption, and development of computer-based rehabilitation programs

TABLE 11A–2   Indications for CAT

Cognition

Concentration	Problem solving
Attention span	Decision making
Auditory memory	Action-consequence
Visual memory	Direction following
Organization	Cause/effect
Sequencing	
Form constancy	Scanning
Figure-ground	Visual discrimination
Position in space	Visual tracking
Direction	Color discrimination
Motor planning	Auditory discrimination

Motor

Hand function	Eye/hand coordination
Arm placement	Response time
Head control	Adapted manipulation

Usage of CAT in a treatment program is at the discretion of the therapist (unless specifically addressed in the treatment orders). Staff, as always, accept the responsibility to determine and use the most effective and efficient means to achieve desired results and functional outcomes. Therapists have long used games, puzzles, and other activities to enhance the patient's perceptual, cognitive, and motor performance. Computers can provide a useful addition to more traditional activities.

REFERENCES

Cognitive rehabilitation survey results. (1984, Nov/Dec). *Cognitive Rehabilitation, 2*(6), 12–15.

Glassman, R. (1970). Contralateral and ipsilateral transfer of a cutaneous discrimination in normal and callosum-sectioned cats. *Journal of Comparative and Physiological Psychology, 70,* 470–475.

Kreutzer, J., Hill, M., & Morrison, C. (1987). *Cognitive rehabilitation resources for the Apple II computer.* Indianapolis, IN: NeuroScience Publishers.

Luria, A. (1948). *Restoration of brain function after war injuries.* USSR, Moscow: Academia Meditsinskikh Nauk.

Rosner, B. (1970). Brain functions. *Annual Review of Psychology, 21,* 555–594.

Part V

Related Issues

Therapeutic Use of Groups

Dorothy Vezzetti, MS, OTR/L

This unit provides a rationale for the use of group treatment as an adjunct to individual therapy. Several examples of specific groups developed at the Rehabilitation Institute of Chicago (RIC) are included. Rehabilitation medicine uses a biopsychosocial model of practice (Licht, 1968). This model relates to the community, social, vocational, physical, and psychological aspects of the individual. The primary goal of the rehabilitative process is to optimize the individual's ability to function independently and assume a productive role in society. Working in groups prepares the patient to meet the social demands of family and community.

Most normal adult human behavior develops through learning and example. The transmission of traditions, customs, skills, mores, and morals, which constitutes the socialization process, takes place through contact with others. Authority figures and peers act as agents of socialization (Berelson & Steiner, 1964). Group treatment provides a supportive setting in which patients with similar problems can relate and begin the resocialization process.

Group treatment can address a variety of deficits frequently associated with head injury (HI). The rationale and goals of groups may differ significantly, however, depending upon whether the intent of therapy is to remediate psychosocial dysfunction or reinforce skill development. These are discussed separately in this unit. The patient recovering from HI is easily confused by group activities unless provided a clear focus. Limiting the goals of a group is usually more effective than attempting to address a number of problem areas at the same time.

TREATMENT OF PSYCHOSOCIAL DYSFUNCTION

There is growing recognition among health care professionals that the major factors that interfere with rehabilitation, family relations, and successful return to work are the psychological and social repercussions that follow HI. The more common sequelae, described in Unit 4, include tension, anxiety, insecurity, withdrawal, apathy, depression, disinhibition, irritability, dependence, egocentricity, feelings of inadequacy, and increased risk of suicide (Lishman, 1978). Group treatment can be used to remediate many of the problems associated with psychosocial dysfunction, and as Mosey (1973) suggests, to "help a patient learn to think, feel, and act in a manner that is more satisfying to himself and others." Through group activities, the patient can develop the psychosocial skills necessary for satisfactory adjustment to disability and good interpersonal relations.

The focus of the psychosocial group is the process by which tasks are accomplished. Both the patient's specific psychosocial skills and group interaction skills need to be evaluated to make an appropriate group assignment. Activities should be graded to approximate the patient's functional levels in two areas: (1) specific psychosocial and related skills, and (2) group interaction level.

To help unify the evaluation and reporting process, the American Occupational Therapy Association has developed a list of psychosocial and related skills. These are included as part of the *Uniform Terminology System for Reporting Occupational Therapy Services* (AOTA, 1979). In *Activities Therapy*, Mosey (1973) discusses five levels of group interaction skills, which can be used as a guide for grading group participation in a psychiatric setting. Relevant information from these references has been adapted to meet the needs of the head-injured population and is a foundation for the material presented in this unit.

Specific Psychosocial and Related Skills

A thorough assessment of the following skills will enable the therapist to identify specific psychosocial and related problem areas for remediation and help her formulate goals for group treatment for the higher functioning patient.

- *Self concept/self identity*: Perceiving the needs of self and others, assessing one's strengths and limitations, and sensing one's competence are frequently problematic after HI. Through group treatment, the therapist can help the patient integrate the changes in self-image precipitated by disability and assist him in formulating new, meaningful goals and in developing sensitivity to others.
- *Situational coping*: The patient may have difficulty managing daily living tasks. The recognition of the need for change may be slow or absent, and reality testing may be impaired. Through the use of groups, the therapist can help the patient direct his energy to overcome problems, initiate and implement decisions, assume responsibility for self and the consequences of actions, and interact with others in a variety of situations.
- *Community involvement*: The patient may exhibit disinhibited behavior and a blunting of social consciousness that interfere with community reintegration. Participation in therapeutic groups can help him relearn the conventions of normative behavior through participation in planning, organizing, and executing social activities.

- *Self expression*: Writing and speaking skills and the ability to interpret and use nonverbal signs and symbols may be impaired. Through group interaction, the therapist can facilitate the patient's ability to communicate effectively.
- *Self-control*: The patient frequently has difficulty controlling impulses and coping with stress. Through appropriate group feedback, he can increase self-awareness and be helped to control undesirable behaviors.
- *Dyadic and group interaction*: Often, the patient has difficulty coping with frustration, anxiety, and failure, and may have problems cooperating and competing. Therapists can help him set limits, develop the ability to compromise and negotiate, and participate in a group in a manner that is beneficial to self and others.

These skills reflect competencies relevant for patients who are alert and oriented. For the patient with more severe cognitive deficits, a modified assessment can be used. Evaluation in the following areas can help the therapist set achievable goals for such patients.

- developing self-concept and self-identity through perceiving basic needs, identifying abilities, building a sense of competence and self-esteem, feeling safe and secure, and formulating simple goals
- developing situational coping skills through an awareness of safety and interacting with others
- developing awareness of the community through understanding social norms and customs, performing basic self-care, and identifying former roles
- developing self-expression through improving verbal and nonverbal skills
- developing self-control through responding to limits and monitoring own behavior.

Grading Group Interaction Levels

Group treatment of psychosocial problems is most effective when the members have similar group-interaction skill levels. Mosey (1973) identified five levels of group interaction skills that represent a developmental framework for grading groups. The criterion for participation in these groups is determined by the extent to which an individual can share a task and feelings with others.

At level 1, the parallel group, the patient learns to work on a task in the presence of others. At level 2, the project group, he learns to share a short-term task in a highly structured setting. A longer-term shared task performed with relatively less structure and assistance from the therapist is characteristic of level 3, the ego-centric cooperative group. At level 4, the cooperative group, the therapist acts primarily as an advisor, and members with common interests learn to enjoy being together on an emotional level. At level 5, the mature group members learn to satisfy their own needs and the needs of others in a task group situation, which integrates the emotional and performance components of group process. It is desirable that mature group skills be developed in a community setting among individuals with disparate backgrounds and interests. This highest level group generally meets outside the health care facility and, therefore, is not discussed further. Group treatment can also be extended to include minimally responsive and awakening patients and provide social readiness experiences for patients with more severe impairments.

Social Readiness Group Experiences

It is essential that even the minimally responsive patient be included in the social milieu. They are often subject to prolonged periods of isolation. With discretion, it may be possible to take the patient to a secure area of the lounge or day room for a brief period each day. In this way, social isolation can be minimized and the individual included in the larger community.

Although awakening patients do not always respond to familiar individuals and may be unable to communicate with others in a consistent manner, social readiness experiences can be provided through modified group treatment. A speech therapist, physical therapist, and occupational therapist may work as a multidisciplinary team to treat a small group. If the therapist-to-patient ratio is kept low, preferably 1:1, a limited number of psychosocial goals can be included, and interaction between members facilitated.

For example, group members can be oriented to the names of others and encouraged to communicate basic needs. A snack time, which reintroduces appropriate social behaviors, such as using a napkin and passing food, may be incorporated. Birthdays, holidays, and special occasions of significance to group members can be celebrated. Patients may help put away supplies and equipment and be assigned simple housekeeping tasks

that help maintain the group space; for example, closing the curtains for privacy.

Awakening patients are usually able to perform only a one-step task. The therapist provides maximum assistance when needed. The psychosocial goals of this group might include recognition of and beginning participation in familiar customs and traditions, and developing the ability to make basic needs known and to communicate with others.

Group activities are inappropriate for agitated patients. They are often combative, easily frustrated, and unable to attend to any activity or delay gratification of needs for more than a very brief period. They frighten others who perceive them (often rightly so) as a threat to their safety.

When the degree of agitation decreases, and the patient can tolerate the presence of others and must no longer be treated in a low-stimulus environment, a trial group session may be attempted. In the beginning, the patient is encouraged to sit quietly in the same room with other group members before task or social demands are made. Several desensitizing sessions of gradually extended periods may be necessary before he is ready to participate. Occasional outbursts may occur as he adjusts to the increased stress of the new social situation. When comfortable in the group, the task or activity selected for the postagitated patient should be one he can accomplish with minimum assistance and enjoys doing. Care taken in initial task selection can help significantly with adjustment to the group. A small parallel group will usually provide the most appropriately graded experience for this patient.

The chronically agitated patient presents a serious behavioral management problem. An intensive behavior modification program may help him gradually regain control. Such a program is usually the treatment of choice for the patient who remains agitated for an extended period and continues to exhibit behaviors that make group participation inadvisable.

Formal Groups

Confused patients are moving from assistance to independence in performing familiar tasks. They are also beginning to initiate true social interaction. Thus, they are usually ready to participate in a parallel group.

Parallel Group. The goals of the parallel group are for members to work at a task in the presence of others and to be aware of and interact with each other appropriately. Individual craft projects, nail care, feeding, and simple meal preparation are examples of activities that can be used. The task should no longer require the patient's full attention. The initiation of social skills, such as greeting other group members, sharing space, taking turns, asking for help, waiting for assistance, asking questions, introducing self to others, listening to others, and following simple rules, can be facilitated by the therapist through modeling and shaping. Specific psychosocial skills developed in this group include:

- knowing one's performance strengths and limitations
- directing and redirecting energy to overcome problems
- observing own and others' behavior
- understanding social and cultural norms of communication and interaction

Oriented patients have usually mastered many familiar tasks and can work independently with growing confidence in a structured, secure environment. Because they can satisfy basic needs more easily, additional energy is available for developing the social skills needed to function independently in the community. It is a difficult passage, however, from the level of dressing independently to the level of assuming household or job responsibilities.

During this phase, the patient must develop the ability to share a task with others and to work with less facilitation and structure from the therapist; that is, develop the skills needed to participate in groups organized at the project and egocentric cooperative level. Groups at this level require members to contribute to group decision making, planning, and task performance; generate ideas and volunteer information; make suggestions to other group members; evaluate alternatives; compromise; initiate action; carry out responsibility; and assume other group roles.

At this level it is increasingly difficult to separate cognitive and social skills. Cooperative work that is not prestructured requires more problem solving. Many patients lack confidence in their task skills and are reluctant to participate in situations where others will depend on them and judge their performance. At this level of interaction, it is more difficult for the patient to deny his deficits by finding excuses to refuse challenging tasks or by ignoring problems when they occur. It is a time for the patient to develop the mature coping mechanisms needed for healthy adaptation to former roles. For many, the transition from hospital to independent living is confrontive and stormy. Through appropriate grading of group experiences, the therapist can help him make this transition gradually and successfully.

Project Group. This group is organized to develop the social skills needed for members to share work on a short-term task. Project activities provide a foundation for higher-level cooperative task behaviors. Other demands should be minimized; therefore, it is important that activities are chosen that can be performed at a relaxed pace where neither speed nor accuracy are crucial. Decorating a room for the holidays, making a fruit salad, simple assembly work, packaging, sorting, or reorganizing supplies are examples of appropriate activities. Specific psychosocial skills for this group include setting limits on self and others, cooperating and competing, responsibly relying on self and others, and participating in a group in a manner that is beneficial to self and others. When the individual is comfortable sharing a task, he is ready for group participation at the next level.

Egocentric Cooperative Group. This group is characterized by the gradual withdrawal of direction by the therapist and the assumption of responsibility for longer-term group tasks by the patients. As the therapist reduces the structure, risks are increased for the patient. Because many group decisions will be made through trial-and-error problem solving, the consequences of these decisions cannot always be anticipated. The therapist, therefore, must make certain that members understand that they will never be permitted to endanger themselves or become involved in a thoroughly disruptive situation although some problems may develop.

Most patients need considerable assistance and support from the therapist when beginning to function at this less secure level. Often, the individual has cognitive deficits that make problem solving difficult and is frequently unaware of the mental energy needed to generate ideas, compare alternative suggestions, examine the consequences of decisions, and plan the details and contingencies of activities. It is usually necessary for the therapist to review these processes with the group using exercises that simulate situations and to give group members time to gear up to these new demands before they assume responsibility for task performance.

Evaluation of group and individual accomplishment is an important function of this group. Group members are encouraged to assess their strengths and weaknesses and the effects of their performance on task outcome. Videotape feedback of role playing, decision making, and planning sessions can also help members develop critical thinking skills. Good decisions and contributions should be recognized, and errors in judgment identified through constructive feedback from the therapist and other group members. The therapist's role is primarily to allow the patient to experience success while maintaining the optimum tension needed for adaptation, growth, and psychosocial skill development. Community trips are especially appropriate. Longer-term projects, such as planning a dinner or party or organizing a rummage sale, can also be successful.

Specific psychosocial skills developed in this group include knowing one's performance strengths and limitations; conceptualizing problems in terms of needed behavioral changes or action; handling competition, frustration, anxiety, success, and failure; responsibly relying on self and others; building a sense of competence and self-esteem; and having a sense of psychological safety and security.

Cooperative or Support Groups. Sometimes, the patient has less difficulty expressing feelings than sharing tasks. Because this group is not task oriented, it places less demand on the individual's cognitive and physical skills than other formal groups. The therapist can foster the development of informal cooperative groups where individuals meet to enjoy each other's company by providing a sanctioned space for congregating and a few catalysts for conversation. A pack of cards, coffee and rolls, or a music area may be all that is needed. These casual meetings can prepare the patient to participate in self-help and support groups after discharge.

Other professionals, including social workers, psychologists, and nurses, often lead formal support groups. State and local chapters of the National Head Injury Foundation sponsor support groups where family members and patients can share personal experiences and express feelings with others who have similar concerns. Therapists working with the head-injured population should be aware of these community resources and make referrals when appropriate.

Specific psychosocial skills developed in this group include clearly perceiving one's own and others' needs, feelings, conflicts, values, beliefs, expectations, sex-uality, and power; and experiencing and recognizing a range of emotions.

PRACTICAL SUGGESTIONS FOR THE USE OF GROUP TREATMENT

- The primary goals of a group should be limited to a specific problem area to help the patient focus attention.
- The patient's group interaction, individual psychosocial, cognitive, perceptual, and motor skills should be evaluated before referring him to an ongoing group.
- A group referral form can be used to communicate information about a patient's strengths and weaknesses to the therapist responsible for the group.
- The referring therapist should be thoroughly familiar with the group's objectives and be kept informed of the patient's progress by group leaders on a regular basis.
- Pre- and post-tests can be used to help measure a patient's change in status.
- Time for planning and processing meetings should be scheduled so that group leaders can organize activities and discuss issues.
- Most patients benefit from continuity and repetition; therefore, for many goals, a group that meets daily is most effective.
- Group treatment requires the skillful use of resources, structuring of the environment, and direction to meet a variety of individual needs.
- The nature of the patient population will determine the kind and variety of individual needs.
- Spontaneous short-term groups can be started whenever the need is recognized.
- Multidisciplinary groups can be quite effective.
- Rotating responsibility for group leadership can help maintain a high level of enthusiasm and encourage innovation.
- Transitions between group leaders can be facilitated by arranging a period of overlap.
- The size of groups should reflect the amount of assistance or supervision members will need to benefit from the experience. Parallel groups with skill reinforcement goals generally tolerate larger numbers than psychosocial groups. The ideal size is usually from three to ten members.

TREATMENT OF OTHER PROBLEM AREAS (SKILL REINFORCEMENT)

Intellectual impairment after HI often interferes with learning. Skills must be repeated frequently in a variety of situations to help the patient compensate for difficulties with the retention of information and generalization of concepts. The patient's struggle to cope with these deficits and meet the demands of the environment may precipitate maladaptive emotional behavioral changes (Goldstein, 1952). Working with others in a cohesive group can provide the individual with the support needed to continue on a productive course of rehabilitation. The encouragement of other group members often acts as a substantial motivating force whose value should not be minimized.

Groups with skill reinforcement goals in areas other than psychosocial performance are frequently organized as parallel groups. Social demands can be kept low, and group members can concentrate their attention and energy on the specific problem area. Skill reinforcement groups can be a cost-effective way to provide the patient with the intensive treatment needed to make steady progress. The following problem areas can be effectively addressed in groups designed to foster skill reinforcement.

- physical daily living skill groups addressing grooming and hygiene, feeding and eating, functional mobility, and functional communication
- work skill groups addressing homemaking, child care and parenting, and employment preparation
- play/leisure skill groups
- sensorimotor skill groups addressing range of motion, gross and fine coordination, strength and endurance, sensory awareness, visual-spatial awareness, and body integration
- cognitive skill groups addressing orientation, concentration, attention, memory, problem solving, and generalization

RIC GROUP PROGRAMS

Independent Living Skills Group

Problem area:	Psychosocial and community planning skills
Tasks:	Planning and participating in a community trip
Level:	Egocentric cooperative
Focus:	Provide patients with the planning and social skills needed for effective adaptation to former roles and reintegration into the community

Prerequisite skills:

- the ability to work with others in a structured group to complete a short-term task
- the ability to
  - write or remember brief messages
  - use the telephone and written material to gather information
  - use landmarks and simple maps for pathfinding
  - communicate with others
  - walk for 3 hours, with brief rest periods, and negotiate curbs and steps independently
- a basic awareness of safety

Frame of reference:	A cognitive model for problem solving
Structure:	The group meets five times per week. Three 1-hour sessions are used to organize the trip, a 3-hour block is for community travel, and the last 1-hour session is used to evaluate performance.
Staffing:	Two staff/six patient maximum

Members decide where they will go for their weekly trip. They are encouraged to use resources to develop a list of possibilities. Decision making should reflect an awareness of the interests and needs of self and others, provide an opportunity for the patient to practice compromise and negotiation, and demonstrate an understanding of performance strengths and limitations, budgeting, time management, and community resources.

Members make reservations, organize a travel plan, confirm bus or train schedules or walking distances, and make arrangements with nursing for passes or medications. Planning should reflect an ability to test goals and perceptions against reality, perceive the need for changes, and direct and redirect energy to overcome problems.

Members travel to and from their destination using public transportation if necessary. Places that have been visited include department stores, restaurants, museums, the beach, public buildings, parks, and other places of interest near the hospital. The experience should provide group members with a sense of competence and achievement, an opportunity to follow through on decisions and assume responsibility for self and consequences of actions, and an understanding of social norms.

Members assess the outcome of the trip and make suggestions for future planning. They are encouraged to discuss anything they learned about themselves, others, or the environment, and how they felt about the experience. Any difficulties that occurred during the trip are viewed as opportunities for the patient to handle frustration, anxiety, and failure, and are treated as positive learning experiences during the evaluation process. It is essential that the therapist maintain a supportive, encouraging atmosphere during these discussions to promote the development of mature coping and functional adaptation. The group discussion can help members identify strengths and weaknesses and set goals for improvement. A group of this type, using a community-based activity, addresses most of the psychosocial components of behavior that are the legitimate concern of occupational therapists and does so in a manner that provides strong incentives for growth.

Meal Preparation Group

Problem area: Work skill reinforcement task: Meal preparation

Task: Members will prepare simple hot or cold meals consisting of three to five items.

Level: Parallel

Focus: Promote the development of safe meal preparation habits for patients returning to semi-independent or independent living environments.

Prerequisite skills:

- the ability to work in the presence of others on an individual task
- the ability to
    - prepare a hot or cold meal with minimal supervision

- work in a distracting environment
- prepare meal and clean-up within 1 hour

- a basic awareness of safety

Frame of reference: Reinforcement of learning through practice

Structure: The group meets for approximately 1 hour daily.

Staffing: One staff/two patient minimum
Two staff/four patient maximum

Meal planning for the week is done by the patient at the beginning of the week. A list of food items needed for the following week is given to the therapist by the patient. The therapist is responsible for ordering supplies.

Members choose to prepare either breakfast or lunch. They consult the menu they have submitted and prepare the meal indicated for the day. Performance is rated according to the patient's ability to observe all safety precautions and demonstrate the proper use and care of a variety of kitchen equipment including the following items: gas, electric range, or microwave oven; electric mixers, blenders, food processors, and dishwasher; knives and other sharp objects. The group activity should provide patients with the opportunity to initiate, implement, and follow through on decisions; manage activities of daily living to promote optimal performance; and practice time management skills.

Avocational Group

Problem area: Cognitive skill reinforcement

Task: Avocational craft activity. The group member will complete one or more therapeutic craft activities, e.g., ceramics, woodworking, macrame, decoupage, latch hooking, selected in conjunction with the therapist to meet cognitive goals.

Level: Parallel

Focus: Promote the reinforcement of the task-related cognitive skills of concentration, attention span, memory, generalization, and problem solving.

Prerequisite skills

- the ability to work in the presence of others on an individual task
- the ability to
  - complete selected project with minimal supervision and exhibit basic safety awareness regarding the use of materials and tools
  - work in a distracting environment
  - work with occasional redirection to task for 1 hour

Frame of reference: Reinforcement of learning through practice

Structure: The group meets for 1 hour daily. The therapist is responsible for selecting appropriate therapeutic craft activities and intervening as needed.

Staffing: Two staff/ten patient maximum

The group activity should provide patients with an opportunity to use a variety of media to make decisions regarding color, size, pattern, shape, and other cognitive concepts; organize tools, work space, and time; plan and sequence components of the activities; follow written and verbal directions; and evaluate and judge own performance.

Perceptual Motor Orientation Group

Problem area: Cognitive/sensorimotor skill reinforcement

Task: Sensorimotor activities; identification and use of familiar objects; recall of basic orienting information

Level: Parallel

Focus: Promote the orientation of the individual to the environment through the integration of basic cognitive/sensorimotor skills for carryover to activities of daily living

Prerequisite skills:

- the ability to work in a small group on a short-term task and be engageable for graded activities with verbal or tactile cueing as needed
- the ability to use compensatory techniques and exhibit some degree of daily carryover, initially with cueing as needed
- the ability to follow simple directions with demonstration or cueing

Frame of reference: Reinforcement of learning through practice

Structure: The group meets for approximately 1 hour daily.

Staffing: Two staff/six patient maximum. Modalities used to meet group objectives include 5 to 10 minutes of reality orientation to self, date, others, and environment; 10 to 15 minutes of gross motor exercises (ball or balloon toss; Lycra band); and 15 to 20 minutes of a specific activity. Group participation should provide members with an improved awareness of body, environment, and others. The selected therapeutic activities should promote purposeful responses to sensory stimulation, reinforce the appropriate use of common objects, improve motor planning and orientation skills, and develop compensatory strategies.

REFERENCES

American Occupational Therapy Association, Inc. (1979). *Uniform terminology system for reporting occupational therapy services.* Rockville, MD: AOTA Commission on Practice, Uniform Reporting System Task Force.

Berelson, B., & Steiner, G.A. (1964). *Human behavior: An inventory of scientific findings* (p. 142). New York/Burlingame: Harcourt Brace World.

Goldstein, J. (1952). The effect of brain damage on the personality. *Psychiatry, 15*, 245–260.

Licht, S. (Ed.). (1968). *Rehabilitation and medicine.* New Haven: Elizabeth Licht.

Lishman, W.A. (1978). *Organic psychiatry* (pp. 191–267). Oxford/London/Edinburgh/Melbourne: Blackwell.

Mosey, A.C. (1973). *Activities therapy* (pp. 122–135). New York: Raven Press.

Family Education and Discharge Planning

Karen Kovich, OTR/L

Rehabilitation begins while the patient is in the hospital and is an ongoing process that may occur over many years. The rate of recovery is generally most rapid during the first 6 months after injury (Miner & Wagner, 1986). However, the length of time spent in a medical facility during this period may be minimal compared with the time the patient will spend recovering in the home or in a long-term-care facility. Studies show that 34 to 40 percent of patients suffering head injury (HI) remain vegetative or severely or moderately disabled according to the Glasgow Outcome Scale (Rosenthal, Griffith, Bond, & Miller, 1984; Jennett & Teasdale, 1981). Because it is likely that continued care after discharge will be required, adequately preparing the patient and family by providing education and support is one of the characteristics of successful long-term rehabilitation.

The team approach that is vital to evaluation and treatment of the patient is also necessary for discharge planning and follow up. Communication between team members should include information on factors that can affect the family's ability to process new information. These include the family's comprehension and level of acceptance of the disability, their learning style, and their ability to interact effectively with the patient. During the initial meetings between the family and therapist, the team members can assess the family's ability to be therapeutically supportive and to participate in the treatment process. Nursing staff can often provide valuable information because they observe patient/family interactions on an informal basis and more regularly than the therapists.

Family education should begin soon after admission and can occur on an informal basis from the first time the family attends therapy. At this time, occupational therapy staff should convey information about their role in the functional remediation of the patient. Information should be presented in general terms and gradually become more specific. The content and amount of material and the way in which it is presented must be carefully graded to encourage the family to integrate it.

To provide such information, the therapist must determine how to instruct the family or caregiver. This can be done through observation of their reaction when information is presented. In the initial stages, it is often beneficial to introduce a simple task, such as application and removal of a splint or passive range of motion (ROM). This can be a valuable method of assessing the family's comfort in handling the patient, their ability to learn and follow instructions and carry them through, their willingness to be involved in the treatment process, and their comfort in asking questions.

Learning styles of family members can be affected by many factors, including their ability to cope with the disability, their level of adjustment, or their familiarity with various aspects of medical care. While some individuals can learn quickly through simple verbal instruction and demonstration, most require significant repetition, both verbally and through demonstration. Many family members require written or pictorial step-by-step instructions to feel secure in performing the task without the therapist present.

Family education should provide the family with an understanding of how HI affects an individual and with knowledge of the patient's present functional capabilities. These should include activities that are expected to be performed daily, such as feeding, dressing, transfers, or wheelchair propulsion. Family involvement in these activities often enables them to look beyond the medical aspects of the disability and establish a nurturing yet therapeutic relationship with the patient. Frequently, from a desire to help the patient, family members are overly willing to provide unnecessary assistance. Others who may be having difficulty accepting the disability or recognizing cognitive and sensory-perceptual deficits may expect the patient to perform more than he is able. Providing the family with specific expectations will assist them to foster independence in the patient.

Once the family is aware of basic capabilities, the therapist can provide instruction about therapeutic activities that can be performed in the patient's free time. It is beneficial to begin with concrete information, such as passive ROM, self-care tasks, or activities related to the patient's premorbid interests. As the family demonstrates understanding of those basic tasks, information such as methods of structuring a task to improve performance is given.

FAMILY CONFERENCES

Multidisciplinary family conferences can facilitate the exchange of information between staff and family members. Held bimonthly from the time of admission, they allow discussion about the current focus of treatment in each discipline, progress, and factors limiting performance. This ensures periodic communication, assists the family in keeping their expectations consistent with those of the treatment team, enables the family to raise questions or concerns, and provides support to the family in recognizing themselves as an integral part of the rehabilitation process. These conferences are beneficial in most cases and are especially helpful when family members cannot attend treatment sessions regularly due to job or home responsibilities. Patient attendance is encouraged but can be determined on an individual basis according to the topics being dis-

cussed. These conferences can also be useful as a method of communicating information to insurance or legal representatives, previous employers, and individuals who will be responsible for the patient's care post discharge.

THERAPEUTIC PASSES

The Rehabilitation Institute of Chicago (RIC) uses a series of therapeutic passes to assist the patient and family with gradual reintegration into the community or family structure.

Day Pass

A day pass is given when the family has demonstrated knowledge of the patient's care sufficient for safely spending several hours away from the hospital. The primary purpose of the pass is to provide a successful opportunity for the family to begin to take responsibility for the care of the patient. The therapist should initially place limited expectations on the family. As much as possible, the family should perform the patient's care while in the hospital to enable the therapist to offer feedback to improve performance. While it is impossible to provide training on every situation that may occur, it is important to provide the family with a sound base of information on which they can problem solve and address new situations. OT should address the following activities prior to the first day pass.

- application of and wearing schedule for splints and orthoses
- management of wheelchair parts or positioning equipment
- management of clothing for toileting purposes or various weather conditions (i.e., coat, gloves)
- equipment and set-up required for feeding
- attention span and appropriate environment for optimal social interaction
- methods of promoting safety and judgment
- suggestions for appropriate games or leisure activities

After each pass, a discussion is held with the family and patient to gain feedback on the success of the experience. Additional goals for the patient and/or educational needs for the family may also be identified.

Overnight and Weekend Passes

Depending on the success of the day pass and the availability of reimbursement, overnight and weekend passes are given periodically until the time of discharge. This ensures continual integration of new information and allows the family to assume responsibility gradually for the care of the patient. Therapists can present additional information necessary for an overnight or weekend pass. This may include instruction in how to:

- perform ROM exercises
- provide the proper amount and type of assistance required for the morning and evening self-care routine
- position the patient in bed
- structure the day
- structure various environments

After all passes, feedback from the patient and family will often indicate their comfort level with the experience. If they appear uncomfortable or overwhelmed, the therapist should provide encouragement and support, highlighting some of the positive aspects of the pass while assisting with problem solving for the stressful occurrences. Repetition of tasks previously taught is essential to insure integration of information before the family assumes total responsibility.

DETERMINING DISCHARGE PLACEMENT

As discharge approaches, the team can identify deficits that will continue to affect the patient's function. Through knowledge of previous roles and responsibilities, the team can anticipate how deficits will affect the patient's ability to function in various living situations. The responsibilities a caretaker or family member may need to assume can also be predicted. With input from the team, the family must decide on a discharge location. This decision can be extremely difficult since it often causes an absolute realization of the permanency of the patient's deficits. Their decision should be based on many factors, including the amount and type of care the patient will require, the cost or reimbursement available for provision of care, roles and responsibilities of family members, accessibility of the home environment, status of relationships before the injury, and comfort level with the caretaker role and adjustments to the disability.

While the physician and social worker are primarily responsible for assisting with this decision, the family often seeks input from other team members. One role of the therapist is to provide the family with objective information about the amount and type of care the patient will require after discharge, as well as the type of environment in which he functions best. Another role is to provide the social worker and physician with feedback on the family's ability to learn techniques that are essential to the care of the patient.

Placement issues for the severely involved patient requiring nursing care, maximum physical assistance, or constant supervision are significant. It is often difficult to determine whether the patient will benefit more from experienced medical care or from being in the familiar surroundings of the home environment. The decision can be equally difficult for the less involved patient when there are issues such as accessibility, behavioral problems, or limited supervision available in the home environment.

The decision to place a patient in an extended care facility is often accompanied by guilt and a conflicting sense of responsibility for family members. They are often concerned with being judged as uncaring or unwilling to accept responsibility by other family members, friends, team members, or even the patient. Having already provided the necessary objective information, the therapist should support the family in the decision.

Whether discharge placement involves a family setting or institutional care, a primary caregiver will need to be identified. Although it is often beneficial for several family members to be involved in a patient's care, teaching should be directed toward one or two individuals who will take responsibility for knowing his total care needs.

If the patient will be discharged to the home, the primary caregiver will often be a family member. Ideally, the primary caregiver has attended therapy and is familiar with the patient's care. For the more severely involved patient returning home, the family may decide that primary care needs will be the responsibility of home health nurses or a personal care attendant. It is helpful for that individual to meet with the treatment team to learn the patient's care regimen. If this is not possible, the family member must learn the regimen in order to convey it to the caretaker. The therapist can assist through provision of written information.

If the patient will be discharged to an extended care facility, the primary caregiver will be the treatment team at that facility. If the patient's care is complex, it is valuable to arrange for members of the new treatment team to come in for teaching before discharge. A family member should be familiar with all aspects of care to assist in the transition.

It must be determined if the patient will benefit from continued treatment in the home or on an outpatient basis. This decision can depend on many factors, including availability of facilities near the home, patient or family preference, or availability of funding. Table 13–1 lists some of the primary criteria in considering therapy needs after discharge.

Regardless of the amount of preparation, the discharge period can be stressful to family members. It is at this time that they must accept full responsibility for the head-injured individual. If teaching has occurred throughout the rehabilitation process, the therapist will have reduced the possibility of overwhelming family members with last-minute information.

HOME PROGRAMS

At the time of discharge, the primary caregiver should be able to perform the patient's care safely and without assistance. To provide the caregiver with a written reference, it is often beneficial to develop a home program. Its content and format will vary depending on whether it is written for the patient, family member, or other professional. When developing the program, the following points should be considered.

- When directed toward family members or nonprofessional caregivers, the home program should include a minimal amount of medical jargon. Statements such as ''proximal upper extremity spasticity limits functional arm placement'' may be written as ''the patient is unable to lift his arms over his head because of muscle tightness in the shoulder.''

- Although the program should cover all areas of treatment, it should be as concise as possible. Having to read through pages of material to find what is needed diminishes the chance of the program being used. Clear subtitles, or bold face type for specific instructions, may assist in organizing the written program.

- A list of goals achieved in treatment and those currently being addressed reinforces therapeutic gains to the patient and family. It also provides historical information to the new therapist if the patient will receive continued treatment at a different facility.

- For severely involved patients for whom many treatment areas overlap, it is often beneficial to

---

TABLE 13–1 Guidelines for decision making for continued treatment

Outpatient treatment	Home health treatment	Discontinue treatments
Complexity of treatment plan requires professional monitoring	Complexity of treatment plan requires professional monitoring	Complexity of treatment plan in home program does not require professional monitoring
Patient's expertise/modalities not available in home treatment	Primary goal areas better addressed in home setting (i.e., homemaking, child care)	Family demonstrates ability to perform home program
Patient requires continued treatment and benefits from change in environment	Outpatient facility unavailable	Patient/therapist has no further goals
Patient requires a multidisciplinary treatment program	Patient performance is better in a consistent environment	Dependent on financial availability
Family/caregiver unable to carry out effective treatment in home program	Family/caregiver continues to require assistance with carrythough of home program	
Dependent on financial availability	Dependent on financial availability	

write a joint home program. This will ensure consistent information, reduce the amount of work to be done, condense the amount of information for the family, and reinforce the interrelation of therapeutic modalities.

- Polaroid pictures or diagrams can be more effective than lengthy written descriptions of equipment use or instructions about tasks to be performed. These may include ROM, splint or cast application, neuromuscular handling techniques, set-up for self-care activities, and use of positioning equipment.
- Home programs can be supplemental to outpatient or home treatment. Patients receiving treatment one or two times a week will often benefit from activities performed with a family member on days not in therapy.
- For patients not receiving treatment after discharge, the program may include general suggestions for upgrading activities and guidelines for when they should be upgraded. This will prevent patients from performing therapeutic activities in which they are already proficient and will give them positive feedback on their performance.
- A home program is not the place to introduce new information. Its purpose is to document what has been taught and what needs to be carried through at home.
- The family should always be given the opportunity to review the home program and demonstrate techniques before discharge. This enables them to ask last-minute questions or clarify written directions.
- All home programs should include the therapist's phone number. General guidelines should also be given indicating when it would be necessary or beneficial to request therapeutic intervention, such as significant loss of ROM.

FOLLOW UP

After discharge, each facility or physician determines a mechanism for ongoing monitoring of the patient's recovery. At RIC, this includes standard rechecks 1 to 2 months post discharge by all disciplines. This provides the therapists an opportunity to assess:

- patient and/or family adjustment to the disability
- follow through with home program or outpatient treatment
- the condition and use of equipment
- the ability to maintain or improve levels of function since the last visit
- the need for change in the home program treatment approach or equipment
- the need to reinstate, continue, or discontinue therapy

After the standard recheck, the therapist may request additional follow-up visits. Therapeutic intervention can also be requested at any time by the physician. Regardless of the mechanism of follow up, the patient and/or family should be encouraged to contact the therapist regarding referrals to other agencies or equipment vendors or to discuss successes or problem areas.

REFERENCES

Jennett, B., & Teasdale, G. (1981). *Management of head injuries*. Philadelphia: F.A. Davis.

Miner, M.F., & Wagner, K.A. (1986). *Neurotrauma: Treatment, rehabilitation and related issues*. Boston: Butterworths.

Rosenthal, M., Griffith, E.R., Bond, M.R., & Miller, J.D. (1984). *Rehabilitation of the head injured adult*. Philadelphia: F.A. Davis.

Treatment of the Head-Injured Child and Adolescent

Christine Morrison, OTR/L

At the Rehabilitation Institute of Chicago (RIC), the pediatric program encompasses infancy, childhood, and adolescence. After head injury (HI), children and adolescents display many of the motoric, neurobehavioral, and emotional sequelae observed with adults. However, some treatment aspects are different. To provide a foundation on which to build occupational therapy (OT) treatment, three concepts are reviewed: (1) the relation between normal development, daily living skill participation, and HI; (2) the difference in the initial level of recovery between children and adults; and (3) the relation between long-term functional outcome and developmental age at the onset of HI.

Therapists must have a good working knowledge of normal development from infancy through childhood and adolescence. They must be familiar with the motor, psychosocial, cognitive, sensory, and perceptual function expected at each stage and identify the implications that it has on a normal child's ability to participate in age-appropriate daily living tasks. This assists therapists in determining the head-injured child's strengths and weaknesses for identification of goals appropriate for his developmental level and aids them in facilitating continued growth along the developmental continuum.

Age is often included as an important factor when predicting recovery and functional outcome (Bruce, Schut, Leonard, Woud, & Sutton, 1978; Eiben et al., 1984; Heiden, 1983; Heiskanen & Kaste, 1974; Storer

& Zeiger, 1976). One study suggests that "functional improvement in the pediatric head-injured population can occur because of several important variables including spontaneous neurologic recovery, normal growth and development, and the effect of intensive rehabilitation" (Eiben et al., 1984). Another study, which included children and adults, found that the best functional outcome occurred in patients under 20 years of age (Tabaddor, Mattis, & Zazula, 1984). A positive correlation between the age of the patient and morbidity and mortality was found; morbidity and mortality increased with age.

Several possibilities have been proposed for this difference in recovery potential. Jennett (1972) suggested that it may be secondary to a "greater plasticity of the child's brain which is not yet as rigidly committed in terms of functional localization." Bruce et al. (1978) suggested a "different pathophysiology of head injury in children as compared to adults" and believe that the threshold for neurophysiological dysfunction may be lower in children. Thus, greater neural plasticity and differences in the effects of HI on a child's nervous system may explain the greater potential for short-term recovery in children.

A study performed at Rancho Los Amigos Hospital that looked at the long-term recovery status of head-injured children found no significant differences in physical recovery among children of different ages but did show a correlation between intellectual evaluation scores and the child's age at the onset of HI. Children who had sustained injury when they were 6 years old or younger had lower scores on the intelligence tests than children injured when 10 years old or older (Brink, Garrett, Hale, Woo-Sam, & Nickel, 1970). One possibility is that the child under 6 years old has not developed the cognitive skills necessary for continued higher-level functioning. This limited foundation may affect his ability to learn, and enhancement of intellectual skills is therefore diminished. While the child's brain may have the potential for greater short-term recovery, the status of his nervous system at the time of injury is also a factor in the long-term functional outcome.

EVALUATION

The first step in the treatment of a child is a thorough evaluation. The areas evaluated are consistent with those stated in Unit 2. In this unit, aspects of the evaluation unique to the pediatric population are highlighted.

Chart Review

For the child, three additional pieces of information will facilitate the evaluation and assist in goal setting and discharge planning: (1) school attendance and performance, (2) parents' working status and availability for teaching, and (3) nature of the injury.

School attendance and performance data can add to the holistic picture of the child and assist in determining his premorbid functional level. The parents' working status and availability for teaching may have implications for their involvement in treatment and discharge placement. In cases of nonaccidental injury, long-term prognosis may vary. Functional outcome of children sustaining a nonaccidental HI is significantly worse because of the potential for multiple head injuries from additional abuse (Brink, Imbus, & Woo-Sam, 1980; Duncan & Ment, 1984). If abuse was involved, parental involvement and support may be lacking and may further complicate the treatment process and the prognosis.

Psychosocial

Evaluation of the psychosocial area must include the parents. For example, if the injury was incurred during a car accident while a parent was driving, the parent may feel guilt, which will need to be dealt with by the therapist as it may interfere with parental involvement in treatment. The therapist should be aware of the parents' understanding of the disability and of their style of coping with the change in their child. This information is used for goal setting regarding parental handling and their ability to provide the environment in which their child functions best. In some cases the child may not return home. This is often the case if the injury was nonaccidental and caused by a parent. The child may be placed in a state institution or foster home. If this is known, expectations placed on the parents will be different, and the therapist may attempt to involve the foster family in treatment.

Parents can provide specific information on how their child's behavior differs from that seen premorbidly. Jennett (1972) suggested that children who incur head injuries are not a random sample of the population. HI occurs more frequently in children already delayed in some areas. At RIC, head-injured children are often described by relatives and teachers to have been impulsive, with decreased attention span, and to have had difficulty in school. This seems to be particularly true for children whose injuries were caused by falling, being hit by a car, or by other accidents that may be related to poor judgment. This information coupled with the child's current status enables the therapist to set realistic functional goals.

The child is assessed in the area of social interaction. The developmental continuum of social interaction is used to identify the age appropriateness of the child's behavior. When observing the child during individual and group treatment, the therapist looks at the following areas in addition to those stated for adults.

- initiation of play
- follow through of play initiated by therapist
- parallel versus cooperative play
- reaction to strangers and new situations
- response to handling and facilitation by the therapist

As the quality of these areas changes with age, they are assessed also for age appropriateness. For example, typically, a 2-year-old demonstrates parallel play; cooperative play becomes apparent at 3 years of age. Therefore, a 2-year-old child would be evaluated on his ability to play in a parallel fashion. With adolescents, peer interactions during group treatment sessions are assessed as related to the patient's overall functional performance.

Cognitive

The therapist evaluates the child's cognitive functioning only as it relates to his ability to participate in age-appropriate activities of daily living (ADL) tasks. Post-traumatic amnesia may be present, limiting attention and cognitive performance. Because of this, the initial assessment is based primarily on observation. Discharge testing may consist of a more formal evaluation.

Specific areas assessed are the same as those in the adult (i.e., attention span, distractibility, ability to follow directions, problem-solving ability, etc.). However, for the child, these skills are evaluated within the context of normal development. At RIC, the Bayley Scales of Infant Development (Bayley, 1969), the Gessell (1940), and the McCarthy Scales of Children's Abilities (1972) are used to provide a baseline for observed behaviors. The tests may also be used for formalized testing when appropriate (Knoblock & Pasamarrick, 1974). Since HI often results in both cognitive and physical impairment, descriptors of behaviors, physical limitations, and other observations made during testing may be used to qualify the findings of the assessment.

Sensory-Perceptual

It is important to look at the child's ability to process sensory information from the somatosensory, visual, auditory, vestibular, olfactory, and gustatory systems. Methods for doing this are described in Unit 5. These techniques are used with children at the minimally responsive, awakening, agitated, and alert confused levels. For children and adolescents functioning at the alert oriented stage, responses are put into an age-appropriate context. At RIC, the Beery Test of Visual Motor Integration (1982), the McCarthy Scales of Children's Abilities (1972), and the Gardner Test of Visual-Perceptual Skills (Gardner, 1982) are used to assist. These tests are standardized on nonneurologically impaired populations but can provide information on the child's ability to attend, process, and functionally use visual and auditory information for motor tasks. As with cognitive testing, descriptions of behaviors and physical limitations should be included in the interpretation.

For the very highly functioning child with minimal motor control problems, the Ayres (1980) Southern California Sensory Integration Tests (SCSIT) may be used with the other tests and with clinical observations. Clinical results from using the SCSIT reveal that many head-injured children have problems similar to those of learning disabled (LD) children. However, the SCSIT was developed for LD children who do not have frank neurological damage. Therefore, results may not be taken literally but can provide information as to which sensory systems the child can use during functional tasks. This is an extremely important area for the therapist to evaluate with the high-level children as they are the ones who frequently go unnoticed in hospital settings and may have subtle deficits that will affect long-term functional performance. By identifying strengths and weaknesses in this area, the therapist can assist the child in improving weak areas or compensating if improvement is not expected.

At RIC, it has been observed that when a child is functioning at a 6- to 7-year developmental level, they can participate in formal sensory testing as described in Unit 2. When he is functioning below this level, the therapist gathers information through observations of him in play and during functional activities. To facilitate this observation, the following questions may be asked.

- Does he respond to touch on either arm by looking at you, pulling the arm away, or changing facial expressions?
- Does he respond differently to stimulation on the right or left arm?
- Does he neglect either arm when moving and not incorporate the extremity into movement?
- Does he allow either arm to be positioned in normally stressful positions and not react (i.e., wrist flexion greater than 90°)?
- Does he use both arms spontaneously during play?

Reflexes

At RIC, formal reflex testing is not done by pediatric therapists. They are examined from a functional standpoint. They are evaluated specifically for the extent to which they interfere with age-appropriate movement and environmental interaction. For this purpose, an understanding of what is normal and the ability to determine when reflexes interfere with motoric performance are required. Refer to Table 14–1 for reflexes frequently encountered and the normal ages at which they are seen. For more detailed information, see Fiorentino (1978).

Strength

For the child or adolescent who is moving within synergy, techniques do not differ from those described for adults. If isolated movement is present in the extremities, the therapist will evaluate the strength of upper extremity musculature.

As with sensory testing, it is often difficult to elicit the participation of young children in formal manual muscle testing. A child functioning at a three- to four-year level can participate when directions are given one step at a time and a game is made out of applying resistance. For example, when testing elbow flexion, begin by telling the child to touch his nose, then joke with him about pulling the arm from the nose. Encourage him to hold, reinforcing him when he resists. This test may need to be repeated two or three times to ensure the child's understanding, which is necessary for an accurate test.

For the child who cannot participate in formal testing because of his developmental level or decreased cognitive level secondary to HI, the therapist must use observation to determine functional strength in movements in both the gravity-eliminated and the antigravity planes. The therapist can encourage the use of different upper extremity musculature through placement of toys for children and by encouraging adolescents to participate in activities within their abilities.

For complete descriptions of isolated muscle use and muscle testing, refer to resources listed in Unit 2 and use these descriptions to analyze treatment activities. Figure 14–1 shows the placement of a toy to examine the functional strength of the shoulder and elbow musculature.

Self-feeding in the sitting position can be used to evaluate the following areas of upper extremity strength.

- shoulder flexion and abduction against gravity
- elbow flexion against gravity
- wrist extension against gravity
- active grasp and release

Postural Adaptation, Balance, and Equilibrium

To evaluate the child and adolescent, a knowledge of when stability and mature equilibrium reactions occur in the normal child in all developmental positions is needed. Refer to standard pediatric literature for this information. The therapist can compare this to what is observed during the assessment. Placement of toys can be used to encourage the younger child to perform transitional movements between positions (Figures 14–2 through 14–6).

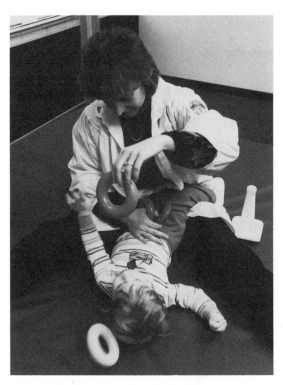

Figure 14–1 Placement of the toy encourages shoulder flexion to 90° and elbow extension against gravity.

TABLE 14–1	Reflexes
Reflex	*Normally present*
Rooting	Birth to 3 or 4 months
Sucking	Birth to 3 or 4 months
Grasp	Birth to 3 or 4 months
Asymmetrical tonic neck reflex	Birth to 4 to 6 months
Landau	5 months
Tonic labyrinthine	Birth to 4 months
Symmetrical tonic neck reflex	Birth to 4 to 6 months

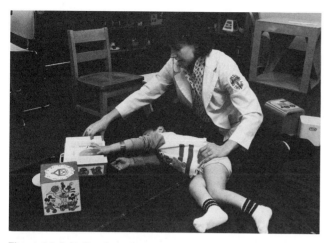

Figure 14–2 Rolling from supine to sidelying is encouraged.

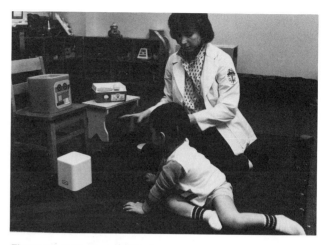

Figure 14–3 Placement of the toy encourages transition from side sit to four-point kneeling.

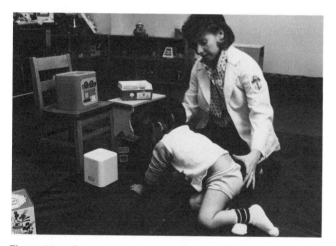

Figure 14–4 Completion of side sit to four-point kneeling

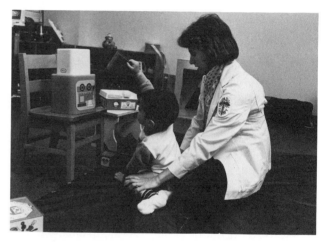

Figure 14–5 The therapist stabilizes the lower extremities to help the patient to kneeling.

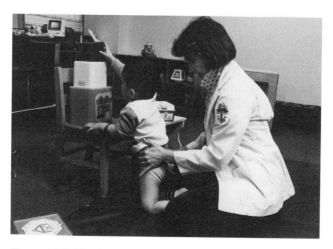

Figure 14–6 The therapist helps maintain hip extension as the patient moves in kneeling.

It is also important to determine which position is the most functional for the individual in performing arm placement and daily living tasks. To assist in this determination, questions similar to the following may be asked:

- Can he Indian sit and reach for toys or does he need to use both hands to maintain sitting balance?
- When in supported short sitting, does he have head control sufficient to look at toys or people?
- When in supine, can he touch his face or abdomen?
- When in sidelying with the arms resting in midline and head and trunk supported, can he reach for toys?
- When in prone, can he shift weight over one extremity and reach for a toy with the other arm?
- When in kneeling or standing, what grasp patterns can he use functionally?

By asking and answering these and similar questions, it is possible for the therapist to identify in which positions the child will be able to use his eyes and hands for the manipulation of objects necessary during play and self-care. For example, if the child requires bilateral upper extremity support to maintain Indian sitting, the arms will not be available for functional use.

Upper Extremity Control and Hand Function

Use of the Erhardt (1982) Developmental Prehension Assessment is helpful in evaluating arm placement and hand function from a developmental perspective. While this entire assessment is not given at RIC, it does contain researched descriptors and age ranges that add objectivity to the therapist's observations. It also contains a section on the development of crayon or pencil grasp. These norms are used to compare information gained from clinical observations to what can be expected based on the child's age. For a description of normal grasp and pinch development, refer to Table 14–2.

Evaluation of specific grasp and pinch patterns is done through engaging the child in tasks that require pincer grasp, lateral pinch, and gross grasp and release, etc., as described in Unit 2. Functional use of grasp patterns is also evaluated. For example, a child may demonstrate pincer grasp within the structure of a treatment activity but use only lateral pinch during most spontaneous grasping of objects.

TABLE 14–2   Developmental grasp and release

Primitive gross grasp	4 months
Release and awareness after sustained grasp	3 months
3 jaw chuck	10 months
Controlled release of 3 jaw chuck	12 months
Fine pincer grasp	12 months
Controlled release of the pincer grasp	15 months

When the child demonstrates isolated movement throughout an extremity and active control of grasp and pinch with no evidence of increased tone, strength measurements of cylindrical grasp and palmar and lateral pinch are taken. Age norms for the grasp and pinch measurements are helpful for comparing performance to that in normal children (Mathiowetz, Wiemer, & Federman, 1986).

Coordination

Assessment of coordination is the same as described for adults. Coordination is still developing and significantly improves with age in children 4 through 6 years old (Denckla, 1974). Younger girls are more coordinated than younger boys, with a plateau at 8, 9, and 10 years of age (Denckla, 1974). Mean scores for these children have been calculated for tasks of repetitive finger touching and forearm pronation and supination movements (Denckla, 1974). While not published as norms, they provide a reference the therapist may use in testing children at the alert oriented level. Knowledge of variations from normal age ranges is relevant to the overall picture of the patient, and delayed areas may be treated. However, it is also necessary to look at the patient in terms of his ability to perform tasks important to him with available grasp patterns.

Activities of Daily Living

For the child under 1 year of age, the emphasis is on mastering the body. Participation in traditional ADLs for infants may be limited to holding a bottle or exploring toys. Around 12 months, the child begins to participate more in self-care. Increasing independence is noted until the age of 7, when all dressing, bathing, and feeding tasks are usually performed independently.

More complex tasks are added to his repertoire, such as going to school and participating in chores around the house. By adolescence, he begins exploring activities such as working, driving, and community participation. At this age, ADLs become similar to those of adults.

With this as a base, the therapist uses the information provided in Unit 9 on adult ADLs and evaluates the child or adolescent in only ADLs they performed independently before injury. As the child matures, other ADLs may need to be evaluated as expectations for ADL performance increase with age. General guidelines for completion of ADL activities are included in Table 14–3. Play is also assessed as an area in ADL for its age appropriateness.

The therapist uses the accumulated information to determine what primary deficits are contributing to the child's inability to perform ADLs and to play at age-appropriate levels. For example, a child who is motorically involved and demonstrates no consistent arm placement may be placed in sidelying with head and trunk supported and demonstrate active arm placement in gravity-eliminated planes. This placement is sufficient only for gross control of toys. If the child can participate in cause and effect or exploratory play, the therapist may provide switch-activated toys. They will capitalize on the child's cognitive strengths while minimizing the physical limitations and facilitate maximal independence in play activities (Figure 14–7).

GOAL SETTING AND TREATMENT PLANNING

After baseline information has been gathered and the child's strengths and weaknesses have been determined in relation to the developmental continuum, initial long- and short-term goals are set, and a treatment plan is established. Units 2 and 3 describe the process of evaluation, interpretation of data, goal setting, treatment planning, measuring of progress, and upgrading of goals. The long-term goals will always be focused on upgrading functional performance, with the short-term goals based upon the component skills of psychosocial, cognitive, sensory-perceptual, and motor performance necessary to accomplish the functional tasks. Goals and treatment plans will depend upon the level of the patient.

Minimally Responsive/Awakening Patients

Patient Characteristics

As this level, the child is beginning to respond to stimulation in one sensory system at a time. The response may be a generalized body reaction or specific to stimuli, such as turning the head in response to a ringing bell. Evaluation reflects the child's ability to respond to various sensory stimulation and the amount of active motor control. At this level, active control is

TABLE 14–3   Pediatric ADL s

Task	Age
Feeding	
Finger Feed	9-12 months
Feed self with spoon with moderate spilling	2 years
Drinks from a cup with one hand	2 years
Feed self with fork	4 years
Cut with knife and fork	7 years
Hygiene	
Wash and dry hands	3 years
Bathing	7 years
Dressing	
Cooperate with dressing by extending arms and legs	15 months
Removes socks	18 months
Finds large arm holes and thrusts arms into them	2 years
Take off all clothes	2 to 2½ years
Put on shoes	4 years
Put on pull-over garment	5 years
Independent in all dressing	7 years

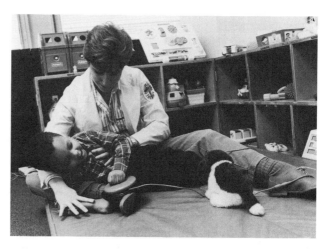

Figure 14–7 The sidelying position may be used to maximize upper extremity movement.

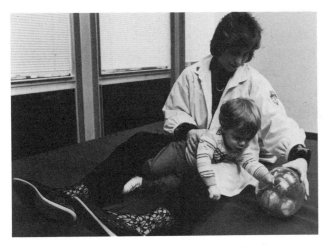

Figure 14–8 Working on head control against gravity

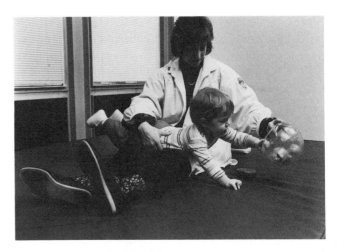

Figure 14–9 Extension throughout the trunk and neck is encouraged.

generally in one body part at a time while the remaining portions of the body are supported. For example, when positioned in supine with head, trunk, and lower extremities supported, the child may demonstrate active arm placement. In supported short sitting, he may have beginning head control. The child may also demonstrate changes in tone throughout the day. These changes are the same as those described for the adult.

Focus of Treatment

Much of the treatment is therapist directed, with the therapist having a more active role than the child. As the child is working on isolated component skills, treatment activities are also being broken down so the focus is on one or two components at a time. Goals are focused primarily in four areas.

1. enhancing responses to sensory stimuli in all modalities
2. upgrading active head and trunk control
3. upgrading active use of the upper extremities
4. preventing deformity and maintaining or increasing range of motion (ROM)

Treatment techniques aimed at accomplishing these goals with children and adolescents are the same as described in the related units in this book. The one area that does vary is handling techniques. While the principles are the same, the use of equipment and the therapist's handling techniques differ because of the smaller size of the patient. In addition to the techniques described in Unit 6, Figures 14–8 through 14–12 outline some handling techniques for use with children.

Parental Teaching and Involvement

It is important to know how the parents are coping with their child's disability and to deal with them at an appropriate level. The minimally responsive or awakening child generally arrives at RIC after an extended stay in an acute care facility. This may have involved use of multiple life support systems, which could have drastically limited the physical contact the parents had with their child. Therefore, parents are often unsure of how to approach him. The therapist must encourage and facilitate their involvement. Initially, therapists promote basic interaction, gradually beginning to teach parents specific techniques. For children who progress through this stage, specific techniques may not be taught. For those who do not progress, parents must learn how to hold their child in ways that will not increase abnormal muscle tone and will provide support where the child needs it. Figures 14–13 and 14–14 show ways to hold children without increasing tone throughout their bodies. The therapist may teach techniques for positioning the patient comfortably. All parents should be taught ways of dressing and undressing the child that will incorporate ROM and relaxation techniques.

The therapist also teaches the parent to observe the child's responses to various stimuli and to interact with their child appropriately within his current functional abilities. As family education occurs, parents frequently feel they are valued members of the team and are often available to follow through with treatment techniques outside therapy sessions. When parents demonstrate an understanding of the child's level of responsiveness, they can also provide the team with

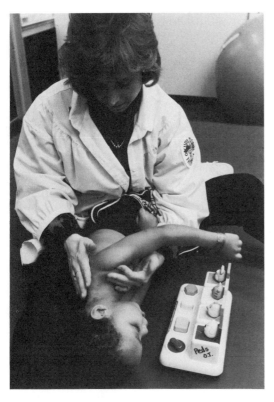

Figure 14–10 Shoulder movement is facilitated as the child actively moves the arm.

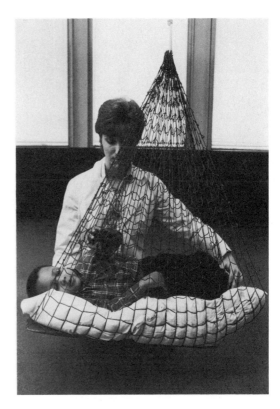

Figure 14–11 In a suspended net swing with pillows to provide support, total body relaxation is facilitated by slow gentle movement.

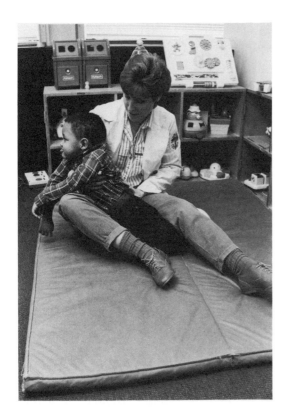

Figure 14–12 Trunk rotation facilitates relaxation of the extremities.

observations from nontherapy hours. This helps create a more thorough picture of the child's strengths and weaknesses.

The importance of grading parents' participation according to their level of comfort cannot be overemphasized. Parents are the child's main resource. The more knowledgeable they are regarding his functional abilities and limitations from the beginning, the better able they will be to care for him. For some children, parents demonstrate little to no involvement during therapy for a variety of reasons. For these children, goals for parental involvement may not be set, but attempts to contact the families and encourage involvement are made. Social work and psychology can also play an active role in this process.

Agitated/Alert Confused Patients

Patient Characteristics

This patient is beginning to put component skills together to interact with the environment more consistently and appropriately. He no longer needs to have tasks broken down to require only one response; he may

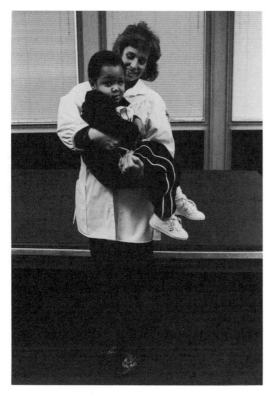

Figure 14–13 The child is held with the body supported and the hips and knees flexed to decrease extensor tone.

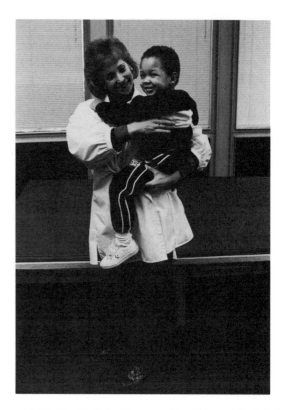

Figure 14–14 The child is held over one hip with legs abducted. Arms are supported in extension.

be able to accomplish two or more components simultaneously. For example, in the physical realm, the child may be able to short sit with good head control and demonstrate active arm placement. Functional examples include hitting a beach ball back to a therapist while the patient is in supported short sitting, or while supported in a standing table, the child may turn pages of a book to look at the pictures.

Confusion or agitation may interfere with participation. They may be displayed in ways different than in adults. For example, the child may be unaware of an unfamiliar environment and not demonstrate appropriate stranger anxiety. The physically active child may roam around the treatment room showing little interest in toys. By the end of this level of recovery, the child should demonstrate self-care and play skills in a structured environment. The ADL tasks and the physical, psychosocial, cognitive, and sensory-perceptual expectations will vary depending on where the child was functioning premorbidly.

Focus of Treatment

At this level, the child becomes a more active participant, with the therapist determining and providing the optimal environment for his participation. The therapist looks at behavioral, cognitive, and perceptual deficits, such as auditory or visual distractibility, decreased attention span, frustration tolerance, internal agitation, and agitation secondary to external stimulation. A determination is made of areas that interfere with participation in various treatment activities and the environments that may minimize the deficits. Because the child can put component skills together, treatment focuses on the combination of skills. Goals are focused on:

- upgrading cognitive skills for participation in functional activities
- maximizing control of movements through all developmental positions
- upgrading age-appropriate unilateral and bilateral arm placement and hand function
- independent participation in self-care and age-appropriate play skills

Activity analysis is performed to determine what component skills are limiting participation in self-care skills, and treatment is focused on those areas. The process of activity analysis, determining limiting factors, and choosing treatment techniques is the same as described in preceding units for adult patients. For example, a 2-year-old at this level may maintain Indian sitting and reach for toys placed at arm's length away. However, he may be unable to move in or out of this position to get toys placed out of arm's length. Play may also be limited to imitating cause-and-effect play initiated by the therapist.

Goals for this child may include independent transitions into and out of sitting to pursue toys and consistent initiation of cause-and-effect play. The component skills limiting the goals would be determined and treatment focused on upgrading them. Techniques aimed at maximizing control of movements through developmental positions are based on principles described for adults. Handling may differ based on the size of the patient. Figures 14–15 through 14–19 demonstrate a treatment sequence focused on upgrading the quality of a child's movement from prone to sitting using a therapy ball.

Parental Teaching and Involvement

The focus of parental involvement at this level is on teaching them how to provide the environment that best facilitates their child's optimum performance. They continue to be included in the setting of goals. Specific treatment techniques are taught, and expectations are expanded within their abilities. When the child is functioning at the higher end of this level, parents are encouraged to allow him to perform self-care tasks within his abilities and to practice them while on day or weekend passes. It is often difficult for parents to allow this independence because task performance at this level may be time-consuming.

Alert Oriented Patients

Patient Characteristics

This patient can put many component skills together and consistently interacts with the environment. In the absence of physical limitations, the child has progressed through the continuum of functional performance and frequently moves independently throughout all developmental positions and performs all self-care independently. The younger child who had not developed complex abilities before the injury may perform at his preinjury level. Intervention may be minimal until

he matures and difficulties emerge in the performance of higher-level ADLs. With the older child or adolescent, deficits may be subtle and require a thorough evaluation of the performance of functional tasks to determine where the breakdown occurs. Several studies (Eiben, et al., 1984; Jennett, 1972; Newcombe, 1982; Newton & Johnson, 1985) suggest that the deficits may lie in changes in the cognitive, behavioral, and emotional characteristics of the child that often remain after physical recovery from HI.

Focus of Treatment

The goals at this level focus on determining the specific deficits limiting age-appropriate ADL participation and on maximizing the child's ability to perform several component skills simultaneously as required in the high-level ADL tasks of the adult. Treatment is similar to that described for adult homemaking and community reintegration tasks. The therapist includes only age-appropriate tasks.

Readiness for participation in school activities must be addressed with the alert and oriented child in school. By evaluating his ability to carry out complex activities

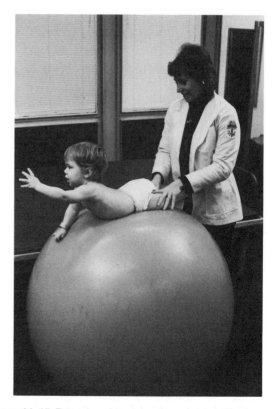

Figure 14–15 Extension of trunk, neck, and extremities is encouraged in the prone position on the ball.

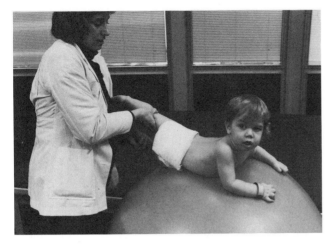

Figure 14–16 Facilitation from the lower extremities encourages trunk rotation and weight shifting.

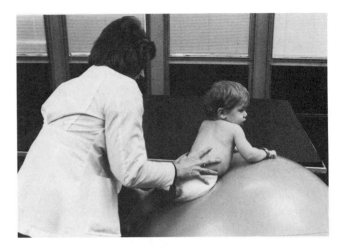

Figure 14–17 Weight is shifted onto the hips.

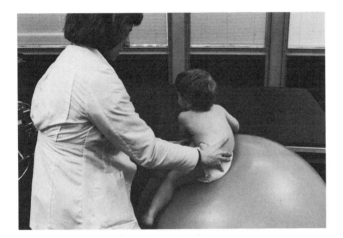

Figure 14–18 Movement of the ball facilitates active control of the trunk.

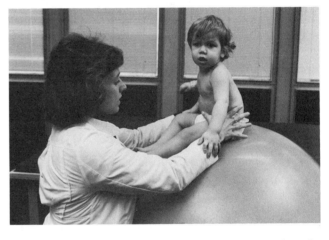

Figure 14–19 The child actively maintains sitting as the therapist releases support.

and to learn new cognitive tasks in a multistimulus environment, the therapist provides the teacher with vital information regarding realistic expectations for him and the environment. This information is used in conjunction with data gathered by the rest of the treatment team to assist with school placement.

Parental Teaching and Involvement

Ideally, the parent or guardian is the primary resource for the child. The therapist teaches this person to be a keen observer of the child during functional tasks and to determine what facilitates an increase in that function. He may improve function when provided with a special environment. The guardians are taught to provide this environment and are encouraged to allow their child to perform within the limit of his abilities.

DISCHARGE PLANNING

Planning for discharge is an ongoing process that begins with the initial evaluation. It is similar to that described in Unit 12.

Home Programs

Ideally, the parents or primary caregivers are involved throughout the child's admission and are familiar with his strengths and limitations regarding functional performance. For these parents, the home program is an extension of what they have been taught. Unfortunately, for a variety of reasons, parents are not always available for teaching on a consistent basis and must learn much new information in the last few days of the child's hospitalization. Regardless of the parental involvement throughout the stay, a home program is written for them to use as a reference.

Recovery is an ongoing process, and many will maintain contact with medical facilities. These children need a safe, supportive environment to encourage them to keep trying when things appear more difficult than for their peers. The home program is written with suggestions for how the parent can assist the child in developing a normal routine at home and school.

Specific exercises are generally not included. Instead, activity analysis of "normal" children's self-care, play, and household chores is provided to show parents how the child can continue to improve by becoming an integral part of the family again. In this way, the parents do not have to assume the roles of therapist and parent and will be available solely as a parent. In some instances, OT treatment is not available to the child, or the parent may request specific treatment activities, which are then provided.

School Placement

In Illinois, regardless of their level of responsiveness, all head-injured children up to 18 years old will attend school. For children functioning up through the agitated and alert confused levels, this will be in a special classroom with teachers and therapists who are usually familiar with treating physically and cognitively involved children. For the child at the alert oriented level, placement is more difficult. Frequently, they are placed in LD classrooms with teachers familiar with the subtle deficits encountered with that population. However, the head-injured child has difficulties different from those of LD children. These differences need to be carefully discussed with the teachers. This may be in the form of written recommendations or school placement meetings between the rehabilitation team and the school professionals. For children who will receive OT in the school, a copy of the discharge note is provided to the therapist. It is also important to have verbal contact with the therapist if possible to increase the possibility of carryover between settings.

RECHECKS

Jennett (1972) speaks of the recovery that head-injured children experience over one year. The importance of the child's maintaining contact with therapists

is emphasized by the Rancho Los Amigos group (Brink et al., 1970). At RIC, medical follow up continues, and physicians may request OT interventions at any time. When additional OT needs occur, outpatient OT is set up either at RIC or in a community facility closer to the child's home. Community settings may include school-based, home health, and hospital outpatient OT. When several multidisciplinary needs are present, an additional inpatient stay may be indicated. Throughout all of these discharge interventions, the primary goal continues to be facilitation of the child or adolescent to perform at his maximal level of ADL independence in the home and school environment.

REFERENCES

Ayres, A.J. (1980). *Interpreting the Southern California sensory integration tests*. Los Angeles: Western Psychological Services.

Bayley, N. (1969). Bayley Scales of Infant Development. New York: The Psychological Corporation.

Beery, K.E. (1982). *Revised administration scoring and teaching manual for the developmental test of visual-motor integration*. Chicago: Follett.

Brink, J.D., Garrett, A.C., Hale, W.R., Woo-Sam, J., & Nickel, V.L. (1970). Recovery of motor and intellectual function in children sustaining severe head injuries. *Developmental Medicine and Child Neurology*, *12*, 565–571.

Brink, J.D., Imbus, C., & Woo-Sam, J. (1980). Physical recovery after severe closed trauma in children and adolescents. *Journal of Pediatrics*, *97*, 721-727.

Bruce, D.A., Schut, L., Leonard, A.B., Woud, J.H., & Sutton, L.N. (1978). Outcome following severe head injuries in children. *Journal of Neurosurgery*, *48*, 679–688.

Denckla, M.B. (1974). Development of motor coordination in normal children. *Developmental Medicine and Child Neurology*, *16*, 729–741.

Duncan, C.C., Ment, L.R.L. (1984). Management of pediatric head injury. *Connecticut Medicine*, *48*, 282–285.

Eiben, C.F., Anderson, T.P., Lockman, L., Matthews, D.S., Dryja, D., Martin, J., Burrill, C., Gottlesman, N., O'Brian, P., & White, L. (1984). Functional outcome of closed head injury in children and young adults. *Archives of Physical Medicine and Rehabilitation*, *65*, 168–170.

Erhardt, R. (1982). *Developmental hand dysfunction: Theory, assessment and treatment*. Laurel, MD: Ramsco.

Fiorentino, M.F. (1978). *Normal and abnormal development: The influence of primitive reflexes on motor development*. Springfield, IL: Charles C Thomas.

Gardner, M. (1982). Test of visual-perceptual skills. Seattle, WA: Special Child Publications.

Gessell, A., Halverson, H., Tompson, H., Ilg, F., Castner, B., Ames, L., Amatruda, C. (1940). *The first five years of life: A guide to the study of the preschool child* (pp. 233–258). New York: Harper & Row.

Heiden, J.S., Small, R., Caton, W., Weiss, M., & Kurze, T. (1983). Severe head injury: Clinical assessment and outcome. *Physical Therapy*, *63*, 1946–1947.

Heiskanen, O., & Kaste, M. (1974). Late prognosis of severe brain injury in children. *Developmental Medicine and Child Neurology*, *16*, 11–14.

Jennett, B. (1972). Head injuries in children. *Developmental Medicine and Child Neurology*, *14*, 137–147.

Knoblock, H., & Pasamarrick, B. (Eds.). (1974). *Gessell and Amatruda's developmental diagnosis* (3rd ed.). Hagerstown, MD: Harper & Row.

Mathiowetz, V., Wiemer, D.M., & Federman, S.M. (1986). Grip and pinch strength: Norms for 6 to 19 year olds. *American Journal of Occupational Therapy*, *40*, 705–711.

McCarthy, D. (1972). McCarthy Scales of Children's Abilities. New York: The Psychological Corporation.

Newcombe, F. (1982). The psychological consequences of closed head injury: Assessment and rehabilitation. *British Journal of Accident Surgery*, *14*, 111–133.

Newton, A., & Johnson, D.A. (1985). Social adjustment and integration after severe head injury. *British Journal of Clinical Psychology*, *24*, 225–233.

Storer, S.L., & Zeiger, H.J.E. (1976). Head injury in children and teenagers: Functional recovery correlated with duration of coma. *Archives of Physical Medicine and Rehabilitation*, *57*, 201–205.

Tabaddor, J., Mattis, S., & Zazula, T. (1984). Cognitive sequence and recovery course after moderate and severe head injury. *Neurosurgery*, *14*, 701–707.

Reading and Resource List

Unit 4

Keilhofner, G. (1985). *A Model of Human Occupation*. Baltimore, MD: Williams and Wilkins.

Manual of behavior management strategies for traumatically brain injured adults. (1983). Members of the psychology department at the Rehabilitation Institute of Chicago. Available through RIC.

Unit 5

Adamovich, B., Henderson, J., & Auerbach, S. (1985). *Cognitive rehabilitation of closed head injured patients*. San Diego, CA: College Hill Press.

Ayres, A.J. (1980). *Sensory integration and the child*. Los Angeles: Western Psychological Services.

Bach-y-rita, P. (Ed.). (1978). *Recovery of function: theoretical considerations for brain injury rehabilitation*. Baltimore: University Park Press.

Brooks, N. (1984). *Closed head injury*. London: Oxford University Press.

Dougherty, P. & Radomski, M. (1987). *The cognitive rehabilitation workbook*. Rockville, MD: Aspen Publishers, Inc.

Gilfoyle, E., Grady, A., & Moore, J. (1981). *Children adapt*. Thorofare, NJ: Charles B. Slack.

Jennett, B. (1984). *Management of head injuries*. Philadelphia: F.A. Davis.

Rancho Los Amigos Hospital. (1979). *Rehabilitation of the head injured adult*. Downey, CA: Professional Staff Association of Rancho Los Amigos Hospital.

Unit 6

Charness, A. (1986). *Stroke and head injury: A guide to functional outcomes in physical therapy management*. Rockville, MD: Aspen Publishers, Inc.

Davies, P. (1985). *Steps to follow: A guide to the treatment of adult hemiplegia*. Berlin: Springer-Verlag.

Ylvisaker, M. (1985). *Head injury rehabilitation in children and adolescents*. San Diego, CA: College Hill Press.

Unit 7

Bell, J.A. (May-June, 1985). Plaster casting for remodeling of soft tissue: 2. *The Star*, 10–14.

Braun, R.M., Hoffer, M.M., and Mooney, V. (1973). Phenol nerve block in the treatment of acquired spastic hemiplegia in the upper limb. *Journal of Bone and Joint Surgery*, *55A*, 580–585.

Hunter, J., Schneider, L., Mackin, L., & Bell, J. (1978). *The rehabilitation of the hand*. St. Louis: C.V. Mosby.

Unit 8

American Occupational Therapy Association, Practice Division. *Seating and Positioning Information Packet*. (1986). Rockville, MD.

Bazata, C., & Jones, K. (1985). *Independent living*. South Bend, IN: Rehabilitation Technology Center, Memorial Hospital.

Carlson, J., & Winder, R. (1978). The Gillette sitting support orthosis. *Orthotics and prosthetics*, *32*(4).

Margolis, S., Jones, R., & Braun, B. (1985). The subasis bar: An effective approach to pelvic stabilization in seated positioning. *Proceedings of the eighth annual conference on rehabilitation technology*. Rehabilitation Engineering Society of North America.

Shaw, G. (1985). Rigid pelvic restraint. *Proceedings of the eighth annual conference on rehabilitation technology*. Rehabilitation Engineering Society of North America.

Silverman, M.W., & Silverman, O. (1983). The contour-u seating system. *Proceedings of the sixth annual conference on rehabilitation technology*. Rehabilitation Engineering Society of North America.

Unit 9

Farber, S. (1975). *Sensorimotor evaluation and treatment procedures for allied health personnel.* Indianapolis: Indiana University Foundation.

Gee, Z., & Passarella, P. (1985). *Nursing care of the stroke patient: A therapeutic approach.* Pittsburgh, PA: AREN Publications.

Logemann, J. (1983). *Evaluation and treatment of swallowing disorders.* San Diego, CA: College Hill Press.

Unit 10

Logue, P. (1975). *Understanding and living with brain damage.* Springfield, IL: Charles C Thomas Publisher.

Rosenthal, M., Griffity, E., Bond, E., & Miller, D. (1983). *The rehabilitation of the head injured adult.* Philadelphia, PA: F.A. Davis.

Trexler, E. (1982). *Cognitive rehabilitation: Conceptualization and intervention.* New York: Plenum Press.

Unit 11

Burkhart, L. (1982). *More homemade devices for severely handicapped children with suggested activities.* Unpublished manuscript. (Available from the author: 8503 Rhode Island Avenue, College Park, MD 20740.)

Closing the Gap. P.O. Box 68, Henderson, MN 56044.

Committee on Personal Computers and the Handicapped. 2030 W. Irving Park Road, Chicago, IL 60618.

McWilliams, P.A. (1984). *Personal computers and the disabled.* Garden City, NY: Doubleday.

Phonic Ear, Inc. (1982 and monthly updates). *The many faces of funding.* (Available from Phonic Ear, 250 Camino Alto, Mill Valley, CA 94941.)

Rehabilitation Engineering Center. (1982). *A guide to controls: Selection, mounting applications.* Palo Alto, CA: Stanford University Children's Hospital.

Rehabilitation Engineering Society of North America. 1101 Connecticut Avenue, N.W., Suite 700, Washington, DC 20036.

Schwejda, P., & Vanderheiden, G. (1982). Adaptive Firmware Card for the Apple II. *Byte, 7*(9), 276–314.

Vanderheiden, G., Bengston, D., Brady, M., & Walstead, L. (1982). *International software/hardware registry,* 2nd ed. Madison, WI: University of Wisconsin Trace Research and Development Center.

Wright, C., & Nomnua, M. (1985). *From toys to computers: Access for the physically disabled child.* (Available from the authors, P.O. Box 700242, San Jose, CA 95170.)

Unit 14

Bly, L. (1983). *The components of normal movements during the first year of life and abnormal motor development.* Oak Park, IL: Neurodevelopmental Treatment Association.

Bobath, B., & Bobath, K. (1982). *Motor development in the different types of cerebral palsy.* London: William Heinmann.

Hinojusa, J., Goldstein, P., Andersen, J., Becker-Levin, M., & Gilfoyle, E. (1982). Roles and functions of the Occupational Therapist in the treatment of SI dysfunction. *American Journal of Occupational Therapy, 36*(12), 832–834.

Index

About the Editors and Contributors

Editors and Senior Authors

Diane E. Bermann, MOT/OTR/L, is currently involved with specialized wheelchair seating and positioning at RIC, where she has worked since 1980 as staff therapist, senior therapist, and acting supervisor. She has worked extensively with head injured patients and was active in the formation of the Brain Trauma Program at RIC. She received her MOT from Western Michigan University and became NDT certified in the treatment of adult hemiplegia in 1982.

Karen M. Kovich, BS, OTR/L, is supervisor of head injury and outpatient services at RIC, where she has worked in the OT department for over seven years. She is certified in Neurodevelopmental treatment of the adult hemiplegic, and was a contributing author to *Spinal Cord Injury: A Guide to Functional Outcomes in Occupational Therapy Management* for Aspen Publishers.

Contributors

Janet Bischof, BS, OTR/L, is a senior OTR at RIC, specializing in SCI, upper extremity amputees, and technical aids including augmentative communication systems, computer access, and environmental control systems. She has been at RIC for six years, including 10 months as acting supervisor of the Spinal Cord Injury team, and has authored a chapter on technical aids for spinal cord injuries and presented numerous lectures on this topic to teachers, therapists, and students.

Anita Van Dam-Burke, BS, OTR/L, has been working with head injured patients at RIC since June of 1985. In 1987 she published an article, ''Guillain-Barré Syndrome: A Unique Perspective,'' in *Occupational Therapy,* and presented a poster, ''Defining Cognitive and Sensory Integrative Components in Relation to Function,'' at a head injury conference in Williamsburg, Virginia. She has also given multiple student lectures regarding evaluation and treatment of head injury patients.

Theresa Bush, BS, OTR/L, was a therapist on the Head Injury unit at RIC and is working toward an MS in Rehabilitation Medicine at the University of Washington. She is co-chairperson of the Research Committee for a chapter of the Washington Head Injury Foundation. From 1986 to 1987 she served as Director of OT at Greenery Rehabilitation Center in Seattle and from 1983 to 1986 was on the outpatient staff at RIC. She presented a paper at the 10th Annual Conference for the Brain Injured Adult and Child in Williamsburg, Virginia, in 1986.

Lorie Cripe, BS, OTR/L, works on the Head Injury unit at RIC where she has been employed as a staff Occupational Therapist for over four years, co-leading a variety of groups specifically for the head injured. She currently co-leads a group focusing on Independent Living Skills in the Community, and has had experience treating all levels of head injured individuals. In 1985 she presented at the national AOTA conference on group treatment for hemiplegics, and was PNF trained in 1986.

Judy Hill, BS, OTR/L, is clinical specialist in spinal cord injury at RIC where she has worked for 11 years as a staff therapist, senior staff therapist, clinical supervisor, and acting director. She has instructed courses on orthotics, casting, and topics related to spinal cord injury in the United States and Canada, and researched the effects of casting on motor disorders in head injured patients. Ms. Hill edited *Spinal Cord Injury: A Guide to Functional Outcomes in Occupational Therapy Management*, another title in the Rehabilitation Institute of Chicago Series published by Aspen Publishers.

Russ Hollander, MS, OTR/L, is Director of the Physical Medicine and Rehabilitation Department at the Chicago Neurosurgical Center. He has worked primarily with CNS dysfunctioned and has extensively studied neuro-developmental and sensory integrative approaches to treatment, with a strong interest in utilizing computers for patient database analysis and in the treatment of higher level deficits. He received his MS degree in Human Services Administration at Spertus College in Chicago, and has previously served as Assistant and Acting Director of Occupational Therapy at RIC.

Marlene Morgan, MOT, OTR/L, is Director of the Occupational Therapy Education Program at RIC, where she has been involved with coordinating and developing continuing education programs for allied health professionals. Previously she was on the faculty of Elizabethtown College in physical rehabilitation, and has had experience as a clinician and administrator in pediatrics.

Christine Morrison, BS, OTR/L, is currently completing her graduate work for an MS in Occupational Therapy at the University of Illinois, and is working as a senior therapist at LaRabida Children's Hospital in Chicago. She was previously at RIC for five years including three years on the pediatric service working primarily with head injured patients. Before leaving RIC she was clinical supervisor of the pediatric OT service for one year.

Jessica Presperin, MBA, OTR/L, is currently in private practice, providing seating evaluations and OT services, and consulting with major wheelchair and seating manufacturers. While at RIC from 1979 to 1986, she co-developed the RIC Seating and Positioning Center.

Vinod Sahgal, MD, is Director of the Brain Trauma Program at RIC, and is a professor in the Department of Neurology and Clinical Rehabilitation Medicine at Northwestern University Medical School.

Dorothy Vezzetti, MS, OTR/L, is a member of the head injury treatment team at RIC. She has been active in program development for group treatment and is a recipient of the Dorothy Donnelley Fellowship at RIC where she has worked since 1980. She received an MS degree in occupational therapy from Rush University.